Health, Safety, Environmental, and Quality Auditing

Wayne Pardy and Terri Andrews

Bernan Press

Lanham • Boulder • New York • London

Published by Bernan Press
An imprint of The Rowman & Littlefield Publishing Group, Inc.
4501 Forbes Boulevard, Suite 200, Lanham, Maryland 20706
www.rowman.com

86-90 Paul Street, London EC2A 4NE

British Library Cataloguing in Publication Information available

Library of Congress Cataloging-in-Publication Data

Includes bibliographic references and index.
ISBN: 979-8-89205-046-3 (cloth)
ISBN: 979-8-89205-047-0 (electronic)

Contents

Acknowledgments

The authors would like to thank and acknowledge a number of individuals and organizations who've played a role in helping bring this HSEQ auditing book to fruition.

First of all, to the authors of the ninth edition of the *Environmental Health and Safety Audits* book, Lawrence B. Cahill and Raymond W. Kane. While we've never met, it's your baseline book on safety and environmental auditing over the past nine editions which has brought us to the first edition of this HSEQ auditing book. We've tried to stay true to your original approach while also acknowledging that the world of work in 2024 is a constantly evolving and changing entity, and auditing processes are getting wider and more inclusive in their scopes on a wide range of management systems and regulatory compliance areas. That said, your book's grounding in audit management principles is standing the test of time, and we thank you for that.

The auditors would also like to acknowledge the contributions of Ron Krebs of Praxiom Research and Sean Scott, executive director of the Construction Safety Association of Manitoba. Ron provided some very fine materials from the Praxiom Research Group related to several ISO management systems and related audit processes. This was a generous offer as part of his retirement decision, and we thank Ron for his contributions to the HSEQ world. Sean provided the CFSA harmonized audit instrument template and audit definitions related to the National COR® accreditation standard. As you read the COR® audit process, you'll see that it's a professional and thoughtful approach to the safety auditing world. We are most appreciative of Ron and Sean's knowledge, expertise, and contribution and think you'll agree that their contributions complement our focus and experiences in professional HSEQ auditing.

We would also like to express our sincere appreciation to Mary Meghan Ryan, who first reached out to us after we proposed a similar idea for a book on auditing. Your patience, assistance, and constant encouragement were most appreciated and invaluable to us as we burned lots of midnight oil and spent countless weekends working hard to bring this final product together.

And to our clients and professional colleagues: Thank you for your friendship and support over the years. We hope you've benefited from knowing us in some small way, as we have most assuredly benefited from all your knowledge and support.

To our family . . . we hope you're just as proud of our most recent accomplishment as we are of yours. You constantly amaze us with your love of life and love of each other.

Chapter 1

Perspectives in HSEQ Auditing

Eyes are more accurate witnesses than ears.

—Heraclitus, c. 540–480 BC

WHY AUDIT HEALTH, SAFETY, ENVIRONMENT, AND QUALITY?

Managing compliance with regulatory requirements and conformance to internal stated requirements, or other requirements like client or contractual requirements, has become what may seem as an overwhelming exercise, involving more and more regulations, more and more client expectations, impacting more and more business practices, and affecting more and more organizations. Throughout the world, issues such as hazardous wastes and materials are now being more tightly controlled, and their discharges are freely and openly reported through community and worker right-to-know regulations. Worker injuries are becoming less and less morally and socially acceptable. Clients are demanding and expect high value and a return for the money they pay to their contractors, subcontractors, service providers, and suppliers.

When we looked at writing this book on HSEQ auditing, we wanted to ensure we provided a practical approach regarding it.

That said, no country can assume that it is at the leading edge of HSEQ management and related regulations. Many countries have either adopted regulations or have written their own regulations and best practices and built even more stringent platforms from there. In North America, the United States–Mexico–Canada Agreement (USMCA), the trade agreement between the named parties, replaced the North American Free Trade Agreement (NAFTA) and included some key environmental obligations.

By way of example, the United States and Mexico have negotiated a separate Environment Cooperation and Customs Verification Agreement that will help bolster efforts to combat trade in illegally taken wildlife, fish, and timber.

Source: https://ustr.gov/usmca

From a labor perspective, the United States, Mexico, and Canada have agreed to a Labor chapter that brings labor obligations into the core of the USMCA agreement, makes them fully enforceable, and represents the strongest provisions of any trade agreement.

Key Achievement: Worker Representation in Collective Bargaining. The Labor chapter includes an Annex on Worker Representation in Collective Bargaining in Mexico, under which Mexico commits to specific legislative actions to provide for the effective recognition of the right to collective bargaining.

- Key Achievement: Labor Rights Recognized by the International Labour Organization. The Labor chapter requires the parties to adopt and maintain in law and practice labor rights as recognized by the International Labour Organization, to effectively enforce their labor laws, and not to waive or derogate from their labor laws. Additionally, the chapter includes new provisions to prohibit the importation of goods produced by forced labor, to address violence against workers exercising their labor rights, and to ensure that migrant workers are protected under labor laws.
- Key Achievement: Enhanced Labor Enforceability. The Dispute Settlement chapter establishes a first-of-its-kind United States-Mexico Rapid Response Mechanism, providing for monitoring and expedited enforcement of labor rights to ensure the effective implementation of Mexico's landmark labor reform at particular facilities while respecting sovereignty and due process.
- Key Achievement: New Labor Value Content Rule. To support North American jobs, the deal contains new trade rules of origin to drive higher wages by requiring that 40–45 percent of auto content be made by workers earning at least USD $16 per hour.

Source: https://ustr.gov/usmca

So, just within North America, the demands of these initiatives can have the potential to impact the efforts and focus of those with environmental or labor responsibilities within their respective organizations.

The traditional approach of regulating only major industry groups is also seen by many as a thing of the past. In this day and age, rules and regulatory requirements can affect anything from small mom-and-pop neighborhood businesses with simple municipal requirements to national and multinational corporations with different regulatory realities in the different countries in which they operate, sometimes with no similarities, and in many cases, completely at odds with one another.

Growth of Regulations

Moreover, the regulatory environment varies significantly from country to country. That said, some might ask the question, "Are there fewer lawyers per capita in other countries because the countries are less litigious by nature, or are other countries less litigious because they have fewer lawyers?" The United States is known to be a very litigious society with an overwhelming regulatory framework. In other countries, the relationship between the regulators and the regulated is generally perceived to be more cooperative and much less litigious, but nonetheless demanding and generally perceived as having a high bar. Some have suggested that European countries are, and have always been, leading the way when it comes to progressive HSEQ regulations and processes. For multinational companies, the need to follow different rule books in different regulatory jurisdictions can be very challenging. The saying, "What you don't know can hurt you" is both real and daunting at the same time.

Growth in Visibility

Not so long ago, an organization's HSEQ information was known only to it and perhaps to its applicable regulatory agencies. We looked inward and, generally speaking, no one else was very interested in what we were doing except our own internal folks, and perhaps by extension, the Board of Directors, if the organization had one. This is no longer true. With the advent of things like community and worker right-to-know legislation, the internet, social and corporate responsibility, annual reporting, and ethical investing and shareholder due diligence, HSEQ data are available to all citizens with the click of a mouse. Just pick any company and go to Google, type the name of the company and then safety or environmental fines or violations, or quality complaints.

Continuing Enforcement

In this regulatory setting, one can only wonder if fail-safe management of compliance is, indeed, an achievable objective. Yet, the penalties for not complying are far too intimidating to risk applying anything but extreme diligence toward meeting standards and applying good HSEQ management practices.

In addition, governmental agencies in North America have reemphasized their enforcement role and have moved toward a policy of taking action against individuals, corporate officials, as well as their companies. We may not like it, but that is the reality.

IMPACT ON THE REGULATED COMMUNITY

What are the implications of these policies and trends for management? With the high probability of continued controversy and complexity in the HSEQ arena, it is very important to avoid complacency and to pay attention to HSEQ compliance matters. Management's ability to anticipate and respond to government, customer, client, and private actions aimed at addressing real or perceived HSEQ problems must remain undiminished. Yet, corporate outlays for HSEQ management, including those for staffing, have generally been reduced, as have expenditures for many other business activities in the competitive economic climate of the last decade. Thus, many companies may be less than ideally prepared to face a future regulatory environment that will continue to be complex, demanding, and onerous.

The task of business, then, in this climate of uncertainty, is to ensure minimal vulnerability in compliance-related matters and to do so in the most efficient and cost-effective way. One solution to this problem is the development and vigorous maintenance of a formal HSEQ audit program that evaluates compliance with regulatory requirements, good management practices, and corporate policies and procedures at all facilities. Of course, the discipline and rigor of these formal HSEQ audit programs should (ideally) be balanced by disciplined and rigorous HSEQ management systems and related processes. But that's another book. This book focuses on the professional and competent auditing of those HSEQ management systems and related processes, and while we will discuss the advantage and value of HSEQ management systems, it will generally be within the context of auditing them for effectiveness.

Our previous books on Integrated HSEQ Management Systems dealt with this on the front end—designing effective HSEQ management systems. In this book, we have now flipped our focus. This book will deal with those issues at the back end—the "pointy end of the stick" many of us have become familiar with through our professional HSEQ audit activities. So why audit? That's the focus from here on in.

DEFINING HSEQ AUDITS

Precisely defining HSEQ audits can be a difficult exercise, in part due to the evolving nature of the concept, its rather recent appearance as a formal management process, and the need to tailor programs to the sponsoring organization. It also has to do with the fact that audit programs are typically designed to meet one or more of the following objectives:

- Assuring compliance with regulations (and determining which specific regulations).
- Determining liabilities.
- Protecting against liabilities for company officials.
- Fact-finding for acquisitions and divestitures.
- Meeting client and related product and service requirements.
- Transferring information among operating units.
- Increasing environmental, safety, and quality awareness.
- Tracking manager and facility accountability for HSEQ performance and compliance.

An alternative definition is that audits verify the existence and use of "adequate . . . systems . . . competently . . . applied." Simply put, an audit program is first and foremost a verification program. It is a variation on the saying, "Say What You Mean, Mean What You Say, and Prove It" cliché. It is not meant to replace existing HSEQ management systems at any level. Indeed, the HSEQ audit program should be designed to verify that these HSEQ management systems do, in fact, exist and are in use. And not only in use, but effective (and that depends on the definition of effective).

These *systems*, whether they are to ensure compliance with customer requirements or define liabilities, need to be *adequate* in that they should acknowledge and respond directly to the regulatory, customer, and internal requirements that define HSEQ compliance or liability. The systems should also be *applied*, meaning that procedures are not simply "bookshelf exercises," out-of-date and out-of-use before the ink dries. Finally, the systems must be applied *competently*. All plant managers and staff, HSEQ staff, and operators must have an awareness of compliance and any related customer requirements and conduct their activities accordingly.

ADVANTAGES AND DISADVANTAGES

Like most things in life, audit programs can have both advantages and disadvantages. On the positive side, audits can result in a number of significant benefits, including

- better compliance and customer conformance with contractual requirements;
- fewer surprises or customer complaints;
- fewer fines and legal actions;
- better public image with the community and regulators;
- potential cost savings;
- improved information transfer; and
- increased environmental, health, safety, and quality awareness.

However, these benefits can be offset by some real and potential costs:

- The commitment of resources to run the program.
- Temporary disruption of plant operations.
- Possible customer or client dissatisfaction with information on how their product or service is being protected (or is not).
- Increased ammunition for regulators.
- Increased liability where one is unable to respond to audit recommendations involving significant capital expenditures.

The last two disadvantages raise a special issue associated with HSEQ audits. Even where programs are operated under legal protections (e.g., attorney-client privilege), there is a chance that audit reports could be "discovered" in a legal proceeding. Thus, it is vital for management to understand that if a program is initiated, the company must be serious about fixing the problems identified in the reports. Otherwise, the report could be most incriminating and embarrassing, in a court case or administrative proceeding.

Notwithstanding these drawbacks, most organizations, when faced with the question of whether to undertake an audit program, have opted to do so. The general theory is that in this day of increased litigation and possible criminal or civil suits, it is better to know your liabilities than to remain oblivious to them. As has been said by many people, many times, "Management ignorance is no defense!"

Want to learn more and have some real-time discussions with those who share your interests and concerns? A quick search on LinkedIn will find hundreds of audit groups available for anyone to join. No matter what your interest or audit discipline, LinkedIn can provide you with a wide range of membership options for sharing ideas and information with like-minded audit practitioners. Every opinion, thought, or industry audit practice you could ever think of is explored on any number of these audit resource groups, and while exhaustive, we would recommend that a little time spent on evaluating the group membership options here can pay positive dividends for those looking to converse with like-minded HSEQ audit practitioners and professionals.

What's In a Name? An Audit by Any Other Name Is Still an Audit

As a purely personal observation, it's interesting to step outside of our professional audit role from time to time to see what other people who are typically on the receiving end of an audit think about the process. One of the more interesting suggestions, which was the theme of a recent LinkedIn debate, was the actual use of the word "audit." It was felt by some of those commenting that the word "audit," in their opinion, carried a lot of negative connotations. Some felt that audit was related to "gottcha" practices and that auditors were only out to find problems or things that were wrong or problems. There were some very negative perceptions about the audit process generally.

And based on their experience, they may have been right. Far be it for us to tell an auditee how their audit was conducted. But for us, there are two main issues here which are important for further discussion, as their focus will determine so much of what the remainder of this book will focus on:

1. What is an audit? (And what are its critical characteristics)
2. What is the role of a (good) auditor?

Many on the LinkedIn thread, when pressed, came up with a wide range of alternatives or replacement words for audit, such as:

- Evaluation
- Assessment
- Measurement
- Scorecard

You get the picture. These words are supposedly meant to appear less threatening, more acceptable, or bland, so as not to invoke any of the perceived negativity around the audit process. But something interesting happened along the way. Regular, run-of-the-mill folks were asked about this audit word and whether they felt threatened by it, or the audit process themselves. Almost universally, folks who responded said that they didn't mind an audit per se, but some of their experiences with auditors were less than positive. In other words, it wasn't the word "audit" as such, but the tone, personality, and approach of the auditor which put them off. In other words, auditors who were "gottcha" artists rather than performance professionals.

And one other thing. Changing out the word "audit" with some other supposed/seemingly less threatening word didn't fool anyone either. One guy even said, "What you're really talking about Is an audit isn't it?" Yes . . . yes, we are. Don't try to bluff anyone with vague or soft language. Folks are tuned in. At the end of the day, whatever you call it, renaming an audit with some other supposedly less threatening name is fooling no one.

TRENDS IN HSEQ AUDITING

In the past few years, several interesting trends have surfaced within the HSEQ auditing discipline, as discussed below.

The Continuing Evolution of Guidelines and Standards

With the advent of several professional auditing organizations, we have seen a push by some segments of the auditing profession toward the development of standards and possibly national and international registration or certification for auditors. International Standards such as ISO 9001 (Quality), 14001 (Environment), and the most recent 45001 (Occupational Health and Safety) are proliferating and gaining both credibility and validity worldwide. The belief is, as validated by recent research, that Standards will help to improve the quality of both audits and auditors and to define more clearly the acceptable HSEQ audit. Given the varying types of audits and the multiple objectives a program can be designed to achieve, the development of Standards has been a challenging exercise. Consensus has never been easy, especially internationally. Nonetheless, there are now some 30 years of history in the development of HSEQ audit and auditor standards.

These are just a few of the more common Standards available and in play today, against which many organizations are auditing to determine their proficiency in these areas:

- ISO 9001 Quality Management Standard
- ISO 14001 Environmental Management Standard
- ISO 45001 Occupational Health and Safety Standard
- ISO 22301 Business Continuity Management Standard
- ISO 27001 Information Security Management Standard
- ISO 13485 Quality Management Standard for Medical Devices
- IATF 16949 Quality Management Standard for Automotive Sector
- AS9100 Quality Management Standard for Aerospace and Defense

Incorporating Security and Social Responsibility

In recent years, security and social responsibility, justifiably, have become critical issues for many organizations. Much like HSEQ programs, or any program for that matter, security and social-responsibility programs require oversight and attention if they are to achieve their stated objectives. Yet, there is some belief that two more independent audit programs could truly hinder a site's ability to accomplish its mission. Thus, organizations are looking at ways to incorporate these additional topics into existing HSEQ audit programs. However, there are some barriers to this seemingly logical approach. The principal one is that most HSEQ auditors are not familiar with the issues of security and social responsibility. Training and education will be required, or audit teams will have to be made larger to include auditors familiar with the topics.

That fact has been recognized in documents such as ISO 19011, which sets forth guidelines for auditing management systems. The standard contains guidance on managing an audit program, the principles of auditing, and the evaluation of individuals responsible for managing the audit programs. The issue every audit organization needs to understand is that the audit consists of both the technical and administrative tools and techniques for the audit, and the technical discipline focus of the audit scope. More on that in later chapters.

Conducting Supply Chain Audits

The supply chain for manufacturers comprises many elements, including raw material, energy, and parts/equipment suppliers; contract manufacturers; construction vendors; IT services, transporters and distributors; waste vendors; and the like. Various stakeholders are beginning to hold companies accountable not only for their own HSEQ compliance and performance but for that of the other participants in their supply chain. A natural outcome has been that companies are now beginning to audit these participants to ensure that they are working with organizations that are ethical and provide their products and services in compliance with a wide range of applicable requirements. This can be a tremendous challenge as some companies have relationships with thousands of suppliers. Innovative and cost-effective approaches, such as using third-party evaluators and teaming with other companies that use the same suppliers, are being explored. More on that later, but the International IOSA audit process is just one example of how synergies can be achieved in a complex, multi-supplier type of audit management program.

Conducting Third-Party Audit Program Evaluations

Commissioning an independent review of the HSEQ audit program is an increasing trend. These reviews help to ensure that the program is meeting its objectives and that those objectives are consistent with current good auditing practices. Moreover, many of the existing auditing standards recognize the need to have HSEQ audit programs evaluated on a periodic basis. This is an important trend. And third-party evaluations of HSEQ audit programs can bring experiences and skill sets from different auditors to your processes, which is a valuable HSEQ audit learning opportunity.

Improving International HSEQ Audits

Conducting international audits effectively has also proven quite challenging. Note we use the term "effectively." The language of the various disciplines being audited is often different, so interviewing and record reviews can be daunting. Also, the local culture must be considered. What might be considered humorous (if an auditor is prone to using humor in the conduct of the audit) in one state, province, or country could be considered an insult elsewhere. Then there is the logistical nightmare of traveling halfway around the world to conduct an audit. We'll speak about the issue of remote auditing later, as brought about in part by the worldwide Covid pandemic. But suffice it to say at this point that remote auditing offers some relief and practical solutions for these globetrotting audit scenarios, as well as cost savings for all interested parties.

Several initiatives have been undertaken in HSEQ auditing to improve the process and outcomes for international audits. Commercial audit protocols, checklists, and regulatory compliance standards have been developed by a wide range of third parties. Also, the Internet is an excellent place to research local HSEQ regulations, requirements, or standards. Overall, technology has made the audit process more professional, streamlined, and transparent (and potentially easier and less expensive). Finally, companies are relying more on third-party consultants from the country, state, or province in which a given site is located. These third parties either make up the entire audit team or supplement an in-house team. And local has its advantages, especially when considering the regulatory realities of the facility in question.

The Use of Digital/Cell Phone Cameras

Anecdotal evidence and surveys have identified that HSEQ auditors are depending more and more on their digital cameras and smartphones in their audits. While this might seem a small matter, it is not. Not so many years ago, cameras were prohibited on audits within most organizations due to concern that the photographs of noncompliance situations would be "discovered" in a legal proceeding and used as evidence by the plaintiff of wrongdoing. Over time, this concern has dissipated. Photographs have been used as stark confirmation of noncompliance in closing conferences with site management and as valuable tools in HSEQ training programs. And who today does not have a smartphone with a digital camera? Few and far between.

While doing more with less may be an understandable attitude and even a worthwhile goal today, any fundamental relaxation of compliance efforts by companies presents an unjustifiable risk. HSEQ auditing is a sound way to prevent damaging situations from occurring. Management should not underestimate its value. Having documented physical evidence by way of a digital image or video clip is akin to the saying, "A picture is worth a thousand words." Written evidence with supporting documentation is always a sound choice. Written evidence with supporting documents, including visual or auditory evidence, is always a safer bet. More on this in later chapters as we find many organizations starting to use digital evidence in the form of audio clips of their activities, rather than stacks and stacks of paper historically doing the same thing.

By way of a more detailed introduction, we want to inform readers that this book is less of a technical tool or cookbook on any specific audit methodology, checklist, discipline, or protocol. We've personally seen too many examples of the following:

- Ten essential steps to auditing.
- Auditing made easy in five simple steps.
- The complete auditing roadmap.
- Audit checklists for every type of audit.
- Auditing made easy—a complete guide.
- Auditing 101—Everything you need to know about auditing.

You get the idea. Everyone with a five-step, or eight-step, or ten-step guaranteed process to make auditing easy and pain-free. A "one size fits all" template. But in our experience, one-size-fits-all fits no one. And we will not tell you that auditing is simple, easy, or painless. In some cases, it is not simple, not easy, and sometimes very painful (for the auditor and the auditee). But when done with integrity, intelligence, and diligence it can provide benefits to both the auditor and auditee. But you need to prepare and prepare well. And even more important, you need to execute well. We cannot emphasize this enough—disciplined, strategic execution.

Audits can be challenging and messy, but they can also be rewarding and satisfying. First, by providing a valuable service and product for your client. Second, by the sense of satisfaction and achievement you can get from helping your clients, their organization, and people perform better.

So, if you're interested in working hard and critically looking at your auditing role with clear and objective eyes, come along on our journey. We promise not to waste your time.

REFERENCES

USMC Free Trade Agreement. https://ustr.gov/usmca

This chapter has been adapted from Lawrence B. Cahill and Raymond W. Kane. *Environmental Health and Safety Audits*, 9th Edition. Government Institutes, 2010. It has been updated for this edition.

Wayne Pardy and Terri Andrews. *Integrated Management Systems: Leading Strategies and Solutions*, 2nd Edition. Bernan Press, 2019.

Chapter 2

Government and Regulatory Perspectives

INTRODUCTION

While government regulators are very good at developing inspection processes for physical environments, their expertise and experience around management system auditing is, in the opinion of the authors, not as strong. That may be because many regulations have their focus on things and physical assets (equipment, buildings, facilities, hardware, physical environment, and materials). The advantage for regulators is that facilities and equipment do not talk back, challenge, have an opinion, question logic or rationale, or disagree. Facilities and equipment just are what they are—passively waiting to be observed and judged.

To generalize that all governments inspect more than they audit might not be completely accurate, but experience has shown that regulators focus more on things and "stuff" more than on processes and management systems. In part, that is because most regulations have been written to be black and white with limited room for interpretation or opinion. And the greyer regulations are, the more they can be subjected to interpretation. And interpretation is not generally the goal of compliance efforts.

Many sound business reasons support having an HSEQ auditing program. Typical reasons cited include the following:

- To help maintain positive public relations and community relationships.
- To satisfy investor criteria and improve access to capital.
- To help secure insurance at a reasonable cost.
- To enhance an entity's image and market share and increase customer confidence.
- To provide the basis for meeting vendor certification criteria.

- To demonstrate reasonable care and prevent workers from getting injured.
- To facilitate the conservation of input materials and energy.
- To improve relations with the government.
- To improve the company's overall HSEQ program and make it more proactive and effective.
- To identify problems internally and correct them before they are discovered by an external regulatory agency or customer.
- To assure management that control systems are functioning as designed.
- To decrease the company's operating, regulatory, and financial risks.
- To provide evidence of meeting customers' HSEQ expectations.

An auditing program is also one of many tools needed to develop and maintain an effective HSEQ management program. But identifying compliance and management deficiencies is only the first step. An organization must be willing to correct nonconformances, other types of regulatory violations and other deficiencies or nonconformances, and root causes to achieve improved results. If an organization is unwilling to act upon the discovered deficiencies, the audits may become a source of damaging evidence of liability. Even worse, they may become a source of cynicism and result in deteriorated performance. People can become very jaded when they see that the actions promised by an audit lack commitment to execute on the audit findings.

An effective auditing program is a very important piece of the overall HSEQ management puzzle. Auditing can serve as a quality-assurance check to help improve the performance of basic management systems and programs by assessing whether necessary control systems and management practices are in place, functioning, adequate, and effective. Effectiveness, some would argue, is perhaps the most important aspect of any audit. Audits evaluate, but do not substitute for, direct compliance and conformance activities such as obtaining permits, installing controls, monitoring compliance, reporting violations, and keeping records. Although they cannot replace regulatory inspections, audits can supplement conventional regulatory and government oversight and point toward more efficient allocation of enforcement resources.

HSEQ auditing has been developed for sound business reasons, particularly to help manage environmental, safety, and customer requirements and expectations over time instead of reacting to crises. Auditing can improve operational or facility performance before the regulatory inspector or client auditor arrives. More importantly, it can help indicate effective solutions to common HSEQ problems, focus operations or the facility manager's attention on current and upcoming regulatory requirements, and can generate protocols and checklists that help operations and facilities better manage themselves. Auditing also can result in improved management of risks, since auditors frequently identify liabilities that go beyond regulatory compliance. The old saying, "Pay me now or pay me later" is certainly at play here.

An effective HSEQ auditing system should include the following general elements:

- *Explicit top-management support for HSEQ auditing and commitment to follow up on audit findings.* Such support could be demonstrated by sanctioning the role of the audit program in a written management policy statement on HSEQ management, buttressed with specific, tangible implementing actions. For organizations that have decided to implement management systems based on any of the more common ISO standards, this is a stated requirement, subject to audit and verification.
- *An HSEQ auditing function independent of the audited activities.* The status or organizational focus of HSEQ auditors should be sufficient to ensure objective and unobstructed inquiry, observation, and testing. Auditor objectivity should not be impaired by personal relationships, financial or other conflicts of interest, interference with free inquiry or judgment, or fear of potential retribution. Simply put, you should not be auditing your own work. Additionally, auditors need to have clear technical competencies in HSEQ discipline areas. Generalists are acceptable; specialists are preferred.
- *Adequate team staffing and auditor training.* HSEQ auditors should possess, or have ready access to, the knowledge, skills, and disciplines needed to accomplish audit objectives. Each individual auditor should comply with professional standards of conduct. Auditors, whether full-time or part-time, should maintain their technical and analytical competence through continuing education and training.
- *Explicit audit program objectives, scope, resources, and frequency.* At a minimum, audit objectives should include assessing compliance with applicable HSEQ laws and evaluating the adequacy of internal compliance systems to carry out assigned responsibilities. Explicit written audit procedures should generally be used. Auditors should be provided with all internal policies and applicable permits and regulations pertinent to operations or the facility, as well as checklists or protocols addressing specific features that must be evaluated.
- *A process that collects, analyzes, interprets, and documents information sufficient to achieve audit objectives.* Information should be collected before and during an on-site visit regarding matters related to audit objectives and scope. This information should be sufficient, reliable, relevant, and useful enough to provide a sound basis for audit findings and recommendations. Sometimes your time as an auditor can be rushed and challenged on-site,

so any opportunity to review any audit evidence before getting on-site is advisable and a definite advantage.

Example: Canadian Offshore Oil and Gas Industry

By way of an example, this is a scenario for the Canadian regulatory environment for the offshore oil and gas industry. In Newfoundland and Labrador, Canada, the offshore oil and gas industry is regulated by the Canada-Newfoundland Offshore Petroleum Board (C-NLOPB). The C-NLOPB was created in 1986 through the Atlantic Accord and its associated, implementing federal and provincial legislation, the Canada-Newfoundland and Labrador Atlantic Accord Implementation Act, S.C. 1987, c. 3 and the Canada-Newfoundland and Labrador Atlantic Accord Implementation Newfoundland and Labrador Act, RSNL1990 c. C-2 ("the Accord Acts"). It regulates petroleum-related activities in the Canada-Newfoundland and Labrador Offshore Area. While the C-NLOPB is an independent regulator that operates at arm's length from the governments, some Board decisions (referred to under the Accord Acts as "Fundamental Decisions") require government approval, as does its annual operating budget.

The C-NLOPB highlights what they feel to be the relevance of audits, albeit somewhat in the same breath as their posted perspectives on inspections:

Audits and Safety Inspections

An audit is a systematic evaluation of all aspects of an operation to determine its overall compliance with regulatory requirements related to safety, environmental protection, and resource management, as well as commitments made by the operator in their application for authorization. Audits include reviewing documentation and records, obtaining samples, conducting interviews with personnel, verifying the quality of information reported to the C-NLOPB, inspecting equipment or other physical aspects of an operation, observing operations, and verifying the qualifications and training of personnel.

An inspection involves the physical presence of an officer at an operation. An inspection focuses on the compliance of the facilities and equipment or on specific physical operations, which require a visit to an offshore facility. Inspections verify that operators are following applicable statutory requirements, which include following their safety and environmental protection plans, and may also verify the completion of investigation of audit corrective actions.

During a safety audit, C-NLOPB Safety Officers can raise a noncompliance against anything that does not conform to the operator's safety management policies and procedures or to legislative requirements. There are two types of noncompliances:

- Observation—A statement of fact related to a noncompliance made during a safety audit or safety inspection and substantiated by objective evidence.
- Finding—A conclusion substantiated by one or more observations, which highlights significant issues with the implementation of the operator's safety management policies and procedures, adherence to legislative requirements, and/or any noncompliance that has significant implications for safety.

Following the issuance of an audit report, an operator has fifteen working days to provide an action plan and time frame that is acceptable to the C-NLOPB. The operator must take action to address noncompliances within the agreed time frame. Failure to comply within that time frame could result in an order to comply or, depending on the seriousness, could constitute an offense under the Act.

So, as you can see, the movement toward an audit process that complements the traditional physical inspection focus of many regulatory enforcement agencies is an item which the authors suggest may begin to gain traction in select regulatory sectors. In this instance, we would suggest that the regulatory agencies have determined that an audit would perhaps help them, and their offshore operators, achieve better outcomes as it relates to the HSEQ management system which many of the offshore operators have implemented.

Of course, there are some questions which regulators would need to consider before they embark upon these audit approaches, not the least of which might be:

- Does doing the audit mean that you've invested yourself in the outcome of the HSEQ processes of the operator?
- If things continue to fail, or not be effective, what responsibility do you as the regulator take in this level of performance?

REFERENCES

https://www.cnlopb.ca/enforcement/compliance/.

This chapter has been adapted from Lawrence B. Cahill and Raymond W. Kane. *Environmental Health and Safety Audits*, 9th Edition. Government Institutes, 2010. It has been updated for this edition.

Wayne Pardy and Terri Andrews. *Integrated Management Systems: Leading Strategies and Solutions*, 2nd Edition. Bernan Press, 2019.

Chapter 3

Legal Considerations

Laws too gentle are seldom obeyed; too severe, seldom executed.

—Benjamin Franklin, *Poor Richard's Almanac*, 1732–1757

INTRODUCTION

Over the past thirty or so years, there has been a veritable explosion of health, safety, and environmental (HSE) laws and regulations at all levels of government. As a result, businesses in all sectors of the economy are subject to requirements that affect a broad spectrum of activities.

Virtually all major HSE statutes vest the government with broad enforcement powers. Those found in violation may be subject to civil penalties, criminal sanctions, and enforcement orders. The potential exposure for relatively minor violations of HSE requirements can often be quite significant. While the costs of penalties might be a factor, equally important in the scheme of incentives for compliance is the potential impact on public profile and reputation.

In response to the broad spectrum of HSE requirements now in place, many businesses have developed new and innovative ways to ensure that their operations are conducted in conformance with applicable HSE requirements. Environmental audits represent a critical tool to achieve these goals in environmental management. Health and safety audits in the occupational setting similarly help to reduce workplace accidents, illnesses, and injuries. Compliance audits at a facility will frequently cover environmental, health, and safety requirements together because the issues are intertwined, and because many corporate programs manage HSE issues in a single unit. In some organizations, the overarching requirements of their quality management system also have relationships to the activities being conducted on an HSE level (corporate oversight and direction for things like internal audits, document control, training and competency, management review, etc.).

FUNCTION OF HSEQ AUDITS

HSEQ compliance assessments or audits are typically designed to evaluate whether specific activities or operations are being conducted in conformance with applicable regulatory requirements and whether associated equipment and facilities meet HSEQ standards, or if the compliance requirement is on documented roles and responsibilities, whether the organization has implemented and executed those roles and responsibilities as required. They may be used to evaluate whether changes must be made in operations or equipment to achieve compliance or whether such changes will otherwise lead to risk reductions. In this regard, compliance assessments may help businesses make informed decisions regarding the appropriate deployment of capital and personnel. They are also useful in identifying opportunities for reducing emissions, minimizing the generation of waste, diminishing workplace hazards, or enhancing services to customers and their requirements. Additional examples of the function of compliance audits can include

- minimizing the potential for governmental enforcement actions or third-party lawsuits;
- evaluating whether nonregulatory standards such as internal corporate HSEQ goals and industry standards are being achieved;
- preparing for due diligence or client business opportunities; and
- satisfying internal or external stakeholder requirements (assuming they have been clearly defined).

HSEQ audits may be performed as part of an overall compliance program designed to meet the family of ISO management systems standards (such as 14001, 9001, and/or 45001) developed by the International Organization for Standardization (ISO). Satisfying these standards may be necessary to participate in certain sectors of the global marketplace or mandated by certain clients who want a higher level of assurance for the money they spend. HSEQ audits may be undertaken for marketing or public relations considerations or to improve relationships with neighbors and customers. Finally, audits may be performed to facilitate compliance with other legal requirements, such as disclosure and reporting obligations administered by select regulatory agencies.

Whatever the motivators may be, HSEQ audits provide businesses with a powerful tool to facilitate compliance; however, they can (and often do) identify areas of noncompliance or other facts that could lead to substantial legal liability. This dynamic potentially creates significant disincentives to performing deep-dive assessments.

For some businesses, concerns over potential exposure to enforcement actions and other litigation predicated on self-identified violations outweigh the benefits to be gained from HSEQ audits, thereby eliminating an otherwise useful mechanism to foster compliance. Getting senior executives to say this publicly is not a common occurrence. Other businesses have sought to strike a balance between these competing considerations by structuring HSEQ audits to maximize the potential to maintain the confidentiality of the assessment results.

ROLE OF HSEQ AUDITS IN REGULATORY COMPLIANCE

One of the principles undergirding regulatory HSE programs is that compliance with HSE requirements represents an important benchmark for evaluating overall environmental performance. You'll note that we left the Q out of this HSEQ equation. Quality is less so governed by multiple regulatory requirements, but often a customer's quality requirements can far exceed documented regulatory expectations.

If these requirements represent societal standards for how members of the regulated community ought to conduct their activities, a critical question then becomes how best to foster a high level of compliance with such requirements. As regulatory programs have matured, agencies have generally recognized that multiple approaches to facilitate compliance are necessary. This is in marked contrast to the view that an aggressive enforcement program, by itself, is the linchpin in promoting compliance. While enforcement actions remain an important component of the overall HSEQ regulatory framework, they can be confrontational, expensive, resource-intensive, and time-consuming.

This is the general backdrop for evaluating the legal issues associated with HSEQ audits. If we assume that performing HSEQ audits is a positive step in assuring compliance and improving performance, then should the results of the audits be promptly disclosed based on the promise of more lenient enforcement, or should they be privileged and subject only to a duty to address areas of identified noncompliance?

PRACTICAL CONSIDERATIONS AND RECOMMENDATIONS FOR PERFORMING SELF-ASSESSMENTS

The overall benefits of performing regular HSEQ audits are clear, and the incentives created by various levels of government, either in the form of legislation or policy, support the process. Below are several recommendations for optimizing these opportunities:

1. Any self-audit should be carefully planned. It is essential that an organization develop the audit process with a full understanding of the available legal protections, whether they are audit policies, statutes, or common law privileges. It will be impossible to retrofit the audit to incorporate the procedures necessary to qualify for these legal protections. In the audit planning stage, care should be taken to ensure that the audit fits within the types of activities covered by the relevant policies. For example, if a regulated entity is setting up a compliance-management system, it should overlay the audit policy criteria and any key terms from any applicable law or policy to ensure that all the various components of the applicable definitions are being met.
2. The team of professionals who will be involved in the self-audit should be identified beforehand and should include, at a minimum, a representative of the regulated entity with knowledge concerning the operations to be evaluated, a technical consultant (or in-house HSEQ staff person), and an attorney, in some cases if it's deemed applicable. Input from each of these disciplines is quite important, especially if the results of the audit report are to be shared with external stakeholders (i.e., regulatory agencies, clients, customers).
3. The time frames for disclosure and remediation set forth in the audit policies and statutes are typically short. This will be very important based on the perceived risk and consequences of not fixing the audit finding within a timeline appropriate to the risk. Therefore, it is critical that the team of professionals conducting the audit be kept directly apprised of the results of the audit. Depending on the information generated by the audit, there may be only a narrow window of time to evaluate the factual and legal predicates to determine whether a violation exists before reporting may be necessary to preserve the benefits of the voluntary-disclosure program. The audit team must also consider carefully the likely period necessary to correct violations found and whether the relevant audit policy or program allows sufficient time to do so.
4. Depending on the circumstances, a regulated entity may wish to conduct audits either in discrete phases or of discrete aspects of its operations.

By dividing an audit into "bite-size pieces," it may be easier to ensure that issues are identified and resolved in a timely and prudent fashion. There also may be less potential for creating paralysis of decision-making resulting from the identification of a host of compliance problems in a single report. Finally, by separating the process into phases, it may be easier to separate legal from business advice and thereby come within the attorney-client privilege.

5. The assessment team should understand the legal framework applicable to the operations being evaluated.
6. Before conducting an audit, the regulated entity must be committed to addressing the issues likely to be identified. Performing an audit and ignoring the results will likely leave the regulated entity in a markedly worse set of circumstances than not performing the audit at all. Once you see something, you cannot "unsee" it.
7. Take care in preparing any written documentation of audit findings and the language used to avoid speculation and unnecessary legal conclusions. Do not use speculative or subjective language. Auditors are (should strive to be) fact finders, which is quite a different function (requiring specific expertise) from drawing compliance and legal conclusions from the identified facts.

HSEQ laws and regulations can be extremely complex and are ever-changing. Environmental, health, safety, and quality audits can serve a pivotal function both in assuring compliance and in establishing protocols to determine areas of noncompliance. These are two different, equally important goals that can be achieved through a thoughtful, well-developed environmental, health, and safety auditing program.

REFERENCES

This chapter has been adapted from Lawrence B. Cahill and Raymond W. Kane. *Environmental Health and Safety Audits*, 9th Edition. Government Institutes, 2010. It has been updated for this edition.

Wayne Pardy and Terri Andrews. *Integrated Management Systems: Leading Strategies and Solutions*, 2nd Edition. Bernan Press, 2019.

Chapter 4

Elements of a Successful HSEQ Audit Program

"For example," is not proof.

—Yiddish proverb

PRINCIPLES OF AN AUDIT PROGRAM

The principles of a Health, safety, environmental, and Quality (HSEQ) audit program are generally thought to be well-known by those who practice HSEQ auditing as part of their day-to-day professional role and responsibility, but may be usefully summarized in the following five points. The audit team, comprising competent, qualified, and knowledgeable professionals (either in-house staff, third parties, or both), carries out such duties as:

1. Understanding and ascertaining the maintenance of schedules and records with respect to all operations having HSEQ compliance requirements.
2. Inspecting facilities, equipment, and personnel performance to evaluate adherence to institutional standards.
3. Submitting written status reports to appropriate senior management.
4. Explaining deviations from the norm and recommending corrective or preventive action, or opportunities for improvement.
5. Operating independently of all audited functions (do not audit their own work) at a peer level with their management.

As these points make clear, the essence of an HSEQ audit program is to provide assurance to top management and key stakeholders that all relevant business and regulatory requirements are being met in accordance with the organization's operating philosophy, policies, procedures, standards, and requirements. Customer and other recognized stakeholder requirements and expectations are also valid here.

To accomplish this goal, an HSEQ audit program must contain certain key elements around which an individualized structure can be developed. The program must be planned carefully and have the appropriate supportive tools and staff. Audits must be conducted on a continuous basis with additional sampling used only when and where necessary. Finally, the results must be evaluated and turned into practical and realistic solutions and corrective actions. Each of these elements is important to the successful implementation of the overall HSEQ audit program. Accordingly, this chapter presents a detailed discussion of each of the elements within the context of the overall program.

PLANNING THE AUDIT PROGRAM

An important first step is planning a program. Among the decisions to be made are the following: What is the objective to be achieved? Who will be involved? How often will audits be conducted? Which laws and regulations will be covered? What standards, procedures, and customer requirements or expectations will be covered? And, should information be kept strictly and completely confidential? As indicated by the list below, the issues to be resolved can be numerous and often complex:

1. Choice of program objectives:
   - Assurance of compliance
   - Management of liabilities
   - Accountability of management
   - Tracking of compliance costs
2. Program organization alternatives:
   - Corporate control with full-time corporate auditors
   - Corporate control with part-time auditors selected from divisions
   - A small corporate oversight group with the delegation of the audit function to the operating divisions
   - A small corporate oversight group with the use of external, independent auditors
3. Legal issues:
   - Written versus oral reports
   - Retained documentation
   - Corporate counsel involvement
   - Protection from discovery
   - Report format and watchwords—including editing or review by legal

4. Program scope and coverage issues:
   - Frequency of audits
   - All HSEQ regulations (other regulations you want considered in scope even though not strictly HSEQ?)
   - All facilities, random sample, or directed sample
   - Past practices
   - Vendor/supplier audits
   - Contractor or subcontractor/supplier audits
5. Process issues:
   - Pre-visit questionnaire
   - Number of auditors
   - Duration of audits
   - Pre-visit, on-site, and post-visit procedures
   - Sampling procedures
   - Interview technique
   - Inspection procedures
   - Use of audit software and systems and related technologies (growing all the time)
6. Auditor selection and training issues:
   - Skills required
   - Just-in-time training provided for previously trained/skilled auditors
   - Training procedures
   - Full-time versus part-time auditor
7. Management issues:
   - Expectations of senior management
   - Measures of successful performance
   - Unannounced visits
   - Reporting protocols
   - Supportive versus combative style
8. Supporting tool alternatives:
   - Pre-visit questionnaire
   - Compliance and conformance checklists
   - Regulatory updates
   - Audit report templates
   - Guidance/procedures manual
   - Follow-up reports
   - Computer and IT support

Although this book and other sources can provide guidance on what might be considered the standard approach to the issues listed above, each organization considering a program must decide for itself the optimal program structure.

There is no one best answer. Other "cookbook" audit approaches will say that there is, but in the author's experience, there is not. There is good and general guidance, but at the end of the day, each organization will choose the approach which best meets their needs and realities.

Most organizations will develop some type of audit guidance manuals or other documents (procedures, etc.) to set the framework for the program and to ensure the consistency, efficiency, and completeness of all audits. Audit manuals or procedures typically address essential programmatic issues and include a variety of audit tools, such as model opening conference presentations, preaudit questionnaires, model audit report templates, and audit checklists or protocols. Essentially, audit manuals or procedures are designed to communicate the structure of the audit program to both the auditors and those being audited (auditees) to remove any mystery from the program. Full and complete transparency is always the recommended approach.

The objective is not to have the audit program as some type of subject-matter expertise issue that only the auditors understand or are familiar with. The objective is to ensure that the audit is a transparent and rational process, and the service of providing the audit helps ensure that the outcome of the audit (report, actions, etc.) is intended to advance the organization or business unit being audited and help them grow and improve.

The next few sections discuss the keys to implementing a successful audit program. They touch upon many of the issues listed above and provide some guidance on preferred approaches. These are the central points that should be addressed in the audit program's guidance manual.

Establishing an HSEQ Audit Policy or Procedure

To demonstrate explicit top-management support for an audit program, most organizations will develop and issue some form of audit policy or procedure. The policy, typically no more than one page in length, will define the auditable site universe, support the conduct of the audits, and make a commitment to the completion of actions needed to correct the identified deficiencies. Support from the top person in the organization goes a long way toward achieving successful implementation. The procedure lays out the processes in support of the policy, which govern and guides the roles and activities of those assigned key roles within the audit process.

Program Objectives for HSEQ Audits

An HSEQ audit program can achieve a variety of objectives. Historically, in many organizations, compliance assurance has been the principal objective, with other secondary objectives evolving along the way. In the occupational safety and environmental management arena, the focus of these compliance-assurance issues has been on protecting people from being injured and the environment from damage. And there's nothing wrong with that, especially when one considers the potential consequences. On the quality side of the house, product and service excellence and meeting or exceeding defined customer or client expectations have been a major focus.

Yet, it is important to note that companies will frame a program to meet individual needs, and these can vary significantly. By way of example, this is a summary of how one fictional organization has framed its HSEQ audit program, with emphasis on the following five objectives:

1. To provide assurance of adequate HSEQ performance and continuous improvement to senior management and the Board of Directors
2. To ensure division and facility compliance with applicable HSEQ regulations and corporate policies and procedures
3. To ensure management accountability for correcting compliance deficiencies identified on audits
4. To increase HSEQ awareness and continuous learning by audited personnel and auditors
5. To transfer HSEQ technological and administrative innovations across the organization

Note that the compliance-assurance objective is one of the five listed. But the additional objectives are quite important as well. For example, the program should also be designed to provide assurance and confirmation of continuous improvement of HSEQ performance to senior management and possibly a Board of Directors. The reason is that these senior and Board members can be deemed to be the "directing mind and will" of the organization, and they can review the outcomes or recommendations of any HSEQ audit to ensure there are no barriers, real or perceived, to the organization meeting its stated objectives. Also, helping keep the organization out from under the target of the regulatory agencies is also positive.

That said, there is nothing to stop any regulatory agency from exercising its mandated compliance verification role. But having objective evidence of efforts and initiatives in support of the organization working to meet its regulatory obligations carries tremendous weight. This objective is very consistent with the international standards discussed elsewhere in this book. It might be said that no one likes having regulatory agencies take a critical and detached look at their operations and compliance commitments. But at the end of the day, it is, in the author's opinion, always better to be prepared for this eventuality than to be caught flat-footed.

Furthermore, the program is designed to hold management, not the audit program manager, accountable for correcting deficiencies. This applies compliance pressure to the appropriate organization and their line management. This helps ensure that those who have the responsibility and authority to address identified issues have the necessary facts and information upon which to base their improvement decisions. Note that it does not hold line management accountable for an excellent rating on any given audit. There is no regulatory requirement or organizational procedure that requires perfection (or at least none the auditors are currently aware of). What it does do is ask of line management that where problems are identified, they be corrected promptly. This approach is supported and reinforced, for example, within the Canadian context for the Internal Responsibility System for workplace safety.

Additionally, the program is designed to be a training tool for rotating auditors, new or inexperienced auditors, and those who are audited. This very common objective for auditing programs is easily achieved. In probably every instance (hopefully), an auditor and those being audited can walk away from the audit and say, "I learned something from that exercise." That said, sometimes the learning might not be positive learning. We'll elaborate on this in further chapters.

Finally, the program is expected to communicate best practices throughout the organization. This also assumes that the organization has identified and rationalized best practices, as using the term "best practice" can be very subjective unless the basis for the best practice has been rationalized, documented, and validated as such. Auditors, especially those who audit multiple organizations, are in a great position to do this as they review practices in many different businesses and geographical regions. Before the advent of communication tools such as email, Zoom, Microsoft Teams, and so on, this kind of communication was quite difficult and posed many challenges. Now even remote auditing using technology tools like Zoom or Teams is part of the landscape.

As mentioned above, these are only a few of the objectives an HSEQ audit program can achieve. Individual organizations must decide for themselves which objectives are appropriate. Whatever is decided, the objectives should be stated in such a way that clear performance measures and expectations can be established. One must be able to evaluate the program's performance periodically to determine where improvements need to be made or where success has been achieved.

And while you might not see this defined as an audit objective, let's address the elephant in the room regarding audit effectiveness. Some might cynically suggest that paper does not save lives or improve product quality, and they may be right. That said, one of the challenges we face with each and every audit program is to consider cause and effect related to your audits. Consider this assertion by Dan Petersen in a 1996 article titled, "Why Safety is a People Problem":

Audits predict results in safety*. Petersen once backed the use of audits, but he said correlational studies between audit results and injury records in large* *companies show very little predictive value. That is because audits "tend to measure regulatory compliance as much as they do the effectiveness of the safety program."*

For example, said Petersen, most audits start with paperwork. "Paperwork doesn't necessarily dictate what the actions have been. There's a little slippage there," he noted. "Also, the more paperwork you require people to do, the less they're out there talking with their people and working on improving their behavior." Nor do the parts of audits that focus on physical conditions prove very helpful, he added, except to ensure regulatory compliance.

Can audits be a good measure of safety effectiveness? Yes, says Petersen, if the audit interviews employees about their perceptions of the safety program. This leads back, he said, to asking employees not only "what is wrong, but how to fix it. That gets back to involvement."

Our challenge to everyone . . . work hard and diligently to ensure that your audit is relevant and is a good measure of the effectiveness of your HSEQ management systems and related processes. The remainder of this book will provide guidance on how you can do that.

Roles and Responsibilities

One of the early keys to developing a successful HSEQ audit program, regardless of the strategy selected, is commitment. Top management's role at this stage is critical. Before any audits are conducted, management must develop and communicate a policy and supporting procedure that supports the concept of an HSEQ audit program. To be successful, the policy must portray the program as a positive move toward helping the organization enhance compliance, conformance, and reduce liabilities. Senior management should explicitly dismiss the notion that the program is designed to be a "gottcha" or "checkup" on facilities or managers. In fact, under a properly designed HSEQ audit program, employees have as much, if not more, to gain than managers do.

In addition, early in the development of the HSEQ audit program, it would be prudent if corporate management designated a senior executive or staff member as the audit program director, manager, champion, or oversight representative. This individual should be senior enough in the organization to establish and maintain the HSEQ audit program's credibility.

The specific structure of the HSEQ audit program will vary depending upon the individual organization, their customer realities, and their regulatory and business/operating environment. Probably the most prevalent—though not the only—approach is to appoint a corporate audit program director/manager and to assign a small group to this individual if resources permit. This group might include a regulatory specialist and one or more, or no, audit team leaders. The auditors and/or team leaders could come from other corporate groups or facility HSEQ staff, and they could conduct a few audits per year while retaining full-time HSEQ responsibilities in their respective organizations. Of course, independence from the process being audited would apply in any event. This might be harder in smaller organizations with limited resources, but it is not impossible.

Quite often, such audit teams are supplemented by outside resources or third parties (e.g., consultants, business organizations) who can provide specialized expertise (e.g., process safety, ergonomics, technical expertise) or added independence or another set of "eyes" to the HSEQ audit program. This "rotating-auditor" approach requires significant "buy-in" from line management but stands a greater chance for success when there is indeed top-management support for the HSEQ audit program.

Keep in mind that the organization's legal resource may provide significant input but is not directly in control of the HSEQ audit program. The audit program director/manager may have organized a small group of audit program managers who serve as team leaders. Qualified auditors can come from anywhere in the organization but must successfully complete any internal auditor-training program, as prescribed, or other HSEQ auditor training or competency requirements determined by the HSEQ audit policy or procedure.

Whatever way it is decided that the audit program is structured, roles and responsibilities should be defined for each of the participant categories, which include, by way of example:

- Senior or executive management
- The audit program director/manager and staff
- The legal department or any other internal or external legal resource
- Business-unit management
- Facility management and staff
- Audit team leaders
- Auditors

A set of roles and responsibilities for the audit program director or manager, for example, might include

- determining, on an annual basis, the sites to be audited, in consistency with the corporate audit frequency policy;
- maintaining and updating program materials, including the program guidance manual, the preaudit questionnaire, and the audit protocols;
- maintaining the auditor-training program, including updating the qualified auditor database;
- reviewing all draft and final audit reports to ensure that they meet quality standards and are submitted on time;

- tracking the status of corrective-action plans and formally "closing out" audits when all findings are corrected;
- providing the audit teams, on an as-needed basis, with country or state regulatory information;
- conducting an annual evaluation of the program;
- reporting periodically on program status to the Board of Directors, if there is a Board; and
- managing, with the advice of counsel, as applicable, and in consultation with document control, the program files, in accordance with the corporation's established record-retention policy.

Roles and responsibilities for other participants can be established in a similar fashion. As with the program objectives, the individual participants' responsibilities should be framed so that performance can be measured.

Legal Protections

The legal-protection issue is one of great concern to most companies; therefore, each organization must decide on the approach that best fits its philosophy or business realities, including its current regulatory operating environment. And the best approach is not always invoking maximum legal protections for the program. Not all companies invoke formal attorney-client-privilege protections for HSEQ audit reports and documents.

Use of the privilege puts the legal department, or outside counsel, at the center of the program rather than in a review and advisory role. Such extensive legal involvement has often led to a more expensive and elaborate program and, perhaps more importantly, can slow down the report-distribution process substantially. It may be said that companies that do not invoke the privilege believe that the risk of disclosure is not improved substantially by attorney-client privilege since the underlying facts are not protected in any event. Moreover, any protections gained are viewed as more than offset by the increased program bureaucracy and the inability to produce and distribute reports expeditiously.

Scope and Coverage

Any audit program must operate within some bounds. Someone must decide which facilities or processes are to be audited, the scope of the audit, what they are to be audited against, and what type of audits will be conducted (which discipline(s): health, safety, environment, quality, and integrated approach of all disciplines, etc.). Risk-based criteria are always a good rule of thumb to follow in these instances.

Quite often, one of the HSEQ audit program director/manager's most difficult tasks is determining the inventory of facilities and related processes subject to the HSEQ audit program. With all the sales, mergers, acquisitions, and divestitures taking place in many organizations these days, the structure of any organization can change very, very quickly. Flexibility is essential. In general, HSEQ audit programs will be responsible for auditing the following facility types:

- Facilities owned and operated.
- Facilities operated on leased property.
  - Supply chain vendors and contractors.
  - Joint ventures with majority ownership and operational responsibility.
  - Joint ventures with minority ownership and operational responsibility.
  - Warehouses and distribution centers owned and operated.
- Administrative and office buildings owned and operated.
- Real estate owned.

For other facility types (such as joint ventures with majority or minority ownership and no operational responsibility or leased warehouses), the organization may attempt to influence partners to participate in the audit program or ensure that partners have an equivalent program—"skin in the game" if you will.

The second audit-scope issue relates to regulatory coverage. Program directors/managers must decide what regulations are to be addressed. Will HSEQ issues be combined into one integrated audit program? There are as many examples of organizations with separate compliance audit programs, based on the regulatory environment they are operating in, as there are of those with integrated HSEQ audit programs.

By way of example, an organization may have operations in many different parts of the world, and while the basis of the HSEQ management system policies, procedures, and processes may be equally applicable wherever in the world that organization is doing business, regulatory realities might not be aligned. In fact, they might be completely different or even in conflict with one another.

A couple of examples based on the experiences of the auditors:

Regulatory Differences to Be Reflected in Quality Audit—Example 1

The authors worked for an organization with its head office in Houston, Texas. The Houston office was given a significant contract by a major Canadian offshore oil and gas company to design and construct some major components for a fixed drilling platform consisting of a concrete gravity structure (CGS) and topsides for oil and gas processing, living quarters, a helipad, and so on.

While the parent company was operating out of Houston, the project office for the CGS project was in St. John's, Newfoundland and Labrador, Canada. The final CGS product was intended for installation and use some 300 kilometers in the waters of offshore Newfoundland and Labrador.

There was a project team assigned to design and build the CGS and related products. This project team consisted of key personnel from the United States and Canada, and even had some support engineering and services from different parts of Europe as well. So, it was truly a multinational project. That said, while the people working on the project were from multiple jurisdictions, the reality for the CGS to be able to operate in Canadian waters meant it had to be designed and constructed based on requirements for which the Canadian government had partial responsibility, so jurisdiction from an HSEQ perspective rested with Canada, despite the main contractor being owned and operated in Houston.

So while the Houston office mandated that their corporate policies and procedures had to be used on the project in Canada, just as they were required to be used in Houston, the local regulatory differences meant that the project team on the ground had to develop HSEQ policies and procedures to meet local, land-based regulatory requirements as well as HSEQ policies and procedures to meet offshore regulatory requirements where the CGS was to operate.

As the Quality Manager and Certification Lead on the project, Wayne was tasked with ensuring that the HSEQ management system and processes for the project would stand the test of an audit, whether it was conducted by the Houston office or the regulatory agencies. The Houston office in question did in fact schedule a quality audit based on the quality requirements of the Houston office, as well as the project-specific quality requirements for the CGS project. Those local quality requirements were mandated by the local regulatory agency with jurisdiction over the CGS project, the Canada-Newfoundland and Labrador Offshore Petroleum Board (C-NLOPB).

The quality audit notification identified the scope of the audit as being a blend of both Houston-based quality requirements and Newfoundland-based quality requirements, based on the Project Quality Plan for the CGS project. Audit focus was placed on the applicable regulatory requirements for the project.

5.0 Applicable Regulations

The Wellhead Platform Certificate of Fitness and prerequisite Certifying Authority's Scope of Work shall be limited to stating and ensuring compliance with C-NLOPB Certificate of Fitness Regulations and the relevant aspects of the following associated regulations.

- *Newfoundland Offshore Installations Petroleum Regulations,*
- *Oil and Gas Occupational Safety and Health Regulations*
- *Newfoundland Offshore Area Petroleum Diving Regulations*
- *Newfoundland Offshore Drilling and Production Regulations*

The Certifying Authority shall confirm compliance with the above regulations for those aspects of the detailed design which impact on the general integrity of the Topsides with respect to general safety and the avoidance of unintended release of contaminants to the environment.

ABC Company shall prepare a certification procedure for their scope of work to detail the coordination of the certification activities described in this plan.

So, as you can see, while the project was being managed by the company based out of Houston, the regulatory realities for the project quality audit were clearly based on the offshore oil and gas requirements of the jurisdiction in question. While the Houston company had very good resources and expertise to ensure compliance with U.S. and Houston-based regulatory requirements for HSEQ, they had to ensure they hired knowledgeable and competent resources here in Newfoundland to customize their corporate HSEQ requirements around the local regulatory realities against which they would be audited.

As can be seen in the project audit schedule, because of the very technical nature and high-risk processes of the project, and the critical nature of all the individual pieces of the project, which collectively would result in over 100 people living on this platform some 300 kilometers offshore Newfoundland, the audit schedule was both thorough and far-reaching in scope over a two-year project period.

Audit Schedule (*Draft*)

Project Name: *Project Name*
Project Number: *Project Number*

Project Manager: *Project Manager*
Project Phase: *Project Phase*

	2013												2014											
Activity	Jan	Feb	Mar	Apr	May	Jun	Jul	Aug	Sep	Oct	Nov	Dec	Jan	Feb	Mar	Apr	May	Jun	Jul	Aug	Sep	Oct	Nov	Dec
Project System Audits																								
PEP/ QMS Requirements																								
Project Management																								
Risk Management																								
Interface Management																								
Project Controls (MoC etc)																								
Information Management																								
Regulatory																								
Training																								
Occupational Safety																								
Procurement																								
Tech Safety																								
Process																								
Mechanical/ Facilities																								
Piping/Layout																								
Civil Structural/ bldgs																								
Intrumentation/ Automation																								
Electrical																								
Subcontractor/Vendor/Supplier (To include review of Inspection Release Certificate)																								
Construction Management																								
Preparedness Assessment for Completion & Close-Out																								
Project Technical Audits																								
Mechanical/ Facilities																								

Project Quality Auditing

To operationalize the above quality audit example, the guidance in place for the project stated that audits were to be conducted or overseen by the project quality manager, with the objective being to judge the compliance of the project's execution to the Project Execution Plan, referenced procedures and contract requirements, as well as the overall status and effectiveness of the project's HSEQ management system. The audit will assess the project execution process to determine project quality status, problem areas, and opportunities for improvement. In some activities, the project quality manager may enlist a qualified and experienced member of the relevant engineering department who is not part of the full-time project team.

The ABC Company procedure titled "Management System Auditing" will be used as a guideline for conducting internal audits. Audits shall follow established protocols and shall be conducted by competent auditors or audit teams, including additional technical assistance where required.

Findings from audits will be recorded, discussed, and agreed with the auditee. The auditee will be required to develop a document action plan to address accepted findings. Audit findings will be tracked, and progress completion will be reported to the project manager.

ABC Company's tracking system (Quality Management Tracking System for Corrective/Preventive Action) will be used to track findings against project quality and contractual requirements. This system will track audit findings through to closure using SMART objectives and send email reminders to the person responsible for closing the finding.

Project Auditing Process

To put the quality audit policy/procedure into practical action, the audit plan documented the following for the quality audit in question:

- Audits shall also confirm the execution of specified quality activities and the existence of quality records. The following audit practices shall be observed.
- Audits of the project are to be scheduled on a regular basis by the project quality manager in consultation with the project manager.
- Written notification announcing the performance of scheduled audit activities will be communicated by the project quality manager.
- Audits of the project are to be scheduled by the project quality manager using the approved audit schedule. Preliminary audit dates will be confirmed two weeks prior to the scheduled date. Actual audit dates may change depending on the progress of the areas to be audited.
- Audits may be rescheduled to allow for variations in the project schedule or allow for the availability of objective evidence.
- Actual audit dates and agendas will be announced by the project quality manager.
- A quality audit checklist shall be forwarded to the auditee two (2) days prior to the audit to enable the auditee to assemble objective evidence. The objective is to reduce the administrative time required for conducting the audit.
- After an audit has been performed, the auditor will prepare an audit report. The report will be provided to the project manager and filed in the project files.
- The project manager will distribute copies of audit reports at his or her discretion.

Project Audit Schedule

Quality audits of the project are to be scheduled by the project quality manager in conjunction with the project manager. Written notification announcing the performance of scheduled audit activities will be communicated by the project quality manager.

The Quality Audit Schedule is a "live" document and as such will be subject to periodic review in line with changes to the contracted scope of work. Actual audit dates may change depending on progress, to allow for variations in the project schedule or allow for the availability of objective evidence. Actual audit dates and agendas will be announced by the ABC Company's project quality manager two (2) weeks prior to commencement.

Quality audits requested by the client or project personnel may be scheduled on an "ad hoc" basis without updating the quality audit schedule. The client shall be included in all formally issued audit notifications.

So, as you can see from this audit example, the entire process was designed and delivered based on the quality and regulatory realities of the audit location in question. It was detailed, specific, applicable to the realities of the auditee, and designed to be a closed-loop process from start to finish, with no gaps or stones left unturned. In the hands of a seasoned, experienced, and qualified auditor, the outcome of the audit process achieved the intended objectives.

Regulatory Differences to Be Reflected in Quality Audit—Example 2

In this example, the client was a U.S. airline that needed to ensure their internal audit process was aligned with the requirements of the International Air Transport Association (IATA). IATA is the trade association for the world's airlines, representing some 320 airlines or 83 percent of total air traffic. The IATA Operational Safety Audit (IOSA) Program is an internationally recognized and accepted evaluation system designed to assess the operational management and control systems of an airline.

The IOSA audit creates a standard that is comparable on a worldwide basis, enabling and maximizing the joint use of audit reports. This has saved the industry over 6,400 redundant audits and continues to lead to extensive cost savings for IOSA participating airlines. All IATA members are IOSA-registered and must remain registered to maintain IATA membership.

Reference: https://www.iata.org/en/programs/safety/audit/iosa/

To ensure their audit program checklists aligned with the regulatory requirements of the Federal Aviation Administration (FAA), as part of the scope of the IOSA audit, author Wayne Pardy, through the HSEQ software company he was vice president of at the time, was contracted to ensure all internal audit checklists were developed in alignment with both FAA and applicable IOSA audit requirements, based on the regulatory focus of the IOSA audit.

While the airline was quite confident of its regulatory compliance obligation to the FAA to be able to continue to operate in U.S. airspace, the IOSA audit presented some challenges, as well as opportunities, for the airline to develop an integrated safety audit based on regulatory and international safety requirements. The author worked with the airline in question to ensure that where select FAA and IOSA audit questions could be combined rather than asking two separate questions, the audit checklist was developed as an integrated audit checklist, thereby "*killing two birds with one stone*" so to speak.

This activity was intended to ensure that whenever the airline conducted a compliance audit, it was assured that the compliance obligations in an industry-standard audit like IOSA were not overlooked.

Once any company has decided on the regulatory scope of the program, it can then decide on the types of audits that can best meet the program's objectives. This may result in the creation of specialized audits, designed to address multi-organizational or multi-jurisdiction/regulatory issues, as well as the more traditional compliance audits. Such specialized audits will be discussed in later chapters.

Facility Audit Schedules

When first faced with the "audit or not" question, many corporate HSEQ departments wonder where the significant additional resources will come from. In an economic environment that shouts, "Do more with less," some initial planning and priority setting can help the compliance manager meet the often-conflicting objectives of (1) increasing HSEQ compliance, and (2) reducing the resources committed to that goal. Fortunately, managers can take some steps to better understand the operations within the company that pose the greatest risks and to design an audit program that addresses those risks within the context of resource constraints. Setting facility audit schedules based on a sense of risk can do much to ensure a cost-effective program.

Many companies with mature audit programs have settled on a two- to three-year frequency for major facilities. Some have moved to a five-year model in instances where the regulatory demands are many and complex. This is after each facility has been audited at least once or twice. Some small facilities might have the time and resources to audit more frequently. Organizations with a single facility have the ultimate flexibility in when and how they intend to audit that single facility.

There are, of course, other approaches to ranking facilities by risk. Generally, site risk factors can be viewed as twofold: inherent and external. First, there are indeed inherent operating risks, which can involve the materials handled, the age of the facility, and the complexity of the process. These risks are important but perhaps more controllable than the second class of external risks, which may include the company's compliance history, the community and environmental setting, customer requirements, or the risks associated with the products or services being offered at that facility. It's always prudent to look to whatever corporate risk-management processes you utilize to help arrive at this risk-based conclusion.

Any facility or unit can be evaluated for its relative risk potential by using the risk assessment process the organization has in place as its main risk-management tool. Corrective-action programs can then be fine-tuned to address the nature and extent of the risk with the most cost-effective solution. One of these solutions could be the development of an HSEQ audit program that uses the material and facility risk-assessment techniques discussed previously as priority-setting tools. The scope, frequency, and resource commitment can be assigned based on an estimate of risks posed by, and the materials handled at, the facility. In this way, resources are committed cost-effectively. That is, the number of auditors and the facilities being audited at any one time are minimized.

Once the organization's inventory of facilities to be audited is established and a frequency, audit duration, and team size are assigned to each facility, the manpower loading for field audits can be determined for any given year. Further, if the number of field hours is increased by 50 percent or so to account for audit preparation and report writing, the result should indicate full labor-cost accounting for the program, except for management and administration time.

Compiling this information on a spreadsheet or some type of similar audit management software will allow the program manager to manipulate critical factors, such as audit frequency, to determine the financial or budgetary impacts of increasing or decreasing the frequency.

Auditor Selection and Training

Thus far, in the history of HSEQ auditing, companies have tended to design their audit function using one of four fundamental organizational approaches. The first of these, appropriate for larger companies, is to set up a corporate audit function. Under this option, full-time auditors are hired or transferred permanently into a corporate staff unit. This staff function alone is responsible for conducting company-wide audits. This strategy can be found in companies where management responsibilities are quite centralized.

The second approach, also most appropriate for large companies, involves establishing audit functions at the division or business-unit levels. Here, the auditors from one division assess the facilities of other divisions and vice versa. Each audit team reports the results of its assessments to corporate headquarters. This strategy is typically used within the operating divisions.

A third tactic is to have each plant audit itself using common guidelines but ensuring that the auditors do not audit their own work. This approach amounts to self-reporting and is used by some larger companies as well as by one-facility organizations.

Finally, some companies use outside contractors or consultants to (1) develop and manage their audit programs, (2) conduct individual facility audits, or (3) complete periodic third-party reviews of their in-house facility audits. Quite naturally, each of the above approaches has its advantages and disadvantages. Choosing among them can sometimes be a difficult exercise, with no clear choice emerging.

Independent of the chosen organizational style of an HSEQ audit program are the questions of how many staff should make up a given audit team and who they should be. Since the assessment team is the heart of each organization's program, the success of the program depends in large part on the skill, judgment, and perception of the team members.

Typically, the size of a given assessment team will depend upon the size of the facility, the complexity of the HSEQ issues, and the time elapsed since the last assessment. Another factor to be considered is if the same auditor has been auditing that same facility for some time. The caution here is that sometimes you don't get, for example, ten different audits over ten years, but you get the same audit ten different times. Experience has shown that four to six people are needed for a week to review complex facilities, with an equal amount of additional time off-site to prepare, write the final report, and respond to inquiries. On the other hand, certain facilities, such as storage facilities or warehouses, can be reviewed by one person in half a day.

Team composition will be dictated largely by the type of facility, the HSEQ issues, and the size of the team. In formulating the team, care should be given to balancing the skills of the team members to include knowledge of

- the audit process;
- the applicable HSEQ regulations;
- corporate policies and procedures; and
- the individual facility operations.

Because of the range of knowledge required, it is not surprising that some organizations will select representatives from among several disciplines, including operations managers, engineers, scientists, attorneys, and accountants (because of their experience with financial audits). However, it is safe to say that the majority of audit teams consist of an operations or HSEQ manager as team leader, supported by engineers and scientists familiar with HSEQ issues. Where a sensitive legal situation dictates, an attorney may provide on- or off-site counsel directly to the audit team. Seldom have the authors seen a member of legal counsel on an audit team.

Audit Reports and Documentation

Audit programs can generate a very large and significant number of documents, many of which can pose significant liabilities to the organization if not managed judiciously, or in conformance with the organization's control of documented information requirements. Thus, document management and retention are critical issues for the audit program manager. Each organization must decide for itself the appropriate document retention procedures.

One of the most daunting decisions with respect to document retention is the question of how long one retains the actual final audit report. Some regulatory requirements can provide guidance here as they stipulate prescriptively how long the document or record is to be maintained. Organizations likely do not want to lose any of the history of the audit program and the audits. They also likely do not want to retain any of the liabilities posed by self-incriminating documents that may no longer be accurate. To each his own.

Audit Program Management and Evaluation

Any management program should be evaluated on a periodic basis. Each year, the audit program manager should report to senior management on the successes and failures of the program. The submittals, concise reports on the status of the program, should contain the following information at a minimum:

- Number of audits completed during the period and the number planned for the next period.
- Highlights of liabilities or nonconformances most affecting the organization.
- Trends in the types of noncompliance items to identify potential corporate-wide issues.
- Trends in the number or percentage of repeat findings.
- Statistics on business success rates in meeting corrective-action plan schedules or the percentage of on-time closures of audit findings.
- Results of formal feedback from those who were audited.
- Development and implementation of an auditor-training program.
- Timeliness and quality of audit reports.
- Periodic information-exchange reports focusing on key findings and root-cause analysis.
- Annual update of the program guidance manual and audit protocols.

Audit program managers often struggle with determining the key metrics for the business units and sites being audited. Often considered are the number of findings, the number of high-priority or high-risk findings, the number of repeat findings, and the on-time closure of action items. Of course, high-priority or high-risk findings can be subjective unless there's a very clear definition of what constitutes the priority or risk. An excellent indicator is the on-time closure of audit findings/action items based on agreed/documented risk. Simply using the number of findings is problematic; all findings do not pose the same or identical risk. Defining what constitutes a high-priority or repeat finding is a challenging task and often leads to controversy. On-time closure of action items is simply a matter of "saying what you'll do and doing what you said."

The audit program evaluation can be done internally or by a third party and should be completed annually and reported to the Board of Directors or executive management.

Audit Program Support Tools

The principal audit program tools include the guidance manual, corporate HSEQ standards, regulatory databases, model presentations and reports, and the auditors' checklists or protocols. The protocols are clearly a critical tool. These are the actual working documents for the auditors. The checklists pose questions relating to the following:

- Compliance with regulatory requirements (the "paper" audit, or perhaps a digital audit).
- Effective organizational controls (the "management" audit).
- Proper on-site and off-site unit operations (the "technical" audit).

These three areas are reviewed to determine whether (1) specific regulatory requirements are known and being complied with; (2) an organization is in place to monitor compliance, respond to upsets or emergencies, and anticipate regulatory changes; and (3) compliance procedures are carried out by unit operators.

Protocols should be developed for key compliance areas to integrate any applicable regulatory requirements influencing the facility. Specific protocols should be developed or obtained for at least the following compliance areas, if they are applicable to the facility.

The following elements should be part of a good audit protocol:

- It should provide the auditor with an abstract or overview of the key regulations and requirements relevant to each compliance area at the facility being audited.
- It should highlight those key definitions that help the auditor conduct the audit without having to refer to the full-text copies of the applicable regulations. The importance of definitions in verifying regulatory compliance areas cannot be overemphasized.

- It should include all the items strictly required by the stated Acts and their associated regulations.
- It should include inspection items that permit evaluation of the plant's vulnerability to "real world" HSEQ problems (e.g., noise, odor, nuisances, community impacts).
- It should provide an opportunity to verify that internal company HSEQ management procedures are understood and adhered to by applicable staff.
- It should give the auditor specific action steps so that compliance can be properly evaluated. Use of action verbs such as "examine," "inspect," "calculate," and the like should be used in the protocol so that the auditor clearly understands what must be done to verify compliance.
- The protocol should provide a space in which comments can be written by the auditor. These notes are then readily available during the writing of the audit report. This also discourages the use of loose paper and notes that could be misplaced. Of course, with the advent of e-auditing technologies, that paper-based process may or may not be in play.

Within these guidelines, individual approaches can vary. Commercially available audit protocols can be purchased (e.g., Dakota Auditor, STP, ENHESA). Protocols can also be obtained for free over the Internet. Or you can create your own. While using a protocol developed by the regulators is by no means a fail-safe approach to assuring compliance, it does provide an internal system of checks consistent with external regulatory expectations.

Remember that in using any protocol, these instruments are designed as aids and should not be considered exhaustive. The auditor's judgment should continue to play a role in determining the focus and extent of further investigation.

The development of an appropriate set of audit protocols is, at a minimum, a challenging task. Prior to the selection of a particular style, the manual developer should think long and hard about the specific objectives of the overall corporate audit program, the demands a particular style may place on plant staff and their willingness to accommodate these demands, and the capabilities of the staff who will be designated, either temporarily or permanently, as auditors.

If one chooses to develop, rather than purchase, a set of protocols, the following steps should be taken:

- *Decide on the scope of the audits.* Which laws and regulations will be reviewed? Will the checklists include federal, state provincial and local requirements?
- *Review your facilities against these standards.* For example, do you have any required permits? Do you have any processes covered by the Occupational Safety and Health Administration's process-safety management regulations? Not all regulations will need checklists if you have no facilities or operations regulated by the standards.
- *Decide on your checklist format.* Use the following sources to choose or develop your checklist style:
  - commercial audit protocols
  - government-available protocols
  - published literature
- *Develop one checklist.* Pick a compliance area (e.g., wastewater discharges, fall protection, control of customer property), and develop the checklist.
- *Test the checklist.* Before proceeding with the remaining checklists, test the first one. It is surprising sometimes how the logic developed in the office is found wanting in the field.
- *Develop and test the remaining checklists.* Complete and test the remaining checklists, looking for a balance between completeness and manageability.

The result of this exercise should be checklists that meet the specific organizational objectives.

A KEY PROGRAM ISSUE: CORPORATE STANDARDS AND GUIDELINES

One of the most useful aids for any audit program is a sound set of corporate HSEQ standards and guidelines. Generally, numerous HSEQ management standards can be developed to enable a company to manage its HSEQ-related activities more effectively. Such standards might involve requiring secondary containment for all drum and tank storage and transfer stations for hazardous materials and wastes, regardless of local regulatory requirements.

Development of a common set of corporate expectations gives the audit team a firm foundation for making risk-based recommendations. For example, in a case with no regulatory or corporate requirements for secondary containment of hazardous materials, auditors might receive significant "pushback" from the site were they to recommend such corrective action, even in cases where the risk clearly justified construction of containment. Several HSEQ management standards or procedures that could be developed in any organization are discussed below. Certainly, many more procedures could be developed as well. Some will relate to administrative requirements, and others might relate to minimally acceptable physical facilities.

HSEQ Record-Keeping/Records-Retention Procedures

The objective of this management procedure is to specify HSEQ-related data, records, reports, and files that should be maintained by the company. HSEQ-related data, records, reports, and files should be interpreted broadly to include all materials strictly required by statute, rule, or regulation, as well as those written materials useful and necessary for the company to manage its HSEQ compliance program but not required by law. The procedure should also identify responsibilities for maintenance and custody of HSEQ records, including minimum retention periods.

In some cases, joint custody of records should be established between departments that share responsibility for compliance activities. Some records and reports must be maintained for specified periods as stipulated in various statutes, rules, and regulations. Many records, however, have no statutory requirements for retention; therefore, considerations of good management practice should be used to establish the retention periods.

Records are normally maintained in a central location. Maintaining them in this manner will aid in the retrieval of HSEQ-compliance-related information and enhance the site's ability to respond to internal audits and external regulatory inspections.

External Regulatory Inspection Procedures

The objective of this management procedure is to specify protocols to be followed when compliance inspections are conducted by external regulatory agencies. Most regulatory agencies have broad statutory authority to conduct inspections at industrial facilities.

Organizations should develop a procedure that includes steps for dealing with these visits. While some might say that government inspectors or auditors can do whatever they want when it comes to workplace audits and inspections, that's not necessarily the case. Others argue that by having steps in place for dealing with inspections or audits of outside agencies only helps create an adversarial relationship with those outside agencies. But prudent organizations recognize that balance and fairness are required, and while the cliché, "*I'm from the government. . . I'm here to help,*" might be met with cynicism by some, prudent organizations will look to develop reasonable and balanced procedures on how internal staff need to deal with these scenarios.

The procedure should deal with items that could be covered prior to, during, and after the audit or inspection. Facility management should have clear guidance on (1) the limits of authority of inspectors, (2) the objective and scope of the audit or inspection, (3) the facility personnel who will accompany the inspector, and (4) legal counsel participation.

During the audit or inspection, facility personnel should have guidance on how they should respond to deficiencies found, what notes they should take during the inspection, and what their general attitude should be in dealing with inspectors. Of course, the general attitude should be one of mutual respect and courtesy. That said, we're sure there are some interesting stories which readers might have, as do the authors, on instances where government auditors or inspectors used their authority in a less-than-courteous or respectful way. After the audit or inspection, facility personnel should have instructions from corporate headquarters on preparing memoranda for the record and developing an action plan for resolving identified deficiencies.

CONTINUOUS REVIEW

Auditing is not done once and forgotten for ten years (or we hope in your organization it's not). Noncompliance and nonconformance can surface quickly. In fact, you can literally be complying one hour and out of compliance the next. Things change sometimes very quickly and dramatically. Therefore, audits should be conducted on a regular basis. What "regular" means will be determined by several factors, not the least of which are available resources to conduct the actual audit. But the audit program should evolve into an integral part of operations, and senior management should periodically review the audit program to ensure that it is continuing to meet its originally stated objectives. In fact, some companies use outside firms periodically to conduct audits as a midcourse review of their program.

EVALUATING THE RESULTS AND IMPLEMENTING THE SOLUTIONS

These two elements must both be included for a program to be successful. Corporations are most vulnerable to potential liability when compliance problems have been identified, yet no solutions are planned. Even worse, having the planned solution but then doing nothing about it, or doing it half-heartedly, is a potential recipe for disaster. These solutions must be documented, even when management initially can only commit to a phased response for a needed major capital expenditure. It is vital that senior management have a system in place to ensure that where violations have been noted, the facility operator is, in fact, on the way toward achieving compliance. History indicates that the corporation and its executives are at great risk when violations have been identified and no plan is in place to remedy the situation. Ignorance or apathy is not a defense of due diligence.

In recent years, there has been a particular trend toward (1) assuring that corrective-action plans are, in fact, just that, and (2) providing formal briefings for senior management, including the Board of Directors, on the status of the audit program. Automated tracking systems have been put in place in most companies. These systems produce monthly status reports for each facility's action plan and, subsequently, produce statistics for senior management on those items completed ahead of, on, or behind schedule. This kind of reporting to senior management has done much to increase the internal credibility of the audit program; after all, senior management can no longer escape the civil and criminal liability associated with noncompliance.

REFERENCES

This chapter has been adapted from Lawrence B. Cahill and Raymond W. Kane. *Environmental Health and Safety Audits*, 9th Edition. Government Institutes, 2010. It has been updated for this edition.

Wayne Pardy and Terri Andrews. *Integrated Management Systems: Leading Strategies and Solutions*, 2nd Edition. Bernan Press, 2019.

https://www.iata.org/en/programs/safety/audit/iosa/.

The IATA Operational Safety Audit (IOSA) Program is an internationally recognized and accepted evaluation system designed to assess the operational management and control systems of an airline. IOSA uses internationally recognized quality audit principles and is designed so that audits are conducted in a standardized and consistent manner.

https://www.iata.org/en/programs/safety/audit/iosa/.

"FAA Approves IATA's Operational Safety Audit (IOSA) Program: A Historical Review and Future Implications for the Airline Industry".

https://digitalcommons.du.edu/cgi/viewcontent.cgi?article=1184&context=tlj.

https://cdn.standards.iteh.ai/samples/70017/559078f9a2634aca84ff0a6aac1498f6/ISO-19011-2018.pdf.

Dan Petersen: "Why Safety is a People Problem", Dec. 31, 1996.

https://www.ehstoday.com/archive/article/21907885/dan-petersen-why-safety-is-a-people-problem.

Note: The reference to any software or IT-related audit software or technology is in no way intended to be an endorsement of that product or the organization providing the product.

Chapter 5

Impact of International Standards on HSEQ Audit Programs

Opinions have vested interests just as men have.

—Samuel Butler, 1835–1902

INTRODUCTION

Many health, safety, environmental, and quality (HSEQ) initiatives have surfaced internationally over the past years. Expectations for corporations are rising even as these initiatives compete for recognition and acceptance. For the past several decades, notable disasters such as the Bhopal and *Exxon Valdez* accidents, as well as more chronic environmental issues such as deforestation and the depletion of the ozone layer, have heightened the world's concerns over the environment by generating support for establishing a "level global playing field" that protects the environment while allowing for sustainable development. In recent years, the "sustainability" and "climate-change" revolution has transformed heretofore recalcitrant companies into leading proponents of the environmental-sustainability philosophy.

"Going green" is an ethic espoused in just about all annual corporate reports today. This fundamental sea change is the underlying driver for all the increased pressure on transnational companies to rethink their performance. Sustainable development in its basic form is the process of meeting the needs of the present without interfering with the ability of future generations to meet their needs.

ISO STANDARDS

The standards with probably the most potential long-term impact for HSEQ audit validity are those crafted by the International Organization for Standardization (ISO). ISO has a long history of developing quality standards (i.e., the ISO 9000 series) that are firmly entrenched in the developed world, including the United States, Canada, Europe, and Asia.

In some industries (e.g., automotive, electronics), becoming a registered ISO 9000 company is almost mandatory. In time, a facility seeking ISO 9001 quality registration may be required to have or be seeking ISO 14000 EMS registration or ISO 45001 SMS registration as well. In fact, there are many organizations already pursuing this integrated, strategic HSEQ management and auditing approach, according to the experience of the authors. And while registration may or may not be mandated, many clients require at least some form of self-declaration or self-conformance to the requirements of these standards. The prudent and practical use of the guidance in these standards can be realized by anyone with a desire for a disciplined approach to helping improve the HSEQ performance of their organization. Full standard adherence is not required.

It might be prudent again to reference just a few of those standards which are gaining traction nationally and internationally:

- ISO 9001 Quality Management Standard
- ISO 14001 Environmental Management Standard
- ISO 45001 Occupational Health and Safety Standard
- ISO 22301 Business Continuity Management Standard
- ISO 27001 Information Security Management Standard
- ISO 13485 Quality Management Standard for Medical Devices
- IATF 16949 Quality Management Standard for Automotive Sector
- AS9100 Quality Management Standard for Aerospace and Defense

Early in 1993, ISO constituted a new technical committee (TC 207) charged with developing international standards in the field of environmental tools and systems. ISO/TC 207 was the result of a two-year study by ISO's Strategic Advisory Group on the Environment, which concluded that international environmental management standards would

- promote a common approach to environmental management, like quality management and the ISO 9000 series;
- enhance organizations' ability to attain and measure improvements in environmental performance; and
- facilitate trade and remove trade barriers.

In mid-1993, several ISO/TC 207 subcommittees were established to address aspects of EMSs. These subcommittees and the countries designated to lead the effort are:

- Environmental Management Systems (United Kingdom)
- Environmental Auditing (Netherlands)
- Environmental Labeling (Australia)
- Environmental Performance Evaluation (United States)
- Life Cycle Assessment (France)
- Terms and Definitions (Norway)
- Environmental Aspects in Product Standards (Germany)

Official ISO 14000 standards related to management systems and auditing were originally finalized in the fall of 1996. ISO 14001 is a specification standard, and companies that wish to have their EMS certified must meet its requirements. The other environmental auditing standards are only guidelines and originally comprised three separate guidelines:

1. ISO 14010: "General Principles of Environmental Management Systems Auditing"
2. ISO 14011: "EMS Auditing Procedures"
3. ISO 14012: "Qualification Criteria for Environmental Auditors"

However, in 2002, a new consolidated guideline document was published by ISO and renamed ISO 19011. This current document addresses fundamental principles of HSEQ auditing. It should be noted that the ISO 19011 auditing guidelines are just that—guidelines. This is to distinguish them from the ISO 14001 environmental management systems specification noted above, which carries with it the "shall" descriptor, as do the ISO 45001 and 9001 Standards. That said, in the opinion of the authors, they are very good guidelines.

ISO 45001

ISO 45001 is an ISO standard for management systems of occupational health and safety (OHS), published in March 2018. The goal of ISO 45001 is the reduction of occupational injuries and diseases, including promoting and protecting physical and mental/psychological health. The standard is based on the old British Standard OHSAS 18001, conventions and guidelines of the International Labour Organization, and national standards. It includes elements that are additional to OHSAS 18001, which it is replacing over a three-year migration period from 2018 to 2021. As of March 2021, companies and organizations should have migrated to ISO 45001 to retain a valid certification, although ISO has extended the transition period for up to six months (to September 11, 2021) for organizations adversely affected by COVID-19.

ISO 45001 follows the High-Level Structure of other ISO standards, such as ISO 9001:2015 and ISO 14001:2015, which makes the integration of these standards easier.

Development

ISO 45001 was proposed at the ISO in October 2013. The committee ISO/PC 283, created in 2013, had direct responsibility for the standardization process. At least seventy countries contributed to the drafting process. Preparation and committee work lasted until December 2015. From 2015 to 2017, a first draft failed to gain sufficient approval from ISO members and was revised in a second draft, which was approved and refined into a final draft. In the final vote, the standard garnered 62 votes in favor, 9 abstentions, and 4 votes against from France, India, Spain, and Turkey. The standard was published on March 12, 2018.

Certification

ISO 45001 replaces OHSAS 18001 over three years following its publication in March 2018. BSI formally withdrew OHSAS 18001 in September 2021, at the end of the extended migration period (due to COVID-19). ISO 45001 uses the management system standard structure guideline Annex SL to allow for simplified integration with other management system standards, such as ISO 9001 and ISO 14001. The International Accreditation Forum has published requirements for migration from OHSAS 18001 to ISO 45001. Also, in March of 2024, ISO published ISO 45004, Occupational health and safety management—guidelines on performance evaluation, intended to assist those who have adopted 45001 on how to measure and evaluate the effectiveness of their management system.

Organizations with a preexisting OHSAS certification that migrate to ISO 45001:2018 can consider both certifications as one. For example, an OHSAS 18001 certification from 2017 that migrated to ISO 45001:2018 in 2020 will be considered as having run from 2017.

ISO/IEC TS 17021-10:2018 is a technical specification setting out competence requirements for auditing and certification of ISO 45001.

Adoption

ISO 45001 was adopted as a national standard by Albania, Argentina, Armenia, Austria, Australia, Azerbaijan, Belgium, Bolivia, Bosnia and

Herzegovina, Brazil, Bulgaria, Canada, Chile, Colombia, Costa Rica, Croatia, the Czech Republic, Denmark, Ecuador, El Salvador, Estonia, Finland, Georgia, Germany, Greece, Honduras, Hungary, Iceland, India, Indonesia, Ireland, Israel, Italy, Japan, Kazakhstan, Latvia, Lithuania, Malaysia, Moldova, the Netherlands, New Zealand, North Macedonia, Norway, Paraguay, Peru, the Philippines, Poland, Portugal, Romania, Russia, Serbia, Singapore, Slovakia, Slovenia, South Africa, Sri Lanka, Sweden, Switzerland, Taiwan, Turkey, the United Kingdom, the United States, Uruguay, and Uzbekistan.

ISO 45001 changes compared to OHSAS 18001

- Context of the organization (Clause 4.1): The organization shall determine internal and external issues that are relevant to its purpose and that affect its ability to achieve the intended outcome(s) of its OHS management system.
- Understanding the needs and expectations of workers and other interested parties (Clause 4.2): interested parties include workers, suppliers, subcontractors, clients, and regulatory authorities.
- Risk and opportunities (Clauses: 6.1.1, 6.1.2.3, 6.1.4): companies are to determine, consider, and, where necessary, take action to address any risks or opportunities that may impact (either positively or negatively) the ability of the management system to deliver its intended results, including enhanced health and safety at the workplace.
- Leadership and management commitment (Clauses: 5.1) have a stronger emphasis on top management to actively engage and take accountability for the effectiveness of the management system.
- Planning: (Clause 6)

Source: https://en.wikipedia.org/wiki/ISO_45001#:~:text=ISO%2045001%20was%20proposed%20at%20the%20ISO%20in,Preparation%20and%20committee%20work%20lasted%20until%20December%202015.

If we were rewriting our book on integrated HSEQ management systems, we would perhaps spend some time on the rationale and logic of the requirement of something like ISO 45001. But we will look at this health and safety management system standard from the other side of the coin. We will profile the requirement as documented by the good folks at Praxiom Research Group Limited but reflected in an audit protocol/checklist which any auditor can use or modify to rationalize an audit approach to 45001 conformance.

The following overview of the 45001 audit requirements is intended to assist any 45001 auditors in focusing on their audit pre-preparation. It provides a high-level view of the scope of the audit and a general overview of the key areas of conformance that must be audited by anyone looking to determine if their OHS management system meets the requirements of ISO 45001.

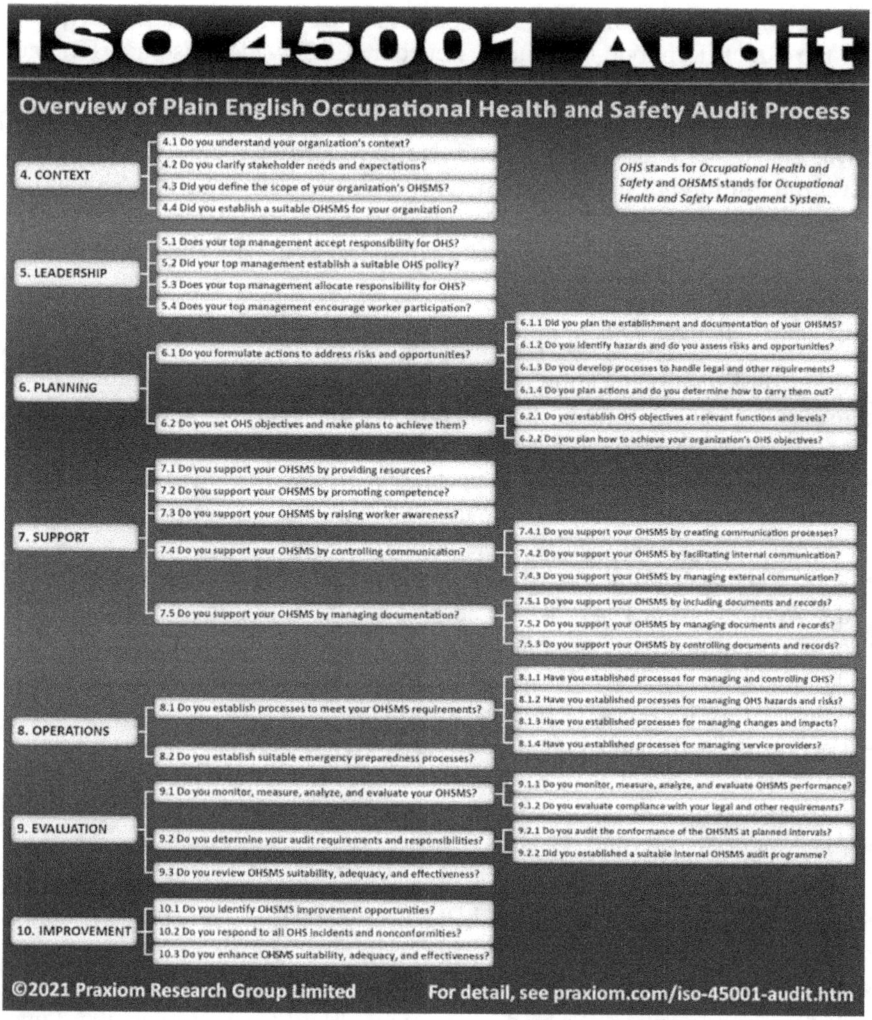

Figure used with permission of Ron Krebs of the Praxiom Research group Limited

CORPORATE RESPONSES

In many ways, the future expectations for the discipline area of environmental excellence can be overwhelming to some corporate executives. Nonetheless, the likelihood that all of this will simply go away is quite remote. Thus, corporations have changed the way they operate, anticipating an increasingly challenging future. Five rather interesting developments are:

1. Appointment of environmental experts to corporate boards.
2. Voluntary public reporting.
3. Third-party program evaluations and certifications.
4. Benchmarking studies.
5. Environmental-performance rating agencies.

Each of these is discussed briefly below.

Voluntary Public Reporting

Public reporting of environmental issues generates great angst among chief executives in major corporations. The Toxics Release Inventory (TRI) is a resource for learning about toxic chemical releases and pollution prevention activities reported by industrial and federal facilities. TRI data supports informed decision-making by communities, government agencies, companies, and others. Section 313 of the Emergency Planning and Community Right-to-Know Act (EPCRA) created the TRI. This is one list that companies will attempt to avoid. And anyone can check it at any time:

Source: https://www.epa.gov/toxics-release-inventory-tri-program

Third-Party Program Evaluations and Certifications

As is consistent with good total-quality-management practices, many companies are now having outside consultants (i.e., third parties) or their internal audit departments (i.e., second parties) evaluate their HSEQ audit programs on a periodic basis. The evaluations help the companies both meet their "continuous improvement" objectives and respond to the increasing pressure by stakeholders, including shareholders, to provide assurances that the company is identifying and remedying its HSEQ issues.

These companies' environmental reports are increasingly addressing the evaluation of HSEQ audit programs. For example, from 1992 through 2010, DuPont provided the results of the third-party evaluation of its Safety, Health, and Environmental Audit Program on its website. Colgate-Palmolive, Sunoco, Eastman Kodak, Bristol-Myers Squibb, and numerous other companies have provided similar information as part of their annual environmental reporting.

Benchmarking Studies

One might ask how environmental expectations should be managed appropriately in the future. Companies have important strategic choices: they can be leading-edge, middle-of-the-pack, or follower companies. Depending on a variety of factors, each of these strategies may be appropriate. One of the key challenges, however, is defining at any given time what each strategy means. The rules and expectations are changing constantly; leading-edge this year could be a follower next year.

Conducting regular benchmarks of comparable companies can help to better define the situation. Conducting simple benchmarking studies can help audit program managers make better decisions about the direction they should take and understand the possible consequences of those decisions.

Many benchmarking studies focus on specific industry sectors. These are useful when a company wants to compare itself to competitors and learn more about the best audit program practices unique to that industry.

REFERENCES

This chapter has been adapted from Lawrence B. Cahill and Raymond W. Kane. *Environmental Health and Safety Audits*, 9th Edition. Government Institutes, 2010. It has been updated for this edition.

Wayne Pardy and Terri Andrews. *Integrated Management Systems: Leading Strategies and Solutions*, 2nd Edition. Bernan Press, 2019.

Praxiom Research Group Limited. Edmonton, Alberta. Courtesy of Ron Krebs.

Source: https://www.epa.gov/toxics-release-inventory-tri-program.

ISO 19011. https://cdn.standards.iteh.ai/samples/70017/559078f9a2634aca84ff0a6aac1498f6/ISO-19011-2018.pdf

Chapter 6

A Review of Some Typical HSEQ Audit Programs

Although many HSEQ audit programs and management systems exhibit the same basic structure, individual program approaches are usually tailor-made to meet the objectives, opportunities, organizational realities, and constraints of the sponsoring organization. Thus, one can find distinctly different audit programs in the same basic industry. But that's a positive thing, as it can help ensure those developing the programs are critical in their thinking and have designed their programs around their needs and realities. Over time, one can even find a dramatically changed program in the same company. The changes can occur due to reorganization, changes in staff, midcourse program evaluations, or, in these days of mergers and acquisitions, a major restructuring of business lines, or in fact, the entire business itself.

PROGRAM NAME

While many organizations use the word "audit" to describe the nature of the program, as we've seen, others use surrogate terms, such as "assessment," "evaluation," "measurement," "surveillance," and "systems review." Some of the reasons given for using surrogates are that (1) audits can connote a more rigorous approach (vis-à-vis financial audits) than is typically the case, (2) the word "audit" (meaning "to examine, verify, or correct accounts, records, or claims") has an accusatory tone, and (3) HSEQ audits are more than the paperwork exercises that financial audits imply.

There has also been some commentary made about the actual use of the word "audit" in some cases and some of the negative perceptions the word "audit" brings. In our experience, this is in part due to negative audit experiences, where the auditee found that the audit experience wasn't a positive one. And in many of those instances, from our experience, they marked that perception down to the personal characteristics of the auditor, not the audit process per se.

Take two exactly the same structured audit plans and put them in the hands of an experienced and inexperienced auditor, and you might get two completely different products. The technical aspects of the audit aside (audit scope, auditor training, etc.), in the hands of an individual who cares little for the product of their activities or is using the audit to further their own ego or self-gratification, an audit can be a very negative or punishing experience. But we'll elaborate further on this.

PURPOSE

More often than not, the stated purpose of the audit program is to attain and maintain compliance with any or all applicable regulatory requirements or conformance to the stated requirements of the organization to the standard or process in question. Many organizations also state explicitly the objective of meeting good management practices and corporate policies and procedures. In the past few years, the widespread development of corporate HSEQ standards and guidelines has emerged in part to take the guesswork and judgment out of good management practices. This has helped to improve the rigor of HSEQ audits, especially in some Third World countries where there are, generally speaking, still fewer HSEQ regulations compared to more developed countries. While most companies recognize there are other benefits (e.g., technology transfer, increased awareness, HSEQ "culture" improvement or enhancement), they are typically seen as the "icing on the cake."

Many companies have redesigned their corporate HSEQ audit programs to emphasize the output of the reviews of their HSEQ management systems as well. This focus attempts to remedy the underlying causes of noncompliance and is consistent with many of the ISO management systems standards, such as ISO 14001, 9001, and 45001. Yet, even more recently, some companies that placed a principal emphasis on systems reviews at the corporate level, leaving detailed compliance audits to the businesses or sites, have pulled back from this approach. They have found that management system reviews alone have contributed to some relapse of noncompliance or nonconformance performance at the sites. Independent audits of actual compliance with HSEQ and related regulatory obligations remain an important part of the current trend toward corporate HSEQ assurance programs.

PROGRAM ORGANIZATION

A certain amount of independence is seen as an essential element of a program, so almost every organization has established a corporate audit function responsible for the program. This function is usually housed in the corporate HSEQ department. Other options include a function in the financial department (where the financial auditing function is located) or in the legal department (ostensibly to provide as much protection from report discovery as possible). Or there may be some strategic partnerships developed between these groups to reflect a holistic approach to any internal audit theme.

The size of the corporate audit staff varies considerably. In some companies, one or two people on staff provide an oversight function, drawing on a pool of facility and plant staff and consultants to conduct the audits. In other cases, a small group (two to five) of corporate staff conduct the audits, but with help from division and staff people. Finally, in a few cases, companies have a corporate staff of as many as twenty to thirty whose responsibility is to run the program and conduct the audits (without assistance). In all cases, however, audit teams comprise staff who are organizationally independent of the plant or site audited.

PROGRAM SCOPE

Many organizations have focused on their head office facilities initially, then broadened the program to all facilities worldwide. That said, some never get out to the "colonies." Many organizations develop checklists and protocols in the native language of their head office location and then expand those audits checklists and protocols to other languages and branch locations. Other organizations have left the implementation of the overseas audit program to regional audit coordinators; audit teams are selected from trained staff within the particular region. This approach can minimize cultural and language barriers. Other companies conduct all their overseas audits using their head office staff who they feel are most familiar with the requirements of the "mothership" and any satellite offices. And still others use local consultants to bolster a mostly local or facility-based audit team. And the proliferation of organizations having integrated and multidiscipline audit teams is growing, helping facilitate true integrated audit teams with functional and technical expertise from several operational areas.

The great number of organizations do perform multimedia HSEQ audits (i.e., hazardous wastes, PCBs) and health and safety audits (i.e., worker safety, occupational health, process safety, ergonomics), and have integrated them with key quality management system processes (customer product or service, customer satisfaction, etc.), but as the programs have evolved and facilities have been audited several times, there has been a tendency to refine the scope of the audit to those media or issues that present the greatest risk or liability at that facility.

PROGRAM METHODOLOGY

Audit Methodology

A "standard" audit methodology, used by many organizations, has evolved over time. It involves the three phases shown in the table below. With some variations and exceptions, in the experience of the authors, organizations with existing audit programs typically use this approach. Some of the more significant exceptions include the following:

- Surprise audits (used by some companies where situations warrant them).
- Effluent/emissions sampling (conducted by a few audit teams independently).
- Ranking of facilities based on a scoring system (used by some companies).
- Vendor/supplier audits (normally the plant's responsibility, but occasionally done by the audit team as well).
- Emergency-response drills during an audit.

STANDARD HSEQ AUDIT METHODOLOGY

Phase	*Steps*
I. Pre-Audit	– Organize the audit team – Assign responsibilities – Notify the site – Review relevant regulations – Review the last audit, protocols, and preaudit questionnaire
II. Audit	– In-brief site management – Meet with environmental staff – Participate in orientation tour – Review records and management systems – Interview site personnel – Inspect facilities – Brief site daily – Debrief site management
III. Post-Audit	– Draft audit report – Respond to reviews – Submit final audit report – Enter report findings into follow-up tracking system – Close-out audit

Although the use of detailed checklists and procedures is pretty much universal, the format for the checklists is typically unique to the organization in question. The main components of the checklists include the basic protocol, a topical outline, a detailed audit guide, a yes-or-no questionnaire, an open-ended questionnaire, and a scored questionnaire or rating sheet. With the evolution of commercially available international HSEQ audit protocols, there has been a trend to buy versus make audit protocols. That said, some have found that by developing audit checklists based on the realities of the facility they plan to audit, they get a better understanding of the facility requirements when they develop or customize their own checklists in the style and language they are most familiar with.

How the checklists are used varies as well. Some auditors use them religiously as they review, inspect, and interview. In other words, they use the checklists to the letter—no variation or flexibility permitted. Other auditors, perhaps those with more experience, use them as references at the beginning and end of each day to assure themselves that they have not overlooked anything. Still, others use the checklists as the source of a one-page list (per topic area) of important items to review during the audit. Each of these approaches has merit; their use must depend on the skill and preferences of the auditors and the audit team leader, and of course, the scope and objectives of the audit itself.

A final point concerns the use of technology. Many organizations now provide their audit teams with laptop computers or tablets. The objective is to have ready access to audit protocols and applicable regulations and to develop both a debriefing document and a draft report before the audit team leaves the site. The more preformatted the audit report, the easier it is to accomplish. And there are many commercial, off-the-shelf software tools that will perform this function quickly and seamlessly. With the technology available today, you can even go so far as to have the audit team submit the debriefing document and draft report to the corporate audit staff and the legal department before releasing it to the site management.

Reporting of Findings

Most audit reports are brief (five to twenty pages), but some can be longer. Increasingly, audit teams attempt to draft a preliminary report before leaving the site, if they have the time and technology to do so. When developed, these are used to debrief site management. At a minimum, many organizations strive to develop a formal list of findings and prepare them while still on-site so they can be inserted into the audit report.

There is no clear consensus as to whether audit reports should discuss good performance as well as out-of-compliance or out-of-conformance issues.

Some do list the positive observations—some don't. Some companies believe that good performance should be incorporated because the report, as a stand-alone document, will provide a more complete and more accurate picture of total compliance. These companies are also concerned that the audit reports are legally "discoverable" and could wind up in the hands of the public. The alternative philosophy is that audit reports should not be subjective, editorialized, political, lengthy, or self-congratulatory documents; instead, they should be straightforward, factual summaries of compliance or conformance items in need of attention. Other audit programs use the exception report format.

Nor is there consensus as to whether audit reports should contain recommendations for how to fix a stated problem. Some organizations include recommendations because they believe the process and report are "cleaner" that way; for every identified problem, there is a solution. This approach avoids the situation in which the audit report is "discovered" without a companion piece stating the company's planned efforts to remedy the problems.

The alternative approach is to include no recommendations in the audit report because this responsibility is thought to be that of the plant manager. Many consider their auditors to be strict auditors and not "consultants" or problem resolvers. The underlying philosophy holds that the auditors are responsible for simply identifying noncompliance or nonconformance and should not dictate to the facility management particular suggestions for how to resolve the problem. One company resolved the "recommendations" dilemma by having the auditors state only their findings in the report but leave room after each finding for the facility manager's proposed solution (to be added later). In this way, auditors do not dictate to the plant staff, but each audit report is a complete document with recommendations.

Finally, many organizations are split once again about whether pro forma legal review of draft audit reports is required. Some companies have their legal department review all audit reports, while others have legal review only when the audit team leader deems it necessary.

Follow-Up Mechanisms

Detailed follow-up systems have evolved rapidly, and the market now has a proliferation of action management software and tools, which can make the follow-up process fast, easy, and accurate. Many organizations, at a minimum, require a formal response from the facility within a defined timeline (i.e. thirty to sixty days). This response should consist of a detailed action plan for remedying all identified problems. The trend presently is to load all action plans onto a database or spreadsheet of some type that generates monthly "tickler" reports, which in turn report on the status of the action plan items. Some organizations go so far as to measure and "score" each plant on its action-item completion rate and submit those scores to senior management. Others employ something similar to a "red tag" procedure, whereby a unit can be shut down if follow-up is deemed nonresponsive. This procedure has been used successfully, albeit sparingly, in the past. Presently, the mere threat of its use seems sufficient leverage to obtain adequate responses.

PROGRAM OPERATIONS

Audit Staffing

Most companies view audits as principally a technical exercise with regulatory overtones. Thus, audit teams consist almost exclusively of experienced technical staff (e.g., engineers, technicians, HSEQ professionals). In some instances, lawyers are part of the audit team, but this is more the exception than the rule. On average, two to four staff make up the audit team, but the range can be anywhere from one to ten, depending upon the audit objectives and the size and complexity of the facility.

Audit Duration

On average, audits will take two or three to four days, but the range can be anywhere from one day to multiple weeks; again, this depends upon the audit scope and objectives and the size and complexity of the facility.

Number of Facilities Audited per Year

The number of facilities audited per year varies considerably. One company may audit as few as six facilities. Another company may audit as many as seventy-five facilities per year, performing audits with ten full-time corporate audit staff members. Of course, the number of facilities audited annually also has a lot to do with the size of the organization, so it is difficult to create a measure of appropriateness.

Frequency of Audits

Generally, organizations aim to audit major production facilities once every two years and to audit minor facilities (e.g., warehouses, distribution centers) once every three to five years. However, there is a trend in companies with mature audit programs to extend the frequency of audits from once every two years to once every three years. And the terms of the registration certificate, if there is one, may dictate audit frequency. Some client requirements may also dictate audit frequency.

CONCLUSION

It is clear that within the overall concept of HSEQ auditing, each organization must design a program to meet its own identified needs and objectives. This program must be structured so that it is consistent with available resources. This "simple" exercise of matching objectives with available resources is, in large part, the reason for the variety of programs encountered today.

REFERENCES

This chapter has been adapted from Lawrence B. Cahill and Raymond W. Kane. *Environmental Health and Safety Audits*, 9th Edition. Government Institutes, 2010. It has been updated for this edition.

Wayne Pardy and Terri Andrews. *Integrated Management Systems: Leading Strategies and Solutions*, 2nd Edition. Bernan Press, 2019.

ISO 19011: https://cdn.standards.iteh.ai/samples/70017/559078f9a2634aca84ff0a6aac1498f6/ISO-19011-2018.pdf

Chapter 7

Benchmarking HSEQ Audit Programs

Best Practices and Biggest Challenges

In the country of the blind, the one-eyed man is king.

—Michael Apostolius, *Proverbs*, fifteenth century

The audit management processes and principles of ISO 9001:2015 have become an important concept in learning how to manage HSEQ audit programs more effectively. An especially useful quality management tool has been competitive benchmarking. Companies use benchmarking studies to identify best practices to incorporate into their programs. In conducting benchmarking studies, evaluators often also identify the biggest common challenges facing audit program managers.

This chapter discusses some of the best practices and challenges associated with HSEQ audit programs. The conclusions are based on several benchmarking studies and third-party evaluations of corporate audit programs. As the sources are necessarily limited to our experiences, no doubt many other best practices, in particular, are not discussed in this chapter. These will surface over time.

OVERVIEW OF BENCHMARKING

The concept of benchmarking HSEQ audit programs has received considerable attention in the past few years. Generally speaking, benchmarking is the process of measuring products, services, and practices against competitors or those who have been recognized as leaders in their fields of practice. This chapter does not intend to provide a discourse on each of the steps involved in the benchmarking process; that task is better handled by other sources. However, based on previous HSEQ audit program benchmarking experiences of the authors, five steps have been deemed key to conducting a successful study. Those five steps are discussed below.

1. Precisely Define the Scope

One can benchmark any and/or all components of an HSEQ audit program. For example, a company in the midst of a reorganization may wish to determine the best reporting relationship for its audit program. Thus, its goal in a benchmarking study might be to determine just that among a dozen or so targeted companies, to whom did the corporate audit program manager typically report?

Broader-based studies can help as well. However, there are many components to an audit program, and it is probably best to define and analyze only the most crucial (e.g., frequency and scheduling of audits, auditor competency and training [in-house vs. external] follow-up systems, software leveraged).

2. Select Target Companies Using a Variety of Techniques

One can select among companies in similar businesses, in the industry in general, or with known "best-in-class" audit programs. Any of these approaches will suffice, depending on the objectives of the study. One can also select companies using financial or business criteria such as company size, return on equity, the percentage of sales in service businesses, and/or the percentage of business in selected locations or countries. The idea is to find groupings of similar companies based on key financial criteria against which to benchmark.

3. Create Participation Incentives

Benchmarking has become a common business analysis technique, so quite often it is not difficult to identify willing participants who are prepared to take the time on their end to be interviewed, and so forth. And some organizations will never be prepared to share their internal practices or processes with anyone, for any reason. However, some incentive will usually be required. This can be a report summarizing the results of the study. Although for a participant to receive the full analysis, some financial participation in the study might also usually be expected.

4. Develop Measurable Criteria

This can be a difficult challenge, especially if one is evaluating the "softer" components of a program. However, developing measurable criteria in advance is crucial to comparing results from disparate companies. These criteria might include the following:

- Frequency of audits for major facilities
- Type of report, if any, left with site staff at the close of the field audit
- Draft and final audit report types (e.g., exception reporting only) and schedules
- Types of technologies leveraged in the audit program
- Frequency and type of follow-up system
- Use of legal protections
- Frequency and type of reporting to management
- Organizational levels between the audit program manager and the chief executive officer
- Budget for audit program per unit of company sales or percentage of the annual operations budget

Each of the above criteria is generally quite measurable and requires short cryptic responses. The evaluator can then make broad conclusions based on the results (e.g., 50 percent of the benchmarked companies use in-house developed software to manage their audit program vs. third-party applications to develop their audit reports).

5. Utilize Focus Group Sessions

Bringing together the participants of a benchmarking study for a day can be an extremely useful exercise. It can help to ensure that individuals are not discussing apples and oranges when addressing complex program issues. The technique can also help to identify subtle nuances in programs that otherwise might not surface during a one-on-one interview. If participants have difficulty assembling in one location, a Webex, Zoom, or Teams meeting can be a suitable substitute, and in some cases, is the de facto audit process for remote auditing for several reasons which we'll profile later.

BEST PRACTICES

In benchmarking audit programs over the past few years, several suggested best practices have surfaced. Not all of these might be applied effectively to a given audit program, but using them selectively can result in an improved audit program that meets the ever-increasing expectations of stakeholders. This section describes a number of those practices.

REPORTS TO MANAGEMENT

Reporting health and safety statistics to executive management has been a common practice in many industries for many years. More recently, overall HSEQ performance is being reported not only to executives but to the public as well, with corporate and social-responsibility reporting gaining traction internationally. Annual environmental or sustainability reports are commonplace among progressive companies. Within these reports, HSEQ audit programs are occasionally, but increasingly, being addressed.

For HSEQ audit programs to be successful, some form of reporting to the company's executives is recommended and strongly encouraged. In some companies, the CEO has shown enough interest that they review every report, and calls are made to line managers when it is perceived that individual issues are not being resolved quickly enough. This demonstrates the top-management commitment that any credible audit management program requires for success. More commonly, senior management might receive a quarterly or semiannual briefing on issues identified by the audits. These issues might be noncompliance problems that cut across the corporation and require a systemic remedy, statistics among business units on the timely resolution of findings, or instances where the audit program saved the company money through, for example, the avoidance of fines or substitution of less hazardous materials.

RELATIONSHIP TO COMPENSATION

To ensure support for an HSEQ audit program, many companies will factor audit results into the bonus equation or annual performance evaluation used for facilities and their management team. This usually gets the attention of the individuals principally responsible for remedying problems; however, some caveats are in order.

First, managers should be held more accountable for fixing identified problems than for the results of the first audit at a given facility. This first audit usually sets the baseline and should not be perceived as a witch hunt or a problem identification/finger-pointing exercise. How well the site staff responds *after* the audit is really what should be evaluated.

Second, one must be careful of falling into the trap of numerically scoring the results of an audit in order to apportion compensation. For one thing, it is difficult to compare facilities and their audit performance. Many factors are beyond the plant manager's control, such as the regulatory stringency of the geographical location in which the plant is located; the type, age, and size of the facility; the toxicity of the materials used; and the nature of the property (e.g., the presence of wetlands).

Also, using a scoring system tied to compensation can heighten the tension of an audit because the plant staff will typically be more argumentative about the number and significance of findings. Where scoring is used, too much time can typically be spent on whether the resultant score is an 81 or a 79, or whether the score is higher than the last audit. This has the potential to take away from the real purpose of the audit—to find and fix the problems. At the end of the day, the audit should not be strictly about numbers, as these numbers can be subjective and arbitrary. It should be about the objective evidence regardless of any number assigned to the final audit conclusion.

That being said, here's some guidance for consideration when looking to develop a scoring system for audits if that's the path you've decided to take. The more you're able to rationalize the basis for your audit scoring process, the better its chance of being able to weather any criticism of the final audit question scores and logic.

Here's an example from Canada based on the Canada Labour Code. Under the Canada Labour Code, there is the provision for what is called an administrative monetary penalty (AMP). An AMP is a financial deterrent to noncompliance with the Canada Labour Code and related regulations. The goal of this penalty is to encourage compliance, serve as a supplement to existing enforcement measures, and offer an alternative to prosecution. As a part of the compliance and enforcement process, the Labour Program will focus on supporting and encouraging employers to be compliant with the code through education and awareness. Generally speaking, an AMP would only be issued after voluntary compliance measures are exhausted and if noncompliance persists.

In some cases, the severity of the violation and the impact on employees, or the reoccurrence of the violation, may require the Labour Program to issue an AMP earlier in the compliance and enforcement process.

The key aspect of this AMP approach for our book is not the penalty process per se, but the risk-based approach to the penalties that can be used by any employer. In Canada, the Labour Program categorizes violations under the code based on how they affect an employee(s) based on the following risk categories:

- ***Classification A****—Related to administrative provisions.*
- ***Classification B****—Related to low-risk hazards that may result in a minor injury or illness that requires medical treatment but does not result in disabling injuries.*
- ***Classification C****—Related to medium-risk hazards that may result in serious injury or illness that prevents an employee from effectively performing their regular work duties.*

- ***Classification D****—Related to high-risk hazards that may result in serious injury or fatality. Noncompliance with a direction. Noncompliance with an order from the Canada Industrial Relations Board.*
- ***Classification E****—Involves immediate life-threatening hazards or hazards known to cause latent occupational disease. These hazards give the employee little to no opportunity to avoid or minimize severe injury, death, or occupational disease.*

As you can see, the entire published list of regulations has been risk-ranked so that anyone can quickly see what the potential consequence of noncompliance with a specific regulation might be. The advantage of having this risk-ranking process already done by the regulator for an employer is that they can create their entire compliance audit approach based on these risks. In other words, if you want to look at only the high or immediate life-threatening risks for a given audit timeline, you can do so.

This provides an opportunity to determine which of your audit questions get rated or scored higher or lower than others based on the defined risks that the regulator has already assigned to those compliance areas. No longer do you have to debate the merits of which issues to focus on to get the best risk-based return for your efforts. And while some might suggest this is intuitive, having the regulator provide you with a risk-based system upon which to base your compliance audit scores is a true gift.

This audit checklist example below, which the authors developed based on the risk-based compliance criteria, is an example of how you can then "*score*" your audit using the rationale of how this audit will align with regulatory risk-based criteria.

EMERGENCY RESPONSE

One of the most important HSEQ compliance areas to audit is emergency response. A good response program can save both money and lives. Moreover, emergency response is now an integral component of regulations promulgated under a variety of statutes, including things like

- spill-prevention control and countermeasure plan under applicable regulations;
- contingency plans;
- hazardous waste operations emergency-response planning under occupational health and safety regulations;
- hazard identification and release reporting; and
- risk-management planning

Table 7.1 Risk-based Regulatory Audit against Canada Labour Code

Labour Canada Violation Type and Risk Ranking	*A= Administrative Provision*	*B=Low-Risk Hazard*	*C=Medium-Risk Hazard*	*D=High-Risk Hazard*	*E=Immediate, life-Threatening Hazard*
Section of the COH&S Regulations	Regulatory Area of Focus	Specific regulatory requirement against which compliance is being assessed	Labour Canada Violation Type and Risk Ranking	Standard or Code referenced in regulatory requirement and guidance regarding method of collecting and verifying information and evidence, including interview, observation, or review of documents, including records	Evidence of ABC Company Compliance: Yes/No/NA
1.5	Records	If an employer is required by section 125 or 125.1 of the Act to keep and maintain a record, the employer shall keep and maintain the record and make it readily available for examination by the minister and by the policy committee or, if there is no policy committee, the workplace committee or the health and safety representative for the workplace to which it applies.	A	Method of collecting and verifying information and evidence related to this requirement includes the review of documents, including records	

(*Continued*)

Table 7.1 Risk-based Regulatory Audit against Canada Labour Code (Continued)

Labour Canada Violation Type and Risk Ranking	*A= Administrative Provision*	*B=Low-Risk Hazard*	*C=Medium-Risk Hazard*	*D=High-Risk Hazard*	*E=Immediate, life-Threatening Hazard*
1.8(2)	Alternate Media	(2) Subject to subsection (5), where an employer or other person is required by these Regulations to give, provide, or make available any information, instruction, or training to an employee and the employee has a special need, the employer or other person shall give, provide, or make available the information, instruction, or training to the employee by means of an alternate medium	D	Method of collecting and verifying information and evidence related to this requirement includes the review of documents, including records	
1.8(3)	Alternate Media	(3) Where information, including warnings, is required by these Regulations to be provided by means of a sign or marking, the alternate medium shall be visible or audible to an employee with a special need	D	Method of collecting and verifying information and evidence related to this requirement includes observations and review of documents, including records.	

1.8(4)	Alternate Media	(4) Where a warning is required to be given by means other than a sign or marking, the warning shall be given to an employee with a special need in a manner that effectively warns the employee of the nature of the danger	D	Method of collecting and verifying information and evidence related to this requirement includes observations and review of documents, including records.
2.2(1)	DIVISION I. Buildings Standards	2.2 (1) The design and construction of every building, the construction of which begins on or after the day of the coming into force of this subsection, shall meet the requirements of the National Building Code.	C	National Building Code

This has made developing an effective emergency-response program a complex exercise. The more progressive audit programs will verify not only that the emergency-response program meets regulatory requirements but, more importantly, that the program will also work when needed, or has been demonstrated to work during real-life scenarios, drills, or exercises. And of course, records of these real-life scenarios, drills, and exercises need to be documented for objective assessment of effectiveness. Interviews with those who have participated in the exercise can also add value. To provide these assurances, firms have conducted "spill or safety drills" during their audits, and many of these take place in the early hours of the morning. As a suitable but less direct alternative, many audit programs will review the results of spill or safety drills conducted during the year, assessing whether deficiencies were identified and remedied. Either way, emergency-response programs should include drills—or simulations at a minimum—and audit programs should assess how sites respond to the results of those exercises.

NEXT-SITE PARTICIPATION

One way to reduce the anxiety of being audited is to have a site HSEQ manager participate in an audit, as a team member, directly prior to the audit of their own site. Some companies use this technique to help individuals better understand the process and prepare effectively for the audits of their own sites.

USE OF LAPTOP AND TABLET COMPUTERS, INTRANETS, AND THE INTERNET

Use of laptop computers is becoming almost mandatory for audits. When one of the authors was with Q5 Systems, the use of mobile technology for field-level auditing was becoming all the rage in the early 2000s. PalmPilots and Pocket PCs led the way initially, eventually giving way to tablets, laptops, and smartphones. Computers are used in a variety of ways. Some companies use commercially available automated audit protocols to directly insert findings generated from a review of the checklists into a report template. The checklists also contain regulatory digests so that the multivolume regulations need not be carried to every audit. In general, computers are used for three purposes on audits: (1) access to an online or cloud/web regulatory database, (2) generation of reports prior to leaving the site, and (3) use of automated checklists in the field. The ability to leave a draft report with the site is especially valuable in that it helps to maintain the momentum of the audit.

Computers are also helpful for keeping in touch with the home office through email, Teams meetings, and so on.

The use of the Internet and company intranets to support HSEQ audit programs has virtually exploded in the past few years. The Internet can be—and is—used to access publicly available regulatory information on a given site. Both the U.S. EPA (http://www.osha.gov) and the Occupational Safety and Health Administration (www.osha.gov/oshstats) and organizations like Transport Canada (https://tc.canada.ca/en) have accessible databases containing large volumes of reporting and inspection information on individual sites. Many firms will access these databases prior to an audit to help the team prepare. This information is also given to the site so that they can review it and, just as importantly, determine whether it is indeed correct and current. Furthermore, the web is often used to obtain the following additional logistical information in real-time, such as

- inexpensive airline tickets;
- weather at the facility site to the time on-site;
- directions to the hotel and facility (Google maps, etc.); and
- information on facilities available at or near the hotel (hotels, restaurants, gas stations, etc.)

Company intranets are also a tremendous resource for audit teams, providing site addresses and phone numbers, audit protocols, procedures and schedules, site plans and reports, lists of best practices identified on audits throughout the corporation, and corporate standards and guidelines.

This availability of critical information on the web and company intranets has truly revolutionized how HSEQ audits are conducted. Organizations not taking advantage will clearly be potentially left behind.

ASSESSMENT OF ANCILLARY OPERATIONS

Most audits rightfully focus on the site's line operations. However, the better programs address certain ancillary operations as well. These can include the following:

- *Off-site hazardous waste treatment, storage, and disposal facilities:* This is an especially important area to review. Audit teams are not typically expected to visit off-site facilities. At a minimum, however, the audit team should check to ensure that the site is using only corporate-approved facilities and/or that the facilities have been visited at a frequency consistent with corporate guidance.
- *Purchasing:* Purchasing staff should be interviewed to determine if they use any HSEQ guidelines in procuring materials. The two relevant audit

questions are, “Is purchasing required to meet any HSEQ guidelines,” and if it is, “Are these guidelines being followed consistently?”

- *Maintenance:* This function is almost always audited; however, the depth of the audit can sometimes be quite shallow. Key HSEQ issues to address include the use and disposal of maintenance chemicals. The safety of the maintenance equipment (e.g., vehicles, welding machines, grinders, lathes, drill presses) should also be reviewed. An area often overlooked is the storage and application of pesticides.
- *On-site contractors:* The audit team should review temporary and permanent on-site contractors, such as general construction and asbestos-removal companies. Their contracts should also be reviewed to verify that appropriate HSEQ provisions are included and that they are being followed.

  Nearby warehouses used by the site: Off-site owned or leased warehouses can create liabilities for companies and should therefore be audited on occasion. If the warehouse is nearby, many audit programs will include it in the site audit.

Addressing these ancillary areas does add time to the audit. However, many companies believe that this is time well spent.

USE OF VERIFICATION AUDITS

One of the biggest challenges associated with audit programs is assuring that problems are corrected in a timely fashion. Companies typically set up sophisticated databases to track the status of corrective actions, either through an in-house or third-party application. How data is entered into these databases, however, is the real challenge. Often sites send quarterly status reports to a central location, and the data is entered there. This approach works reasonably well, except when site management's perception of a “fix” diverges from that of the audit team.

These audits help to “*verify*” the accuracy of the data being submitted and assist in resolving any problems the site might be having with interpreting a finding. They also help to “keep the responses honest” because sites recognize that each year they might receive a verification audit.

SITE-SATISFACTION QUESTIONNAIRE

One way for the audit program manager to ensure that the program is achieving its objectives is to have the site staff being audited complete a questionnaire evaluating the audit team's performance. Brutal honesty is essential here. This questionnaire is typically given to the site management at the close of the audit, and it is mailed back to the audit program manager, not the team leader. Online survey services like SurveyMonkey can now make this process faster, easier, and more meaningful. Survey topics include the competency and reasonableness of the team, the adequacy of the interpersonal skills of the team, the depth of the audit, the perceived value of the audit, and any improvements that could be made.

Companies often keep extensive statistics on the returned questionnaires, which are used to adjust the program. It should be noted, however, that the completed questionnaires must be reviewed very carefully. One should be cautious if the site responses are overly positive or negative. While a high-scoring questionnaire might be a good result, it could also mean that the audit team was quite lenient in its dealings with the site management. Conversely, a questionnaire that comes back with excessively low scores could mean that the team was ineffectual, but it could also mean that there were numerous serious (and justified) findings, and the plant staff took their frustration out on the auditors when completing the questionnaire. It is only human nature to react emotionally in these situations. That said, while this is subjective feedback, if collected, it should be carefully examined and considered as part of any audit program.

PERIODIC THIRD-PARTY EVALUATIONS

As is consistent with good quality management practices, many companies are now having outside consultants (i.e., third parties) or their internal audit departments (i.e., second parties) evaluate their HSEQ audit programs on a periodic basis. The annual or biennial studies help the companies meet their "continuous improvement" objectives and also relieve the increasing pressure from stakeholders to provide assurances that the company is identifying and remedying its HSEQ issues.

Third-party evaluations usually include a review of program documentation, including audit reports and corrective-action plans, interviews with key program participants, and observation of a representative number of audits. Programs are typically compared with any external audit management protocol or process, as well as with other companies' programs and internally developed standards and policies.

DEVELOPMENT OF AN AUDIT PROGRAM NEWS OR CHAT GROUP

This is an option for many larger or multinational organizations. There should be no secrets about the objectives, implementation, and operation of an HSEQ audit program. Most programs have guidance manuals that describe the workings of the audit process. The manuals provide much-needed program consistency, should the audit program manager be reassigned. Some companies take this one step further and develop program newsletters or email groups. A newsletter or email group can do much to put the HSEQ audit program in a very positive light and to communicate important information, such as new corporate standards, chronic deficiencies, and exceptional HSEQ programs that might otherwise go unrecognized.

BIGGEST CHALLENGES

Benchmarking studies and third-party evaluations identify not only best practices but usually the biggest challenges as well. Discussed below are a few items that seem to recur time and again as deficiencies in HSEQ audit programs.

THE PROGRAM MANUAL

Putting together an HSEQ audit program manual can be an onerous task, especially for smaller organizations with limited resources and expertise; as a result, it is quite often not done formally. Some programs will have no written guidance document whatsoever, while others might use a presentation package describing the program in audit opening conferences. The lack of a program manual does not necessarily mean that a given program is not operating well; however, a manual does help document and communicate the program's objectives and procedures. Furthermore, it is difficult to assess the relative successes or failures of a program without some written guidelines against which this evaluation can be made. To be consistent with quality management principles, all HSEQ audit programs should be evaluated on a defined, periodic basis. Finally, a manual or very detailed procedure helps to guide the program during the resulting transition when the program manager vacates their position, or new auditors are brought onto the team.

PROTOCOL AND CHECKLIST UPDATING

The problem with audit checklists or protocols is that they can typically be out-of-date once they are created. This poses a problem because auditors who rely heavily on checklists, rather than fundamental knowledge of regulations, may not be evaluating a site based on the most recently applicable requirements. Many audit program managers find it difficult to allocate the resources or the time to update protocols more than once every couple of years. An update, at least annually, is consistent with good audit practices. This is where having someone designated as a regulatory subject-matter expert can yield positive dividends for the HSEQ audit program.

Use of commercially available automated checklists can help to avoid the problem of outdated program documents. These checklists are updated automatically by the company providing the product. The initial investment in the checklists may seem high, but this updated service can be very cost-effective. Keep in mind that this area of intellectual data, customized for client use, is growing every day. A simple Google search of the phrase, "safety or environmental audit checklist" will give you an indication of the size and scope of this market.

The authors have also started to experiment with Artificial Intelligence (AI) through the use of several of the free AI tools on the market. While still in its infancy, there are potentially many different applications for the new AI tools for your HSEQ audit needs. Want to try it out? Simply go to an AI platform like ChatGPT and give some thought to the question or content you would like it to generate for you. By way of an example, here's a sample question:

> *I am a HSEQ professional, and my company is embarking on a project to implement an integrated HSEQ Management system. I need a checklist to use to both develop a gap analysis and then eventually conduct an integrated HSEQ management system audit against the requirements of ISO 14001, 9001 and 45001. And I also need to align this with the requirements of the Newfoundland and Labrador OHS regulations which are applicable to these 3 ISO Standards. Develop this checklist for me.*

Of course, you can type in your own regulatory requirements instead of the Newfoundland and Labrador OHS regulations to suit your needs, but just look at the results.

I put in the query above and got the following in less than 1 minute. Now that's some powerful technology! In fact, it took the authors about 15 minutes to edit and format what ChatGPT generated in less than 1 minute. Suffice it to say that AI will hold much more potential for HSEQ audits in the coming months and years. And while we were tempted to lessen the burden of editing/rewriting this entire book by using AI, we can honestly say the only AI used for this book is in the example below.

ChatGPT response to our query:

> *Certainly! Here is a comprehensive checklist designed to help you develop a gap analysis and conduct an integrated HSEQ management system audit*

against the requirements of ISO 14001, ISO 9001, and ISO 45001. This checklist also aligns with the Occupational Health and Safety (OHS) regulations of Newfoundland and Labrador (NL).

Integrated HSEQ Management System Checklist

- *General Information*
- *Project Name:*
- *Audit Date:*
- *Auditor(s):*
- *Location:*
- *Department:*

Part 1: Context of the Organization

Understanding the Organization and Its Context
Have external and internal issues relevant to the organization's purpose and strategic direction been identified? (ISO 9001, ISO 14001, ISO 45001)
Are these issues documented and reviewed regularly?

Understanding the Needs and Expectations of Interested Parties
Are the needs and expectations of workers, clients, regulators, and other interested parties identified and documented? (ISO 9001, ISO 14001, ISO 45001)

Determining the Scope of the HSEQ Management System
Is the scope of the HSEQ management system defined and documented? (ISO 9001, ISO 14001, ISO 45001)

Part 2: Leadership. Leadership and Commitment

Is there evidence of top management's commitment to the HSEQ management system? (ISO 9001, ISO 14001, ISO 45001)

Policy
Is there a documented HSEQ policy that includes commitments to compliance, prevention of pollution, continual improvement, and worker safety? (ISO 9001, ISO 14001, ISO 45001)
Is the HSEQ policy communicated within the organization and made available to interested parties?
Organizational Roles, Responsibilities, and Authorities
Are roles, responsibilities, and authorities related to the HSEQ management system defined, assigned, and communicated? (ISO 9001, ISO 14001, ISO 45001)

Part 3: Planning. Actions to Address Risks and Opportunities

Are risks and opportunities related to the HSEQ management system identified and documented? (ISO 9001, ISO 14001, ISO 45001)

Are actions planned to address these risks and opportunities?

HSEQ Objectives and Planning to Achieve Them

Are measurable HSEQ objectives established at relevant functions and levels? (ISO 9001, ISO 14001, ISO 45001)

Are plans developed to achieve these objectives?

Planning of Changes

Are changes to the HSEQ management system planned and implemented in a controlled manner? (ISO 9001, ISO 14001, ISO 45001)

Part 4: Support

Resources

Are resources needed for the establishment, implementation, maintenance, and continual improvement of the HSEQ management system determined and provided? (ISO 9001, ISO 14001, ISO 45001)

Competence

Are the necessary competencies for personnel affecting HSEQ performance determined, provided, and maintained? (ISO 9001, ISO 14001, ISO 45001)

Awareness

Are workers aware of the HSEQ policy, their contribution to the HSEQ management system, and the implications of not conforming to the requirements? (ISO 9001, ISO 14001, ISO 45001)

Communication

Are internal and external communications relevant to the HSEQ management system determined and implemented? (ISO 9001, ISO 14001, ISO 45001)

Documented Information

Is documented information required by the HSEQ management system determined, controlled, and maintained? (ISO 9001, ISO 14001, ISO 45001)

Part 5: Operation

Operational Planning and Control

Are processes needed to meet HSEQ requirements planned, implemented, and controlled? (ISO 9001, ISO 14001, ISO 45001)

Are criteria for processes and the acceptance of products and services defined?

Emergency Preparedness and Response
Are procedures for responding to potential emergency situations established and maintained? (ISO 14001, ISO 45001)

Part 6: Performance Evaluation

Monitoring, Measurement, Analysis, and Evaluation
Are HSEQ performance indicators determined, monitored, measured, analyzed, and evaluated? (ISO 9001, ISO 14001, ISO 45001)

Are the results of monitoring and measurement documented?

Internal Audit
Are internal audits conducted at planned intervals to provide information on the HSEQ management system? (ISO 9001, ISO 14001, ISO 45001)

Are audit results documented and reported to relevant management?

Management Review
Are management reviews conducted to ensure the continuing suitability, adequacy, and effectiveness of the HSEQ management system? (ISO 9001, ISO 14001, ISO 45001)

Part 7: Improvement

Nonconformity and Corrective Action
Are processes in place to handle nonconformities, take corrective actions, and prevent recurrence? (ISO 9001, ISO 14001, ISO 45001)

Continual Improvement
Are opportunities for improvement identified and implemented? (ISO 9001, ISO 14001, ISO 45001)

Alignment with Newfoundland and Labrador OHS Regulations. Legal and Other Requirements
Are all applicable NL OHS regulations identified, documented, and taken into account in the HSEQ management system?

Risk Assessment and Control
Are risk assessments conducted according to NL OHS regulations, and are control measures implemented and maintained?

Worker Participation

Are workers involved in OHS decision-making processes as required by NL OHS regulations?

Health Surveillance

Are health surveillance programs in place to monitor worker health in compliance with NL OHS regulations?

Incident Reporting and Investigation

Are incidents reported, investigated, and documented in accordance with NL OHS regulations?

Training and Competency

Are workers provided with training and competency development as required by NL OHS regulations?

Emergency Preparedness

Are emergency procedures in place and compliant with NL OHS regulations?

Inspection and Maintenance of Equipment

Are regular inspections and maintenance of equipment conducted to ensure safety and compliance with NL OHS regulations?

By following this checklist, you can ensure a thorough gap analysis and audit of your integrated HSEQ management system, aligned with the requirements of ISO 14001, ISO 9001, ISO 45001, and the Newfoundland and Labrador OHS regulations. Regular reviews and updates of this checklist will help maintain its relevance and effectiveness.

Source: https://chatgpt.com/

So, this is the other question we asked ChatGPT. Take a look at what it created for us in a matter of minutes—*"I am an HSEQ professional auditor. I need a comprehensive audit checklist developed so that I can conduct a comprehensive, integrated audit against the requirements of ISO 9001, 14001 and 45001."*

ChatGPT:

To develop a comprehensive, integrated audit checklist that covers ISO 9001, ISO 14001, and ISO 45001, we will focus on common themes and requirements from each standard. Below is a high-level checklist that integrates key elements from all three standards, followed by detailed sections from each standard for more specific audit points.

INTEGRATED AUDIT CHECKLIST

1. Context of the Organization
   - Identify internal and external issues relevant to the organization's purpose and strategic direction (ISO 9001: 4.1, ISO 14001: 4.1, ISO 45001: 4.1).

- Determine interested parties and their requirements (ISO 9001: 4.2, ISO 14001: 4.2, ISO 45001: 4.2).

2. Leadership and Commitment
   - Verify top management's commitment to the management systems (ISO 9001: 5.1, ISO 14001: 5.1, ISO 45001: 5.1).
   - Ensure the establishment of policies for quality, environment, and occupational health and safety (ISO 9001: 5.2, ISO 14001: 5.2, ISO 45001: 5.2).
3. Planning
   - Assess risks and opportunities that could affect the management systems (ISO 9001: 6.1, ISO 14001: 6.1, ISO 45001: 6.1).
   - Verify objectives and planning to achieve them, including environmental and OH&S objectives (ISO 9001: 6.2, ISO 14001: 6.2, ISO 45001: 6.2).
4. Support
   - Check the provision of necessary resources (ISO 9001: 7.1, ISO 14001: 7.1, ISO 45001: 7.1).
   - Review competence, training, and awareness programs (ISO 9001: 7.2, ISO 14001: 7.2, ISO 45001: 7.2).
   - Verify communication processes (ISO 9001: 7.4, ISO 14001: 7.4, ISO 45001: 7.4).
5. Operation
   - Ensure operational planning and control, including emergency preparedness and response (ISO 9001: 8.1, ISO 14001: 8.1, ISO 45001: 8.1).
   - Verify the processes for product/service realization and operational controls for environmental and OH&S risks (ISO 9001: 8.2, ISO 14001: 8.2, ISO 45001: 8.2).
6. Performance Evaluation
   - Review monitoring, measurement, analysis, and evaluation processes (ISO 9001: 9.1, ISO 14001: 9.1, ISO 45001: 9.1).
   - Verify internal audit processes and their implementation (ISO 9001: 9.2, ISO 14001: 9.2, ISO 45001: 9.2).
   - Ensure management review meetings are conducted and documented (ISO 9001: 9.3, ISO 14001: 9.3, ISO 45001: 9.3).
7. Improvement
   - Check processes for nonconformity and corrective action (ISO 9001: 10.2, ISO 14001: 10.2, ISO 45001: 10.2).
   - Verify continual improvement processes (ISO 9001: 10.3, ISO 14001: 10.3, ISO 45001: 10.3).

DETAILED AUDIT CHECKLIST SECTIONS

ISO 9001:2015 SPECIFIC CHECKLIST POINTS

1. Quality Management System
   - Establish and maintain a quality management system (QMS) (Clause 4.1–4.4).
2. Customer Focus
   - Ensure customer requirements are met, and satisfaction is measured (Clause 5.1.2).
3. Performance Evaluation
   - Monitor customer perceptions and analyze data for QMS effectiveness (Clause 9.1.2–9.1.3).

ISO 14001:2015 SPECIFIC CHECKLIST POINTS

1. Environmental Management System
   - Establish and maintain an environmental management system (EMS) (Clause 4.1–4.4).
2. Environmental Policy
   - Ensure the environmental policy is appropriate and communicated (Clause 5.2).
3. Evaluation of Compliance
   - Evaluate compliance with legal and other requirements (Clause 9.1.2).

ISO 45001:2018 SPECIFIC CHECKLIST POINTS

1. OH&S Management System
   - Establish and maintain an OH&S management system (Clause 4.1–4.4).
2. Hazard Identification and Risk Assessment
   - Identify hazards and assess OH&S risks (Clause 6.1.2).
3. Incident Investigation and Corrective Action
   - Investigate incidents and implement corrective actions (Clause 10.2).

ADDITIONAL REFERENCES FROM STANDARDS

- Internal Audit Requirements

- ISO 9001: "The organization shall conduct internal audits at planned intervals" (Clause 9.2) (ISO 9001 Standard).
- ISO 14001: "The organization shall establish, implement, and maintain an internal audit program" (Clause 9.2) (ISO_14001).
- ISO 45001: "The organization shall establish, implement, and maintain a process for internal audits" (Clause 9.2).

This comprehensive checklist should help you conduct an integrated audit covering the essential requirements of ISO 9001, ISO 14001, and ISO 45001.

So, we then took the baseline audit checklist that ChatGPT developed for us, reviewed it, and then enhanced it to make a more complete audit tool for field use.

While this HSEQ auditing book was written using old-school methods, the world of work is rapidly being changed and challenged by the proliferation of AI tools and products. And it's getting more and more evolved. While we don't have a crystal ball, we predict that in the coming months and years, the HSEQ auditors' job will be impacted (hopefully in a positive way) through the efficiency and productivity gains that the AI world might bring. To give everyone just a quick glance, here's how your HSEQ audits might be impacted in the coming years by AI.

We asked ChatGPT this question: *"What impact might ChatGPT have on the world of HSEQ auditing in the future, and how can ChatGPT be used by professional HSEQ auditors to conduct and deliver their HSEQ audit programs?"*

Here's what ChatGPT told us:

IMPACT OF CHATGPT ON HSEQ AUDITING

1. Enhanced Efficiency and Productivity:
   - **Automating Routine Tasks:** ChatGPT can automate repetitive tasks such as scheduling audits, sending reminders, and generating preliminary reports, freeing up auditors to focus on more critical tasks.
   - **Document Review:** ChatGPT can quickly review and summarize large volumes of documentation, highlighting key points and potential areas of concern.
2. Improved Data Analysis:
   - **Real-Time Data Analysis:** ChatGPT can analyze data from various sources in real-time, identifying trends, patterns, and anomalies that may not be immediately apparent to human auditors.
   - **Risk Assessment:** By analyzing historical data and industry benchmarks, ChatGPT can help identify potential risks and suggest mitigation strategies.

3. Enhanced Decision-Making:
   - **Knowledge Integration:** ChatGPT can integrate knowledge from multiple standards (ISO 9001, ISO 14001, ISO 45001), helping auditors make more informed decisions during integrated audits.
   - **Continuous Learning:** ChatGPT can stay updated with the latest regulations, standards, and best practices, providing auditors with the most current information.
4. Streamlined Reporting:
   - **Report Generation:** ChatGPT can assist in drafting detailed audit reports, ensuring that all relevant points are covered and the language is clear and professional.
   - **Customizable Templates:** It can use customizable templates to generate reports tailored to the specific needs of different clients or industries.
5. Enhanced Communication:
   - **Stakeholder Engagement:** ChatGPT can help in communicating findings and recommendations to stakeholders in a clear and concise manner.
   - **Training and Development:** ChatGPT can be used to create training materials and modules for auditors and employees, promoting continuous learning and development.

HOW CHATGPT CAN BE USED BY PROFESSIONAL HSEQ AUDITORS

1. Pre-Audit Preparation:
   - **Document Review and Summarization:** Upload documents such as policies, procedures, and previous audit reports for ChatGPT to review and summarize key points.
   - **Checklist Generation:** Create customized audit checklists based on the specific requirements of ISO 9001, ISO 14001, and ISO 45001.
2. During the Audit:
   - **Real-Time Assistance:** Use ChatGPT to look up specific clauses or requirements of the standards during the audit.
   - **Data Entry and Analysis:** Input findings and observations into ChatGPT for real-time analysis and initial categorization of nonconformances.
3. Post-Audit Activities:
   - **Report Drafting:** Have ChatGPT draft the audit report, including executive summaries, detailed findings, and recommendations.

- **Action Plan Development:** Use ChatGPT to develop corrective action plans based on audit findings, including timelines and responsibilities.

4. Continuous Improvement:
   - **Trend Analysis:** Periodically analyze audit results to identify recurring issues and areas for improvement.
   - **Training Programs:** Develop and update training programs for auditors and employees based on the latest standards and best practices.
5. Regulatory Updates:
   - **Stay Informed:** ChatGPT can monitor and inform auditors of changes in regulations and standards, ensuring compliance and up-to-date practices.

PRACTICAL EXAMPLES

1. Automated Checklists and Reports:
   - After uploading audit criteria and previous reports, ChatGPT can generate a comprehensive checklist tailored to specific audit needs.
   - Post-audit, ChatGPT can compile findings into a structured report, saving time on documentation.
2. Real-Time Query Resolution:
   - During an audit, auditors can query ChatGPT about specific standards or best practices, receiving instant and detailed responses.
3. Training and Onboarding:
   - New auditors can use ChatGPT as a learning tool to understand auditing processes, standards, and methodologies through interactive Q&A sessions.
4. Data-Driven Insights:
   - By feeding audit data into ChatGPT, auditors can receive insights on compliance trends, common issues, and potential risks, allowing for proactive management.

FUTURE DEVELOPMENTS

1. Integration with IoT and Data Systems:
   - **Seamless Data Collection:** Integration with IoT devices and enterprise data systems can provide real-time data for audits.
   - **Predictive Analytics:** Advanced analytics can predict potential issues before they become noncompliances.

2. Advanced Natural Language Processing:
   - **Contextual Understanding:** Improved NLP capabilities can provide deeper insights and more accurate interpretations of audit findings and documentation.
3. Customized AI Models:
   - **Tailored Solutions:** Developing industry-specific AI models to address unique challenges in different sectors within HSEQ.

By leveraging ChatGPT, HSEQ auditors can enhance the efficiency, accuracy, and effectiveness of their audit processes, ultimately leading to improved compliance and safer, more sustainable operations.

Stay tuned . . . it's going to be an interesting ride.

JURISDICTIONAL REGULATORY REVIEW

It is imperative that audit teams independently evaluate a site's compliance with any applicable regulatory requirements. Because many audit checklists and protocols emphasize only the federal or national requirements, auditors too often rely on the site HSEQ manager's knowledge of applicable state or provincial requirements, and this is clearly not an independent assessment. Several available regulatory databases and audit protocols allow for an independent review of state regulations prior to an audit. State and provincial requirements must be addressed, and they must be addressed independently. And just to reiterate, consider doing an AI query to see what benefit AI might have for you.

UNCLEAR OR UNKNOWN CORPORATE STANDARDS

Many, if not most, companies audit compliance with both applicable regulations and corporate standards, procedures, policies, or guidelines. Audit teams quite often have a difficult time with the latter. Corporate standards may be vague, unclear, or poorly written or communicated throughout the organization. Moreover, often a distinction is not made between mandatory standards and optional guidelines. Make sure you get clarity here before issuing your audit scope.

MISLEADING CLOSING MEETING AND CONFERENCES

The closing meeting or conference can be one of the most difficult elements of the audit process. There is sometimes a strong tendency to sugarcoat the findings in order to avoid antagonizing site or facility management and to make the meeting go smoothly. All too many closing conferences begin with an extended discourse on how cooperative and wonderful the site staff is and how well the site is being operated. On one particular audit, the team leader opened with the statement that the plant "was found to be in compliance with applicable rules and regulations." At that point, the plant manager left the meeting, leaving the HSEQ manager to deal with the forty or so compliance findings that the audit team subsequently raised. Audit team leaders must have the fortitude to make sure that plant management gets the right message. Any significant findings should be raised early in the meeting and given their rightful emphasis. Misinformation is just as bad as no information.

A recent example by one of the authors dealt with a medium-sized construction and fabrication company which had to maintain its COR® certificate of recognition to be able to bid on and secure government-related contracts. The certificate of recognition program was based on the requirements of the Newfoundland and Labrador Construction Safety Association:

> Our key offering is the Certificate of Recognition® (COR®) program, which is specifically designed to help companies institute an effective health and safety management program. In addition, the program emphasizes current safety training, legislative, and due diligence obligations that both employers and workers have under the OH&S Act and Regulations.

Due to a number of changes internally with their Health and Safety staff, they did not have a local resource to conduct their annual re-certification audit, so the authors were called to conduct this COR® audit on behalf of the client.

Long story short, after a 2.5-day audit, it became clear that the client had a number of nonconformance/noncompliance issues that needed attention. To set the tone and focus of the closing meeting, this fact is important: the last individual they had brought in to perform their COR® audit had scored the audit 100 percent. Our audit only scored around 80 percent, based on the objective evidence, interviews, and observations over this 2.5-day period.

Of course, management asked how this could be possible. How could one auditor identify everything as perfect just twelve months earlier, and another auditor find so many deficient issues? Of course we could not comment specifically on the question, partly since we have no objective evidence upon which to base an opinion. All we could do was show the auditee the objective evidence upon which our findings were based and let them come to their own conclusions. To make any other assertion without having clear evidence upon which to make that assertion would be very unprofessional. But as you can see, it's issues like this which can cause credibility issues with auditing. That said, we have some suspicions, but as of the writing of this book, that suspicion and issue remain unanswered. Perhaps for another time.

In the closing meeting, we just stuck to the facts as they were documented and didn't "assume" anything about the previous audit or auditor. To do otherwise would have been unprofessional and subjective in that meeting. But this is just one example of how different auditors, supposedly looking at the same processes, may come out at the back end of the audit with completely different conclusions.

TIMELINESS AND QUALITY OF THE AUDIT REPORT

Considering the emphasis that most companies place on the audit report, one would think there would be few problems in this area. However, this is not the case. Established programs generally have more problems with late reports than with anything else. Late reports can destroy the momentum gained by the audit and create liabilities for the organization. Quality is always an issue with any program; yet, after a few reports have been developed, there are typically adequate models to follow. But be careful if you are using a cut-and-paste template. Make sure you only cut and paste the generic template and not any previous audit findings from another audit you might happen to overlook in the cut-and-paste process. It can be embarrassing to find another location's information in a different audit report. A good technique used by many companies is to develop an audit program writing manual, which provides general guidance and samples of acceptable findings and complete reports. Finally, any audit training conducted as part of the program should stress the written report and findings as much as anything else. Proofread critically and judiciously. We can't make it any clearer.

INSUFFICIENT FOLLOW-UP

This has the potential to be a chronic problem in any HSEQ audit program. Audit reports are developed, corrective action plans followed, and then many systems break down. There are no systematic assurances that findings are being corrected in a timely fashion. This, of course, can create major liabilities for the organization.

The development of a sound database or IT-based systems (even spreadsheets), which allows periodic (e.g., monthly, quarterly) tracking of corrective-action status, can help to alleviate this problem. Verification audits are another useful technique but a little more labor-intensive. One should not wait until the next scheduled audit, which might be two, three, or more years away, to verify the completion of corrective actions, although the closure of findings from a previous audit should be a formal part of any audit.

A good action management tool and related process are essential requirements here, preferably in some type of database or other digital-based tool. We'll speak about this in later chapters.

LACK OF PROGRAM METRICS

It is ironic how few HSEQ audit programs have developed performance metrics for their activities, given that the operations these programs audit are routinely evaluated against innumerable metrics. Today, metrics should be the rule, not the exception. Good examples of metrics to consider include

- scheduling audits so that established frequencies are met;
- completing scheduled audits on time (on average);
- issuing reports on time;
- assuring that all auditors have received audit training;
- soliciting and receiving formal site feedback;
- developing and reporting statistics on findings closure; and
- maintaining up-to-date protocols and procedures.

Of course, other metrics can also be developed based on your defined audit management processes and requirements. Suffice it to say that HSEQ audit programs should be viewed like any other program. There should be a way to measure success or failure. *Note:* Any discussion of a company's individual HSEQ audit program approach in this chapter is based on information provided to the public at large through technical papers, presentations, and the like. Any discussion of a commercially available audit product does not imply an endorsement of that product.

REFERENCES

This chapter has been adapted from Lawrence B. Cahill and Raymond W. Kane. *Environmental Health and Safety Audits*, 9th Edition. Government Institutes, 2010. It has been updated for this edition.

Wayne Pardy and Terri Andrews. *Integrated Management Systems: Leading Strategies and Solutions*, 2nd Edition. Bernan Press, 2019.

https://chatgpt.com (query for audit checklists based on the requirement of ISO 9001, 14001, and 45001)

Newfoundland and Labrador Construction Safety Association: https://nlcsa.com/about/.

Labour Canada: https://www.canada.ca/en/employment-social-development/corporate/portfolio/labour/administrative-monetary-penalties.html

Labour Canada: https://laws-lois.justice.gc.ca/eng/regulations/

Chapter 8

Competencies, Characteristics, and Training of HSEQ Auditors

The vanity of teaching doth oft tempt a man to forget that he is a blockhead.

—George Saville, Marquess de Halifax, 1633–1695

THE NEED

Auditor training is an essential element of any HSEQ audit program. Correction—an essential element of any "*successful*" audit program. Sending poorly trained staff to conduct audits at operating facilities can create technical, legal, and organizational problems, particularly when companies or institutions are attempting to establish the credibility of a corporate or headquarters HSEQ audit program. It can be embarrassing for these auditors. Don't do this to them.

Generally speaking, you will want to determine if your audit team is able to demonstrate the personal attributes and skills that include, but are not limited to, the following:

1. Competence in clearly expressing concepts and ideas, orally and in writing.
2. Interpersonal skills conducive to the effective and efficient performance of the audit, such as diplomacy, tact, and the ability to listen.
3. The ability to maintain independence and objectivity sufficient to permit the accomplishment of auditor responsibilities.
4. Skills of personal organization necessary for the effective and efficient performance of the audit.
5. The ability to reach sound judgments based on objective evidence.

6. The ability to react with sensitivity to the conventions and culture of the region in which the audit is performed.

There are externally driven, as well as inherently logical, reasons for assuring that an organization's auditors are formally trained. Fortunately, with a modest investment of effort up front, management can feel comfortable knowing that the auditing staff is at least trained in the fundamentals of operations, regulatory requirements, interviewing and inspection techniques, and, perhaps most importantly, dealing effectively with facility management.

The choice of the best training approach must be made by management for its particular organization. No one solution fits each and every case. However, the audit manager can go through the following analytical process to define the training needs of the organization, and whether the resources to deliver that training reside in-house or outside the organization. The steps typically include the following:

1. Diagnosing the situation
   - What is the status quo?
   - What discrepancy exists between the current proficiency of the trainees and what is desired?
   - What are the realistic goals for training?
   - What methods are needed to achieve the instructional objectives?
2. Developing the instructional plan
   - Title?
   - Trainer(s)—internal or external?
   - Sponsoring organization?
   - Participants?
   - Dates and times?
   - Places?
   - Overall training objectives?
   - Training plan?
   - Time period
   - Goal
   - Method
   - Materials needed
   - Evaluation procedure?
3. Implementing and monitoring
   - Frequency?
   - Updating?
   - Annual evaluations?

COMPETENCY FRAMEWORK

Before these factors can be addressed, a fundamental question must be answered: What specific competencies should HSEQ auditors have (or do you want your auditors to have)? Foundational competencies are the basic human behavior skills fundamental to auditors being able to work effectively in the audit environment. Many of these are self-taught core social skills learned from life and business experiences and even from parents and teachers. Functional competencies include skills that focus on the audit process or methodology and relate to conducting audits with due professional care. Finally, the technical skills should relate to the specific HSEQ regulatory knowledge or technical content of the audit scope.

The second element of the competency framework deals with the question, "Do all audit practitioners need the same skills and at what level of proficiency?" This is addressed by recognizing that individuals involved in an HSEQ audit program play different roles. Most audit programs involve the following key functions:

- Audit program director or manager
- Lead auditor
- Auditor(s)
- Subject-matter auditor
- Guest auditor or observer

The audit program director or manager, or the individual given responsibility for the HSEQ audit program, is usually a senior staff person who may have other responsibilities in the company in addition to the HSEQ audit program. Or they may be dedicated to that role. When one of the authors was the quality lead for Husky Energy's East Coast Operations, his role was supplier/contractor HSEQ audit coordinator. His sole role was the coordination of every and all aspects of the audit process for Husky-approved suppliers and contractors.

This individual is normally responsible to top management for the implementation, staffing, and budgeting of the audit program. The audit team leaders or lead auditors are the individuals who direct the audit activities in the field. These staff need to have most of the foundational and functional audit skills, depending on the audit scope, and a good grasp of the technical competencies required for the scope in question.

The HSEQ auditor will need to have many, but not necessarily all, foundational, functional, and technical skills. For example, the resolution of conflicts, which can and often do occur on audits, will usually be handled by the lead auditor, so it is not necessary that auditors have proficiency in that competency.

Subject-matter expert auditors are typically assigned specialty areas that require a technical competency that other auditors do not have. These individuals will not necessarily need to have the full range of audit skills because their contribution relates more to a technical specialty within the scope of work.

Finally, a guest auditor may be involved as an "auditor in training" or as an observer from another company division. While this person may assist other members of the audit team, they will not necessarily need a high level of proficiency in most audit competencies while functioning in this role. The fact of the matter is, most of them are there in a learning capacity and, in our experience, don't want a lead role to play in the audit. They are quite content to sit back, listen, and observe.

The third element of the competency framework is the level of proficiency required by various audit practitioners for each audit competency. Four levels of proficiency are typically established for this:

- *Level 1:* required skill or knowledge (must have)
- *Level 2:* important skill or knowledge (should have)
- *Level 3:* helpful skill or knowledge (preferable to have)
- *Level 4:* skill or knowledge (not required or not necessary)

Putting this all together in a matrix will show the interrelationship between the HSEQ auditor competencies, the required audit functions, and the required level of proficiency. A few points should be emphasized regarding the competency framework. Training in all the competencies noted above is neither mandatory nor required. Auditors may function solely as environmental auditors, health and safety auditors, or quality auditors, or all three, (or perhaps have other discipline scopes), and the technical competencies required will depend on their role and the audit scope. It is important, however, that all auditors have some degree of proficiency in the foundational and functional competencies for auditing and general auditing principles.

Auditor training can take many forms other than formal classroom training. On-the-job training, professional development seminars, and HSEQ auditing textbooks, videos, and cloud or web-based training are available to help auditors learn audit skills. Finally, one-on-one coaching and mentoring by senior, experienced auditors or other HSEQ auditors is sometimes the best way for new and prospective auditors to master several of the competencies needed to perform effectively on HSEQ audits. Some training lends itself well to online learning. Others benefit from face-to-face learning and interactions. We would suggest HSEQ auditor training is a quintessential face-to-face learning opportunity.

Now that we have a better understanding of the specific auditor competencies and skills, the remainder of this chapter attempts to provide some insight into how management might go about answering HSEQ audit program questions. The discussion below addresses issues such as who should/could do the training, who should/could be trained, where the training should take place, and what techniques should be used. Several suggestions for ensuring that the training is effective are included.

SELECTING THE TRAINERS

There are three basic choices involved in selecting the trainers for an HSEQ audit program:

1. Using experienced in-house auditors to train junior staff.
2. Sending inexperienced staff to publicly available courses on HSEQ auditing.
3. Hiring qualified consultants to come in to train staff in groups.

Alternatively, there may be some variation or an approach using all three processes, but generally the three processes highlighted above are consistent with what the authors have experienced.

The first option can be done formally, or it can be provided on the job. That is, junior staff can be teamed with more senior staff on actual audits. As they gain experience, they can be given additional responsibilitics. Using the in-house training option has the advantage of giving the auditors company-specific training. However, it can be taxing on the lead auditors. It also does not expose trainees to how other companies handle the variety of issues that auditing presents and thus may stifle program advancements and improvements.

Publicly available courses can be used as training vehicles for auditors. In fact, the authors would suggest that this book can be considered a possible text for any HSEQ auditing course (shameless self-promotion).

The external-course approach has merit because it exposes auditors to other organizations' programs and to the wide variety of strategic and operational approaches they use. However, in order to cram a considerable amount of material into one, two, or three days, these courses cannot tailor the program to an individual company's needs and typically cannot include field exercises as part of the agenda, unless a particular venue is more accommodating than most.

A third approach is to contract with consultants experienced in HSEQ auditing. The consultant can conduct a one-, two-, or three-day training seminar that not only highlights the broad issues but is tailored to meet specific program requirements of the company in question. The consultant can also take photographs in advance of typical facility scenarios or physical conditions, or customer-owned equipment, to add realism to the training. This seminar can be held at a facility, site, or, in larger companies, during an annual HSEQ management meeting, and it might include several field exercises as well as classroom instruction. As worthwhile as this approach is, it is also probably the most expensive, and it is beneficial only if there is a sufficient number of auditors to train on an initial and ongoing basis, and if the cost is within the budget of the organization in question.

SELECTING THE TRAINEES

Obviously, those staff members who will be conducting the audits should (some would say, "must") be trained prior to their first audit. In addition, however, refresher training for all auditors should be considered. This ongoing training can be accomplished through conventional courses or through participation in organizations. Management should also consider including those people who will be on the receiving end of the audit (e.g., facility managers, HSEQ coordinators) in the training programs so that they are aware of the objectives of the HSEQ auditing program. Having an individual trained, having them conduct one audit, and then not doing anything else for one to two years before you assign them to another audit is a disservice to that individual.

SELECTING THE SETTING

With instructional courses and on-the-job training, management has little control over the setting in which the training is conducted. That setting is either in the cities where the courses are offered or in the plants where the audits are conducted. However, when a formal in-house classroom approach is selected, there is a choice of venues:

- Corporate headquarters
- A facility or satellite site
- A training center, off-site hotel, or other suitable training facility

Each of these options has its advantages and disadvantages. The corporate headquarters location is usually more accessible to most staff than a particular facility site. Moreover, there are often periodic meetings of one kind or another at headquarters, which could provide a forum for a training program. However, a facility offers a real-world setting for incorporating field exercises into the training program (e.g., conducting a mock audit of the facility, fabrication shop, hazardous waste storage area). Some larger companies have regional training centers that provide effective locations and facilities for a program, particularly if they are close to a facility site. One of the real advantages of a training center, regional or otherwise, is the resources it offers in the way of rooms, audiovisual equipment, and other amenities.

SELECTING THE TECHNIQUES

A variety of teaching techniques can be used to structure an HSEQ auditor-training program. The most appropriate are discussed below.

Lecture

Probably the most used technique, the lecture, can be useful in explaining the fundamentals of HSEQ auditing. Lectures can be supported by audiovisuals to make them more interesting. In particular, photographs and slides portraying typical situations an auditor might find in a plant can be especially informative, as can videos of typical physical conditions or facilities. The biggest risk with lectures is overusing them. In other words, the instructor may talk too much. And as much as very experienced auditors like to talk about their experiences, the communication that occurs during a lecture is typically only one way. Lectures need to be supported by more interactive techniques to make the entire training experience valuable. This is where the skill of a seasoned HSEQ auditor/instructor comes into play. They have experience in getting engagement and participation out of course participants, even though the "lecture" remains a key part of the training.

KEYS TO MAKING IT WORK

Developing and implementing a successful HSEQ audit training program is not always easy. Some of the keys to making the program are as follows:

- *Be prepared.* Diligent preparation is essential. The program planner needs to outline the objectives, develop the agenda, select the trainers and audience, select the methods, and develop the training tools in advance. Do not be afraid to perform a dry run of the materials. If there are field exercises, survey the facilities before the training session. Attend to details; make sure audiovisual equipment is available, is in working condition, and has all the necessary spare parts (e.g., light bulbs).

- *Make it fun.* Do not rely too heavily on lectures. Use interactive techniques such as in-class problem-solving, role-playing, and field exercises. Engage the students and get their active participation.
- *Evaluate the program.* Always prepare an evaluation sheet to assess the program. Training programs should not be static. Improvements should be made constantly. Feedback is essential.
- *Leave the trainees with a to-do list.* In many training programs, the trainee receives a barrage of materials and can easily become overwhelmed by the volume and complexity of the issues. It is important to sum up the training by focusing on the most important points a trainee should take from the training. Examples could include the following:
  - Develop a checklist for yourself to keep track of what you need to accomplish during the preaudit phase.
  - Develop a list of the materials you need to take with you on any audit.
  - Spend at least four hours a week reviewing the HSEQ literature to keep up on things like regulatory trends.

These exercises can help trainees identify the most important techniques to be learned from the training. Some may have a sense that the competency-training requirements discussed so far are complicated and burdensome. However, this will not prove true if some perspective is maintained. Learning how to audit effectively takes time. It is a continuous improvement process. And as noted above, not all audit staff need to master all HSEQ competencies.

For example, regarding the onerous area of environmental, health, and safety technical regulatory knowledge, HSEQ auditors only need to have a working knowledge of the applicable regulations. This knowledge can certainly be acquired through courses, textbooks, and the review and application of audit checklists or protocols. This last way of learning about regulations brings up an important point. Regulations do not have to be—more importantly, they cannot be—committed to memory.

The term *working knowledge* means just that. Auditors should be familiar enough with the regulations to be able to use a protocol effectively, and the protocols need to be detailed enough to support the auditor's efforts.

There is a secondary issue related to regulatory knowledge. Auditors too often limit themselves to their very defined area of expertise. We all have our own levels and areas of comfort. It is important that auditors also become comfortable reviewing areas related to those in which they are not experts. This makes them more valuable and flexible as team members and allows them to "pinch-hit" should one of the team members become indisposed during an audit.

The auditor should also be familiar with the facilities being audited and comfortable in a plant setting. This does not mean, however, that to be effective, every auditor of a chemical plant must be a chemical engineer with twenty years of facility experience. Or, just because it is a fabrication facility doesn't mean that you must be a welder. In fact, a good, solid, smart professional with an unabashed, natural curiosity and some familiarity with the facility being audited is probably the best candidate to do a good quality HSEQ audit. Further, no single educational background is best suited for auditing. Engineers, scientists, lawyers, managers, financial auditors and, yes, even English majors trained as auditors can bring valuable skills to the table.

Computer literacy is also a necessary core skill for several reasons. First, it has become routine for a working draft report to be prepared on a laptop, tablet, or desktop computer before the team leaves the site, especially if they are leveraging any of the many audit software products on the market today. Also, some companies are now using automated checklists or protocols loaded onto laptop, desktop, or tablet computers. Further, cloud-based or computerized regulatory databases provide additional field support to audit teams. Finally, facility data files (e.g., training records, inspection and maintenance reports, customer feedback surveys, meeting records) are now more frequently automated or put in a digital record of some kind. Thus, it is presently difficult to get by on an audit without some familiarity with computers and working with automated information technology.

By way of an example, when one of the authors was working with the electric utility company, Newfoundland Power, it was a common practice to audit the records of tailboard talks (sometimes called toolbox talks). Crews would take these forms/checklists out to the field, write up the site risk assessment/job plan, and review it before starting the job. All the paper or digital records would then be filed for future reference or eventual audit. Now, these tailboard talks are recorded via audio on a smartphone, and the WAV. file of the discussion. Digital audit records are maintained, date-stamped, and saved in their safety management system software, and anyone, at any time, can listen to what was discussed in that pre-job meeting. Brilliant.

CHARACTERISTICS AND QUALIFICATIONS OF GOOD AUDITORS

All of the above skills can be acquired with a little effort and dedication. However, some other core skills are more difficult to attain unless fundamental "building blocks" exist within the auditor's personality. The two that come to mind are interpersonal traits and, believe it or not, physical and mental stamina.

Good interpersonal skills go a long way in conducting quality HSEQ audits. In fact, of all the core skills required, these are clearly the most important. Such skills include being able to interview people effectively, having a high degree of curiosity, adjusting smoothly to changes in schedule, responding professionally to challenges to your verbal and written statements, working well under pressure, and generally keeping a cool head when everybody around you is panicking. The bottom line is that an auditor must be both a good communicator and an excellent listener. This takes sincerity, patience, and, at times, a great sense of humor.

While these skills can certainly be learned through experience, many individuals will never attain them to a sufficient level to work effectively as an HSEQ auditor. Remember that audits, unlike regulatory-agency inspections, are meant to be a supportive function; therefore, individuals who are inherently brusque, volatile, argumentative, and overly egocentric will not be successful. And when we say successful, we mean that their personal attributes contribute to the success of, and the perception of, the success of the entire audit process.

It may sound ludicrous to place a strong emphasis on physical and mental stamina as an important trait for auditors. However, any of us who have participated in audits know how important this can be. Consider the pace of an audit. Auditors often travel on the weekends or late at night. They climb towers and buildings all day, which can be exhausting. Or they may enter confined spaces or be required to wear PPE like a full-face respirator. They are under constant pressure to "perform" and to ensure that they are being diligent and thorough in the investigation. Think it's not important? Try auditing in an iron ore mine with a full-face respirator on for the full day and then looking for ways to engage folks who don't want to be engaged.

The most taxing tasks of all can be the daily late-night team meetings to discuss observations and findings. When a draft report is to be prepared prior to the team's leaving the site—a general trend these days—the night before the day of the closing conference can flow into the early hours of the morning if the data-gathering phase has not been completed sufficiently early. Attempting to craft an articulate, accurate, and precise finding at 1:00 a.m. is no simple feat.

And quite simply, auditing means you have to be "on" the entire time. While both authors are actors in their other lives, this is not to say that auditing is contrived or staged. But your behavior, and perceived behavior as an auditor, is closely observed by everyone. Being down or subdued in your auditing activity does nothing for the integrity of the audit process. At least show enough respect to the auditee to keep them remain awake during your auditing process.

OBSERVING AUDITORS IN THE FIELD

Now, how do these skills and attributes contribute to or hinder the quality of an audit? As an audit team leader or program manager, what should you be looking for or watching out for in an auditor. Examples of the worst and best behaviors are discussed below.

The Worst Attributes

No auditor is perfect. However, certain characteristics and behaviors should clearly be avoided:

- *Insufficient records review:* Too many auditors want to do a field inspection immediately upon beginning an audit. Records must be reviewed first to determine the applicable requirements. This problem often results from a lack of familiarity or comfort with the regulations or corporate standards. An auditor should take the time early on to determine the requirements.
- *Excessive records review:* This often occurs when auditors are intimidated by the size or complexity of the site and just do not know where to begin. They will bury themselves in the records and never come up for air. A better approach would be to first take a "windshield" tour of the facility, then cut off small chunks of the operation and visit appropriate locations in a modular fashion.
- *Captivity to checklists:* A very common problem arises when the auditor becomes too dependent on the checklist: he or she focuses on symptoms instead of causes. This might also be a problem caused by an external audit organization only concerned with its own audit protocol. Auditors add value when they address underlying or root causes. They should take some time to think through what really might be happening at the site to cause the identified problems. Answer the why as well as the what question. Compliance and conformance are fine . . . adding value to the business and its related processes is even better.
- *Jumping to conclusions:* This is the opposite of the problem discussed above. Some auditors tend to draw broad conclusions before all the evidence is in. Auditors can sometimes let their egos get in the way of doing a thorough analysis and verifying their findings. They have seen it all before, and they simply "know" what is causing the problem. This results in statements such as, "The hazardous waste management system or the fall protection program or the objective setting process at the site is deficient," which is not a very articulate or helpful finding. Auditors need to take a step back and make sure that there is evidence to support their conclusions. What do you mean by "deficient." Deficient "how"?

- *Poor time management:* There are auditors who never seem to finish on time. This often occurs when they are given more than one compliance area to cover and spend 90 percent of their time in the area where they feel the most comfortable. Make sure that auditors attack compliance areas in parallel, not in series. It is risky to leave one area for the last day of the audit. Learning how to pace yourself and place adequate emphasis on all assigned topics is an important characteristic of a good auditor and a characteristic of good planning. We execute well what we plan well.
- *"In my experience" syndrome:* Nothing annoys site staff more than having auditors preach to them about how things are done in their "experience" or at their location. Auditors should research the appropriate site-specific regulations for the site and audit the site against those regulations. They should, of course, tactfully report on what is being done at their site if it might be a helpful suggestion for improving performance.
- *Being too easy/too tough:* Auditors must strike a balance between being supportive and providing an honest assessment of the site's performance. Over the years, auditing programs sometimes tend to swing back and forth between "good cop/bad cop" scenarios. When the facilities scream that the program is becoming punitive, then the "white hats" go on, and the reports become so vague that management cannot tell if there is a problem or not. There is no easy solution here—nor should there be. Auditors should not, however, pull any punches in the closing conference or report if they have objective evidence upon which to base their conclusions. Site and facility managers need to understand all the ramifications of their actions.

The Best Attributes

What makes an individual a good auditor? Communication skills certainly count, but other characteristics contribute as well:

- *An even disposition:* People with volatile personalities do not make good auditors. This very stressful occupation requires a level head and the ability to adjust to new people, surroundings, and constant change. People (auditees) can be fickle.
- *Flexibility:* Audits never go quite as planned. An auditor needs to be flexible to adjust to changing dates, schedules, situations, and the like.
- *Natural curiosity:* Mentioned previously, this is an important trait. Some would say that the better descriptor would be "healthy skepticism." In either case, a natural inquisitiveness is important.
- *High energy level:* There is no time to relax on an audit. Days typically start for many site audits at 7:00 a.m. with a breakfast meeting and end at 9:00

p.m. or later with a discussion of findings. This can be very taxing, and an auditor must enter the process understanding that.

- *Grace under fire:* Site staff constantly challenge auditors during an audit. It is simply the nature of the process. Auditors must be able to handle this with tact and professionalism. This is especially true during the closing conference when those doing the challenges are more likely to be senior staff. And sometimes they may, and do, take things personally.
- *Under-control ego:* A healthy ego is probably an asset for an auditor, who must present his findings confidently, but a "know-it-all" attitude is not helpful.

MAKING GOOD THINGS HAPPEN

How does one ensure that auditors do indeed have the appropriate skills? Most firms accomplish this through a variety of techniques.

First, certain individuals can be eliminated because of their personalities. This does not necessarily mean that they are not good performers, just that they might not be suited to be auditors. Second, most firms require that auditors attend a formal training program. These programs can be tailored to address those issues most in need of attention. In fact, some companies have both basic and refresher seminars. The best basic programs usually include a "mock audit" of an actual plant so that auditor candidates can get a true feel for the experience. Such programs feature simulated opening and closing conferences and actual interviews, records reviews, and facility inspections. Improving communication skills through role-playing and group exercises is usually an essential element of the program.

The refresher programs can focus on historical problems experienced in the field by the audit teams. These problems can be identified using several techniques. For example, audit team leaders can—and do—critique both the process and the auditors. And they should be confident enough to do this during the audit, as well as after it is complete. On-the-spot constructive feedback is one of the best ways to improve performance. Further, as part of a quality-assurance program, some companies will have an oversight auditor participate as a select member of the audit team during the year to evaluate the process. Lastly, site feedback questionnaires are used to identify problems from a "customer" perspective.

CONCLUSION

Attaining and maintaining good HSEQ auditor skills is a challenging and never-ending task. To be effective, auditors need more than just knowledge of the regulations. Training should include the required foundational and functional competencies discussed in this chapter, as well as the technical knowledge required by the audit scope. The challenge is to ensure that auditors are trained properly and receive continuous feedback. Numerous techniques can be employed to deliver a good training program, all of which should be evaluated so that companies invest time and resources wisely in the most cost-effective manner.

Third-party certifying organizations must ensure that auditors whom they certify have the full arsenal of skills necessary to conduct a quality audit and require continuing education to maintain auditor skills. In addition to having audit skills, regulatory knowledge, and competencies, good auditors should learn and demonstrate certain characteristics and attitudes. A helpful reminder for HSEQ auditors is to keep in mind the sometimes delicate balance of what to be and what not to be when conducting an HSEQ audit.

REFERENCES

International Organization for Standardization (ISO), *Guidelines Auditing Management Systems*, ISO 19011. https://www.iso.org/obp/ui/en/#iso:std:iso:19011:ed-3:v1:en.

ISO 19011: https://cdn.standards.iteh.ai/samples/70017/559078f9a2634aca84ff0a6aac1498f6/ISO-19011-2018.pdf

This chapter has been adapted from Lawrence B. Cahill and Raymond W. Kane. *Environmental Health and Safety Audits*, 9th Edition. Government Institutes, 2010. It has been updated for this edition.

Wayne Pardy and Terri Andrews. *Integrated Management Systems: Leading Strategies and Solutions*, 2nd Edition. Bernan Press, 2019.

Chapter 9

Conducting Third-Party Evaluations of HSEQ Audit Programs

On March 24, 1989, the Exxon Valdez ran aground in Alaska's Prince William Sound. Ever since then, this notorious incident continues to have unexpected consequences, and it is not confined to the folks at Exxon, and not all negative. One of these consequences is the emergence of independent, third-party evaluations of corporate health, safety, environment, and quality (HSEQ) management systems and their related audit programs. These evaluations are being conducted by leading companies to provide additional assurances to stakeholders and shareholders that the regulated community is responsibly and proactively achieving its compliance obligations.

Consider Exxon for a minute. One of the consequences of the Exxon Valdez Incident was the development of what Exxon calls OIMS, their Operational and Integrity Management System. In the words of Darren Woods, chairman and chief executive officer of Exxon Mobil Corporation:

> *ExxonMobil is committed to producing products that are essential to modern life and economic development, in a way that helps protect people, the environment and the communities where we operate. We are steadfast in our commitment to excellence in Safety, Security, Health, and Environmental (SSH&E) performance, referred to overall as Operations Integrity.*
>
> *The ExxonMobil Operations Integrity Management System, or OIMS, establishes a strong foundation and sets clear expectations for managing the safety, security, health and environmental risks inherent in our business, and guides the daily activities of our global workforce. Operational excellence requires strong leadership at all levels. It also requires each ExxonMobil employee and contractor to be an effective risk manager. It is everyone's responsibility to make management of hazards, risks and safeguards a key focus in their daily activities. This ensures we are upholding our core value of care—operating*

in the best interests of each other, our families, our communities and our shareholders.

As Exxon notes:

The 1989 Valdez accident was one of the lowest points in ExxonMobil's long history. . . . In the aftermath of the accident, we also undertook significant operational reforms and implemented an exceptionally thorough operational management system to prevent future incidents. This system has been deployed globally and in the years since the accident, we have had nothing similar occur. We believe our subsequent record of safety stems primarily from disciplined and systematic improvements that we have made. We are particularly proud of the spill prevention performance of our global marine transportation affiliates since the Valdez spill. We consider this strong performance encouraging and it serves as a solid platform for continuous improvement efforts.

WHAT ARE THE HSEQ PROGRAM CRITERIA?

1. Explicit Top-Management Support

It is generally expected that an HSEQ audit program will receive support and commitment from the highest levels of an organization. This includes a written policy articulating upper management support for the auditing program and an explicit written commitment to follow up on audit findings to correct identified problems and prevent their recurrence.

The program should be positioned properly in the organization with sufficient support so that audit findings and recommendations receive very serious consideration by line management. Management commitment also presumes attendance at opening and closing conferences by the most senior on-site manager and timely responses to audit findings. Managers at all levels should cooperate fully with audit teams.

2. Program and Auditor Independence

Both an audit program and the auditors themselves must be sufficiently independent of audited activities to ensure that objective reviews are conducted. This expectation does not necessarily mean that external, third-party auditors must be utilized. It does mean that auditors should not generally audit programs for which they provided development and/or implementation advice or assistance.

3. Appropriate Audit Team Staffing

"Auditors should have completed auditor training that contributes to the development of knowledge and skills. This training may be provided by the person's own organization or by an external organization" (ISO 19011). What is appropriate means can be subjective, but ISO 19011 offers good guidance here.

4. Comprehensive Written Audit Procedures

Audit protocols, checklists, and/or guides that reflect the scope of the audit must be used when auditors review operations against audit criteria in order to ensure consistency and reliability. Such materials must be kept "up-to-date" to ensure that they address changes in regulations, organizational policy, operational activities, or any other criteria about which the program is intended to provide assurance.

5. Defined Program Objectives and Scope

The scope and objectives of an audit program should meet certain expectations, as defined by management and generally accepted audit practices. At a minimum, audit objectives should include assessing compliance with applicable HSEQ laws and evaluating the adequacy of internal compliance policies, procedures, and personnel training programs to ensure continued compliance. The objectives of an audit must be clearly established and fully communicated beforehand to the auditee.

6. Adequate Program Resources

An audit program must have sufficient authority, resources, and personnel to carry out its mission. This essentially implies that the required number of audits must be conducted at the established frequencies, utilizing the appropriate number of qualified auditors, who are provided with the necessary auditing tools (e.g., regulatory information, audit protocols). Further, there should be a strong management commitment to ensuring that sufficient resources are available to attain the efficient closure of identified deficiencies.

Audit teams must be of sufficient size to complete audits of sites in the time allotted. The team makeup should be such that all compliance areas are addressed fully and competently.

The words "adequate" and "sufficient" can also be subjective, so make sure you design your processes around your realities and limitations of what "adequate" and "sufficient" mean to you and your organization.

7. Audit Frequency Based on Risk

In general, most organizations will audit sites with a frequency based on some evaluation of their stated priorities, or the risks posed by the organization or the facility. Although it should be noted that most of the external guidelines are notably silent on any quantitative expectations for audit frequency, the commonly held expectation for audits is that major facilities generally are audited no less frequently than once every two to three years.

8. Documented Audit Process

The information should be sufficient, reliable, and useful to provide a sound basis for audit findings and recommendations. Audit procedures, including the testing and sampling techniques employed, should be selected in advance to the extent practical, and expanded or altered if circumstances warrant. Any written procedures should be consistent with actual practice.

9. Documentation of Audit Findings

The written audit report is one of the most important elements of an audit program. Producing accurate, understandable, and timely reports poses a significant challenge for most organizations. Each finding of noncompliance or nonconformance shall be based on appropriate supporting evidence and stated clearly to identify both the applicable requirement or criterion and the noncompliant or nonconforming condition or activity. Written reports should be handled in a manner consistent with written document management procedures.

10. Resolution of Corrective Actions

Ensuring adequate follow-up for each audit is a crucial element of any audit program and one that is quite often deficient. Procedures should be in place to ensure that information is communicated to managers, including facility and corporate management, who can evaluate the information and ensure the correction of identified problems. Corrective-action procedures should include monitoring mechanisms to verify progress toward the ultimate completion of the plan.

11. Appropriate Quality-Assurance Measures

Quality assurance may be accomplished through supervision, independent internal reviews, external reviews, or a combination of these approaches.

HOW ARE THE EVALUATIONS CONDUCTED?

In order to evaluate an HSEQ audit program, a third party should undertake three fundamental tasks:

1. Review program documentation and systems, including audit reports, corrective-action plans, and tracking databases.
2. Interview program staff and customers.
3. Observe a representative number of field audits.

As with a facility audit, the evaluation team typically begins with a review of the program documents. This provides the foundation for subsequent interviews and field observations.

Once the review of the program's paperwork is complete, interviews with key staff are conducted. Candidate staff include senior management, audit program staff, auditors, and line staff and management who have been audited. Many of these interviews are conducted face-to-face, but others are conducted by telephone. Approximately fifteen to twenty individuals are typically interviewed.

One of the most crucial evaluation techniques used during third-party reviews is for the evaluator to actually observe a representative number of audits. This allows the evaluator to verify that the program's established procedures and protocols are used correctly, by the audit teams. This field verification also enhances the credibility of the evaluation tremendously, an important factor for outside parties and/or the Board of Directors.

The number of audits observed varies substantially, but a minimum of three is considered representative. Factors to consider in determining which particular audits will be observed include large versus small sites, domestic versus overseas facilities, and variances in types of business units.

Completion of the above activities should provide the information necessary to draw a conclusion about the effectiveness of the audit program.

REFERENCES

This chapter has been adapted from Lawrence B. Cahill and Raymond W. Kane. *Environmental Health and Safety Audits*, 9th Edition. Government Institutes, 2010. It has been updated for this edition.

Wayne Pardy and Terri Andrews. *Integrated Management Systems: Leading Strategies and Solutions*, 2nd Edition. Bernan Press, 2019.

https://corporate.exxonmobil.com/who-we-are/technology-and-collaborations/energy-technologies/risk-management-and-safety/operations-integrity-management-system

Note: This discussion attributes what the authors consider to be unsubstantiated "best practices" to particular organizations where they have been observed by the authors. Commentary is not attributed to any given company and simply reflects the recollections and experiences of the authors.

Chapter 10

Leveraging Information Technology for HSEQ Audits

> Information is not knowledge. But knowledge can come from various sources or information.
>
> —Wayne Pardy, 2024

Ensuring HSEQ compliance and conformance status has become an information challenge of great proportions. Let's face it. You can be in complete compliance one minute and, because of the actions or inactions of an individual or several individuals, be completely out of compliance the next. Compliance is not a static process but a very dynamic one, especially when it comes to the actions of people. Facilities can be a bit more static and reliable but not exclusively so. Companies typically need to generate and track a variety of documents such as permit applications, manifests, monthly and annual operating reports, incident reports, audit action-item reports, and the like. In addition, they need to manage the incoming information stream generated by potentially many different regulatory agencies in their continuing efforts to communicate and enforce standards, regulations, and guidance.

In response to this ever-increasing flood of information, corporate HSEQ auditing staff are developing in-house, or purchasing from vendors, computerized or cloud/web-based data-management systems. For audit programs, these systems generally fall into three classes:

1. Management system software integrated with local and international regulatory databases/checklists.
2. Commercially available audit software and protocols.
3. Information management databases, which include software to manage all aspects of an HSEQ management system, including HSEQ audits and related action management—an integrated HSEQ software solution.

This chapter discusses these systems, focusing on the factors that should be considered when evaluating any given package or approach.

Because the HSEQ software field is so dynamic and has exploded in scope over the past ten to twenty years, this chapter does not evaluate individual products or online services. For detailed reviews and comparisons of current products, the reader should refer to HSEQ software buyer guides that can be found on the Internet. One particularly useful site is Capterra. Individuals can do their own research at https://www.capterra.com/

REGULATORY DATABASES

More and more auditors are using commercial, off-the-shelf information systems, both in preparation for an audit and during the on-site activities. This on-site use means, of course, that the audit team must have access to a computer or some other technology (tablet, smartphone, etc.) during the audit and that the computer must have the ability to connect to either the Internet (web, cloud, Wi-Fi, etc.) or a CD drive. The regulatory databases are especially important in identifying applicable regulations, as many audit protocols will address a wide range of regulations.

Automated regulatory databases should incorporate the following characteristics:

- *Coverage:* All major federal, provincial, and state HSEQ regulations should be a part of the system. As discussed above, this federal, provincial, and state coverage is essential. Some of the products also offer international coverage (e.g., the European Union, individual countries). As audit programs have gone global, this added feature has become more important, especially if audit teams travel internationally and not all team members might be familiar with local regulatory requirements.
- *Currency:* The systems should be relatively current; updating should occur at least every six months, if not more frequently. More frequent updating at the federal or national level should be expected. In the United States, the *Federal Register* provides an expedited means of doing so. Updating of individual state regulations is more problematic since many states are not as systematized in codifying their regulations. That said, most regulatory agencies the authors are familiar with make their requirements available online, which are updated accordingly.
- *Ease of use:* These systems should be, and for the most part are, user-friendly. Moreover, they should be friendly to both the casual and the power user.
- *Flexibility:* Systems should be designed for single-user applications, local-area networks, and wide-area networks. A user should be able to access the

database from other software such as Microsoft Office, Mac, and so on. The provider should be willing to arrange for a corporate license that responds to these varying needs without breaking the corporate bank, as some of the content can be very expensive.

- *Powerful search capabilities:* The programs should incorporate some kind of search engine that allows for easy and powerful searching in a variety of ways, including searches by keyword, acronym, citation number, and subject. The user should be allowed to search across multiple jurisdictions simultaneously.
- *Notation of changes:* Some of the databases have incorporated a feature that marks text to show the user exactly what has been added, deleted, or amended since the last update. This is especially useful for auditors who need to keep abreast of changing requirements in an efficient manner.
- *Online help:* The database should have online help that is easy to access and simple to understand.
- *Speed and more speed:* With tens of thousands of pages of regulations now in the books, the database should work very quickly in its searches. Or try an artificial intelligence application and see what you get.
- *Ease of exporting or printing:* Although this certainly is the computer age, it is still sometimes helpful to be able to print a hard copy or otherwise output the regulations being researched. Some folks are still more comfortable with a physical, hard copy of information rather than a digital version (check the age bracket here). The database should have a print and/or export function that will allow regulations to be printed in a high-quality format (including tables) and/or be directly inserted into reports.

Although computerized regulatory databases are powerful tools for auditors, sometimes it is still helpful to talk to a fellow human being for interpretations of requirements. For particularly complex issues, it is probably a good idea to call the applicable contact number twice and determine whether the interpretations are consistent. This is a good quality-assurance step.

COMMERCIALLY AVAILABLE AUDIT PROTOCOLS

Auditors' checklists or protocols are a key component of any audit program. The checklists typically contain hundreds, if not thousands, of questions related to applicable government regulations, company standards and guidelines, and good management practices. Historically, checklists have been fairly large, hard copy documents, making it difficult and costly for companies to both develop and routinely update these checklists. Because of this and other difficulties associated with maintaining audit checklists, several software companies have developed comprehensive audit checklists. These checklists can be used online or loaded onto a laptop computer and used as the principal audit protocol tool in the field. The automated checklists have their uses but come with some disadvantages.

ADVANTAGES

The commercial checklists or protocols offer a number of key advantages:

- *Regulatory coverage:* The checklists typically cover the major HSEQ regulations that would be of concern to almost any organization. In many cases, state, provincial, and international requirements are addressed as well.
- *Regulatory searches:* The checklists are generally contained in a linked database that provides the actual regulations that drive the audit requirement. The user can quickly access these regulations by using a "hot key." The user has access to a detailed interpretation of the requirement without having to refer to a separate document, system, or regulatory database.
- *Currency:* A real advantage of the commercial checklists is that they are kept current by the supplier. Most checklists are updated every three to six months, incorporating new regulatory requirements. Updated files, cloud-based access, and/or CDs are routinely distributed to customers. CDs, we predict, will eventually disappear.
- *Consistency:* By providing each auditor with a comprehensive set of audit protocols, the company is likely to achieve more consistent auditing over time.
- *Training:* The checklists can be an invaluable training device. They contain a wealth of information on regulatory requirements, and particular areas of interest can be accessed quickly. The checklists are often used as part of site self-assessment programs in which site HSEQ coordinators select one or more compliance areas to audit every other month or so.
- *Report generators:* Some of the commercial checklists contain report generators, which can automatically incorporate findings through "red flag" triggers. That is, the audit questions are structured so that certain answers will trigger a finding, and these are imported into the report generator automatically. Some advanced users have been able to use this powerful red-flag tool in a Windows environment and have transferred the findings to more traditional word-processing software.

DISADVANTAGES

The commercial checklists bring with them a number of potential challenges that must be considered and overcome:

- *State, provincial, or municipal coverage:* Not all the checklists contain the HSEQ regulatory requirements at every regulatory level. This can be a significant drawback because ensuring adequate regulatory coverage is a key component of any HSEQ audit. The programs do allow for incorporating additional questions in each module to address corporate standards and guidelines, as well as multiple regulatory requirements. Adding these components to the checklists will increase their value, but updating them will burden the purchaser of the product.
- *Small-site applicability:* In order to be comprehensive, the checklists can contain several thousand questions. This comprehensiveness can be a problem when auditing a small manufacturing site, a warehouse, or a laboratory. An auditor does not usually have the time to review several thousand questions on a one- or two-day audit of these smaller facilities. As a consequence, the programs often provide for an initial screening of the areas in need of review and also have the ability to follow up with a more focused audit. Nonetheless, auditors sometimes feel more comfortable with a paper checklist so that screening and culling can be accomplished more quickly and effectively.
- *Multiple-user costs:* Like any software product, commercial checklists have become much more cost-competitive over the past few years. However, if a large corporation adopts one of these packages as a universal audit tool, the costs can become significant because each user often requires a separate license. Software companies will work with purchasers of multiple systems to develop a corporate license that can significantly reduce the cost per user.
- *The occasional user:* Comprehensive, commercial checklists work best when auditors use them often enough to become very familiar with their capabilities. The packages are more of a challenge when auditors use them only occasionally. Such occasional usage is very common with audit programs that employ part-time auditors from divisions and plants. It is difficult to become facile with a software package when one uses it only once or twice a year, as many of these part-time auditors do.
- *Interference with the audit:* One of the most often communicated problems associated with computer-based audit checklists is that they can interfere with the normal audit process. Sometimes auditors become so engrossed in interacting with and completing the checklists that they do not spend sufficient time interviewing staff, reviewing records, or inspecting the facility.

It should be noted here as well that the Internet provides competitive products—and for free. In sum, commercial checklists are definitely worth exploring, especially for programs in which self-audits will be expected. There are some risks in adopting this approach, however. Careful planning can do much to mitigate these risks. You need to decide if you have the time, expertise, and resources to do the required work or whether to contract it out to external subject-matter experts.

HSEQ AUDIT SOFTWARE—INFORMATION MANAGEMENT DATABASES

Audit Management Systems and Technology

In the past ten years, there has been an explosion of integrated management system software solutions, including HSEQ audit management technology. Not only is the market more crowded, but the level of functionality of many of the technological solutions available has become leading-edge and innovative. The integrated management system practitioners and auditors of today have significant opportunities and advantages over their colleagues of even five short years ago. The proliferation of software solutions to take the mundane and drudgery out of management system and audit coordination (documentation control and management, data analysis, root cause/hazard analysis, action tracking, auditing, risk assessment, customer communication) is almost essential for today's management system practitioner and HSEQ auditor.

On second thought, it is essential. Having said that, the authors have been amazed at the number of large, medium, and small businesses which have no technology tool available to them to manage HSEQ or operational integrity, other than word-processing software or spreadsheets. Old school—yes. Ineffective—yes. Shortsighted—absolutely. And cost is no longer a barrier or a reason for not integrating and leveraging technology for your management and HSEQ audit systems.

There are a wide range of products on the market with a wide range of price points—from the inexpensive to the very expensive—depending on budget, functional requirements, and resources available. For years, management systems were, and some would argue, still are, characterized by unending volumes of paper records, checklists, binders, and documentation. So much so, in fact, that much of the negative debate about management systems was centered around the perception that they can be nothing more than a massive paper chase. In other words, an endless list of procedures and documented processes. And in some respects, for some organizations, that assertion was correct. The role of an effective management system and audit technology should be to help add significant value to an organization through the use of timely, accurate, and meaningful information and data management.

And most organizations generate tons and tons of information and data, but with no meaningful endpoint or conclusion. Looking at stacks and stacks of paper piled high on a desk may tell you that you and your colleagues have been doing something, but there is typically a gold mine of data in that pile of paper that you can never extract due to the nature of paper-based documentation. Great for the paper industry—unfortunate for the management system and HSEQ audit community.

Many management system practitioners are familiar with the continual improvement cycle model: Plan—Do—Check—Act (PDCA). This model basically follows the guideline of "say what you do, do what you say, and prove it." And whatever you've proven, or determined, take that information and use it to enhance, improve, add more value, or innovate to bring you to the next level. While pure conformance to management system requirements is only one aspect of an effective management system, the effective management of information and data is also crucial. If management by fact is to have any relevance, those facts must be discernible from just mundane information. If we are to make decisions to better our business or enhance performance, we had better be as sure as possible that the basis upon which we are making those decisions is based on good evidence and is factually correct. Of course, the "Act" aspect of the PDCA model lends itself well to the HSEQ audit model and related processes.

For some organizations, especially those with the financial resources to both develop and maintain such systems, the decision to build in-house software is rationalized, while many prefer to contract the development of a management system software solution to third-party, proven technology providers. In looking at technology-based solutions for the management system, the authors are not advocating one approach over another. Nor will we speak to any one commercially available system or product; however, as the authors have had significant experience in designing and building in-house solutions, as well as custom, off-the-shelf management system and HSEQ audit software solutions, we will profile the pros and cons of both approaches.

The objective, however, should be to ensure that whatever route you choose (in-house vs. contracted out, commercial off-the-shelf, hybrid, etc.) you have some confidence at the end of the day that the technology solution you've chosen can add value to your management system audits that you and your management team expect. Also, the data you generate from your management system audit initiatives should generate information to help you and your management team manage better, make better and more informed decisions, and ultimately improve the value of your integrated management system.

Let's take a brief look at some of these management system opportunities that can be further enhanced by some of the leading-edge technology solutions that are on the market today.

CONTROL OF DOCUMENTED INFORMATION (DOCUMENTS AND RECORDS)

As previously noted, one of the complaints against structured management systems is the amount of information and documentation required to maintain the system to a level deemed appropriate by management system practitioners, internal and external auditors, regulatory agencies, and customers. For most activities associated with your management system, there can be a wide array of policies, practices, and procedures that need to be managed, updated, communicated, and made available for ongoing revision and update.

Interested parties might also require access to this information. For those of you who bid for jobs and respond to formal tenders, you've perhaps noticed that the level of due diligence and vetting of those to whom they may be giving large contracts is getting (is already) greater. Major employers want assurance that the systems, including documented information, are a critical aspect of the project or tender award. The review of policies and procedures demands that those policies and procedures be well documented and readily available.

Many in-house and third-party applications currently available on the market use some variation of a server or cloud-based data warehouse to enable a document repository for the maintenance and coordination of management system documentation. Using a cloud-based or intranet data warehouse with the ability to store, sort, and manage management system documents provides an easy-to-access site for everyone within the organization. Further security-based access can ensure that only those who have a need to access the documents can do so, and read/write-only access can help protect sensitive data from accidental deletion.

Take 10 minutes to run a search on Google, and you'll come to quickly realize that many of the third-party applications currently on the market have migrated from old, client-based technology solutions to completely cloud or web-enabled solutions, whether through a client's own intranet or available through the vendor's website through an ASP web-hosted solution. The critical issue here is for the integrated management system to be designed in such a way as to make access for critical documentation readily available in an easy-to-access/read format. Generally speaking, HSEQ audit software typically generates the following types of documents. Check with your preferred vendor to see if their audit management solution offers these features:

- Audit scheduler (including scheduled vs. planned, etc.)
- Audit notification templates
- Audit planning templates
- Audit team logistics templates
- Audit checklists/templates and guidance features
- Opening and closing meeting templates
- Audit conclusion/presentation templates
- Audit report templates
- Action management templates or modules
- Analytics module for custom query and report writing, and data analysis

CONFESSIONS OF A VICE PRESIDENT OF HSEQ MANAGEMENT SYSTEM SOFTWARE

It wasn't all that long ago (at least it feels that way) that one of the authors, Wayne Pardy, was vice president of marketing for Q5 Systems Limited. Q5 is an international leader in software management applications for integrated management systems, with a specific emphasis on audit, inspection, and action tracking software solutions. It was in this role that Wayne got to see the management system business from a different perspective—that of the management system practitioner looking for a technology solution for their unique management system and HSEQ audit requirements, while at the same time looking for every modification possible (usually for no cost!) and that was created in the image of the respective culture and administrative requirements of each and every company. And yet while they were all different, they were all generally the same.

Most management system practitioners have little or no experience in technology solutions for their management system requirements. This is not surprising, but it can be frustrating to both a management system technology vendor, who, while sometimes trying, cannot be all things to all clients, and it can be frustrating to the customer who wonders why "your" software doesn't do what they want it to do. While many software vendors will assume a "take it or leave it" attitude, other management system software vendors are very willing to work with a customer to try, as much as reasonably possible, based on their technology platform and available resources, to "customize" the one-size-fits-all technology solution to your respective audit requirements.

For those looking for technology solutions for their audits, a word of advice from a former industry insider—make sure you define your functional requirements as clearly and definitively as you can "before" you ever consider going to the market and speaking with a software salesman. Don't take the approach of, "When I see it, I'll know it." You need to do just as much research on an audit technology solution as you did in the research and design phase for your audit program. Technology solutions are not inexpensive, and like the saying goes, "You get what you pay for." But it is critically important that you not let the vendor define your clearly defined requirements. You must be crystal clear on your defined functionality. And you must try to ensure that, though cost is a factor, it should not be the most critical factor. You don't want to get stuck with a moderately priced technology solution that everyone complains about, and which doesn't provide good information and value. The more flexible the software, the more you as the user can define select features, fields, and reporting options, the better the software solution will complement your existing management system.

AUDIT MANAGEMENT TECHNOLOGY

This is the area in which those management system technologies that have a mobility application win hands down over paper checklists and word-processing software. The most advances in management system auditing over the past five years haven't necessarily been with systems or standards, but with technology solutions. The ability to capitalize on a field-enabled audit management system, with integrated action tracking, puts those organizations that leverage this technology leaps and bounds ahead of the paper-based, word-processor devotees. Here's a typical scenario. Take any management system audit you can imagine (checklist-based, open-ended questions, etc.). You design your audit in the software, do your audit in the field, and "synch" it back when you have access to a network connection. Finalize your report and the audit is finished. But wait. The client wants a copy of the report before your audit team leaves the site. No problem . . . use the offline feature and print feature on the mobility solution, and you can leave a complete audit report with your client without ever having to return to the office. The drawback with most paper-based audit systems is that the data cannot be mined, sorted, or queried.

Many still use word-processing software to prepare the audit report, and while the audit is available for reading, over the course of time (and a multitude of audits) the data amassed from numerous audits doesn't tell you anything. You must manually sort through all that data and try to manipulate it to identify issues, trends, or problem areas. If you're looking for a value-added audit technology, look for one that can analyze and trend by sections and actual questions in your audit. This will also satisfy the requirement of some standards that require you to demonstrate analysis of data, and audit data can generate meaningful information about issues and trends.

CUSTOMER COMMUNICATION AND FEEDBACK

There are many options available on the market today for management system specialists looking to implement a technology solution to add value to their current management system. We thought we would provide you with a small overview of some of the products that are currently available on the market which, in the opinion of the authors, offer good potential for complementing the strategic approach to management systems and system practices. (Author's note: The following is not meant to be a complete overview of the many and varied types of management system software solutions available on the market today. Like most organizations, if you are looking for a software solution to enhance the effectiveness of your management system processes, your first prudent step is a functional requirement assessment of what you want the system to do.)

Not knowing the functionality you desire from a software solution can have you running in circles. Worse still, functionality will become very subjective, and you'll simply be responding to the sales tactics and spin of software salesmen whose job, rightfully, is to sell software. Whether what they are selling is right for your management system should not be left up to a software salesman. If the company is as forward-thinking and progressive as it needs to be in today's software market, most of the functionality you desire will be available, with the ability to customize in-house.

While it is very rare to get 100 percent user-defined functionality in a commercial off-the-shelf (COTS) software solution, if the solution has been designed by those who know the management system business, you should at least get a software solution that will enable you to adapt it to your current business realities. The reference made to these select management system software vendors in no way constitutes an endorsement by the authors of these software vendors. There may be other management system technologies available on the market as well. As with any purchase of software, always do your homework.

A simple query in Google will provide you with plenty of options for consideration.

HSEQ SOFTWARE—MODULES AND PROCESSES

Capterra describes itself as the leading online resource for business software buyers. Founded in 1999, Capterra features validated user reviews and independent research across hundreds of software categories. Capterra is a free service that helps organizations find the best software for their needs. Capterra is free for users because vendors pay them when they receive web traffic. Capterra lists all vendors—not just those that pay us—in our comprehensive directories so that you can make the best-informed purchase decision possible.

Another good source is the National Association for Environmental Management (NAEM) report, which provides some practical information and insights that can be used in your HSEQ software selection process. The report indicates it can be used to:

- Identify signs it's time to replace your current Environment, Health, Safety, and Security (EHS&S) system
- Key criteria to look for when shopping for a new system (in addition, you need to be very clear on your functional requirements—in other words, what you want the software to do for you).
- How to structure your selection process and prioritize your requirements
- Best practices to gain leadership support and ensure user engagement
- Lessons learned on how to buy EHS&S software right the first time

DEFINING YOUR FUNCTIONAL NEEDS FOR HSEQ SOFTWARE

With so many different HSEQ audit software products and applications on the market today, it's becoming more and more challenging for the average HSEQ auditor to know where to begin in their evaluation and selection of an HSEQ audit technology solution. That said, it's often the best course of action to start at the beginning. The beginning is the answer to this question: What do you want your software to be able to do? It's easy to be swayed by a software salesperson who is spinning out the latest and greatest they believe only their software solution can offer.

Remember the last time you went to buy a computer and were bombarded by the technical jargon of a twenty-something salesperson who seemed to be speaking some foreign language you can't understand? No? Then perhaps it's just me. But what I suggest anyone do first when looking at an HSEQ audit technology solution is to be clear on what you want the technology to be able to do for you. You first need to define your "functional requirements."

Simply put, the audit technology needs to be able to . . . ????—well, you fill in the blanks and question marks based on your defined needs. In an HSEQ audit software evaluation, with the guidance of an audit software evaluation team, you first come up with a functional requirement document which is issued to all potential vendors and asked them to indicate whether their software product matches your defined needs, and how it meets those needs. Then, after shortlisting a number of vendors who pass the first test of addressing your defined functional requirements, you should then use that document in the demo evaluation period of the software to validate that the software is indeed able to mirror what you desire the solution to do for you. This process will be as unique as the organization and software vendors who are being considered; however, here is an example of the type of functional needs assessment which can be used as a guide in the identification and selection of an HSEQ audit software vendor.

HSEQ AUDIT SOFTWARE FUNCTIONAL NEEDS ANALYSIS

ABC Company is seeking to identify an HSEQ audit management system software solution, which has the following modules:

1. HSE compliance module (regulatory management)
2. Internal Audit and Inspection module
3. Action Management module (HSE and Quality)

1. HSE Compliance Module Essential Features

- Ability to manage compliance-based directives/stop-work orders.
- All compliance data is viewed in dashboards with compliance performance status.
- Ability to manage compliance-based checklists for use in inspections/audits, and so on.
- Ensure regulatory compliance is managed as required and accomplished consistently throughout the organization.

2. Internal Audit and Inspection Module Essential Features

- Ability to accommodate an audit schedule and assign auditors.
- Ability to print an entire audit schedule.
- Ability to capture audit reports/link audit report to audit records.
- Ability to link to action module.
- Compare results across the organization with consistent reports, audit checklists, and processes.
- Identify audit or inspection trends that reveal areas for improvement and best practices.
- Ensures regulatory and corporate standards compliance.
- Ensure corrective actions are completed on time and linked with action management module features.

3. Action Management Module Essential Features

- Ability to accept multiple actions associated with a single event.
- Ability to segregate HSE and Quality actions and the ability to roll up into a single corporate report.
- Ability to report on action status by individual/department/company-wide roll-up, including status by date, status of completion (open or closed), and actions that are past their due date.
- HSE to include actions from OH&S Committee meetings, workplace inspections, internal and external HSE audits, incident investigations, safety meetings, or toolbox meeting actions—essentially any HSE-related event.
- Quality includes actions from internal/external audits, CAR and PAR, non-conformances, management review—essentially any Quality event.
- Ability to add ad hoc actions not related to any HSEQ process per se.
- Ability to escalate overdue action emails to others based on lack of completion.
- Individual dashboard/reporting for everyone who has been assigned actions so they can see/track their individual performance.

4. General Considerations

- Ability to be installed in-house on a local wide-area network, or licensed as a cloud-based option.
- Field-level mobility (tablets, smartphone, network disconnected laptop enabled).
- Robust audit and action status reporting modules and data mining are required.
- Username- and password-protected modules and access.
- Options for annual maintenance.
- Training considerations for in-house staff. Note that we're looking for the application to do some very specific things. These things that we feel are important in the application based on our reporting needs, data needs, and analytical needs. The objective is to try and find the best product that best matches our needs.

This can be a challenge. Finding a commercial off-the-shelf product that meets 100 percent of your functional requirements can be challenging; however, without ever defining your needs, it will be almost impossible to find a system that's right for you. As the saying goes, "If you don't know where you're going, any road will get you there." If you don't know or define what you want in an HSEQ software solution, any software will do—or not.

And as you can see, this is just a basic example. Many organizations will have quite detailed technical requirements which, in many cases, their IT departments will help lead and structure. The bottom line—define what you want your audit technology to do. If you don't, who will?

A REAL WORLD HSEQ SOFTWARE STORY

The world of HSEQ audit software has exploded with a wide range of products and vendors, with the current trend being cloud-based solutions with field mobility applications for smartphones and tablets.

To give you a sense of how and why HSEQ audit software products get developed, here's a little bit of an old-school history lesson about Wayne Pardy's move from a full-time safety professional to the vice president of sales and marketing with an HSEQ software company he cofounded with two other coworkers back in late 1997. Back then, they had an idea for a software product which, when they were employees of Newfoundland Power, they could not seem to be able to find on the market.

In retrospect, it seems amazing that there was nothing on the market similar to what they were looking for, but they couldn't find good safety audit/inspection and action tracking software anywhere. Keep in mind as well that the world of search engines and product development was not as mature as it is in 2024.

Long story short, after finding nothing and feeling that perhaps others would need and pay for a similar solution, they quit their secure, full-time jobs and founded a software company, Creative Business Solutions Inc. (later to become known as Q5 Systems). Longer story short, they spent two years in product conceptualization, design, and development before they had a product. Full of zeal and excitement about what they thought they would develop, to what they eventually did develop, they can honestly say that over that two-year period, from thinking about a product on a napkin in a Tim Horton's coffee shop to their first product sale, was like night and day. When they first developed their Q5 system, there was no such thing as smartphone or tablet apps. In fact, software was still used on a desktop or laptop computer in an office for the most part. And cell phones were available, but smartphones were still years away.

When they were finally ready to commercialize their software, they started to market it as an inspection and audit tool. Conventional sales approaches were used, and they took out magazine ads, went to several trade shows, sent lots and lots of emails, but sales were very slow. How come? Was the price point right? Was the competition better? Was their product any better? And then, as often happens in the technology world, the landscape changed overnight with the introduction of the field mobile device, the PalmPilot.

Here's a history lesson for all you smartphone kiddies. The PalmPilot PDA (personal digital assistant) devices were produced by Palm Inc. (then a subsidiary of U.S. Robotics) and launched on March 10, 1997. Palm devices are often remembered as "the first wildly popular handheld computers." So, what difference did PalmPilot make to their software? They decided to configure their software for the PalmPilot and suddenly, the software became popular, due in part to the ability of a user to conduct an audit or inspection out in the field without paper.

And did the software sell after that? Not really, but there was one small marketing innovation they settled on. What they did was increase the price of the software by the same amount as the price of a PalmPilot, and then offer the software with a "free" PalmPilot. The product flew off the shelf (or at least their digital download site). So now they were off to the races. And when they sold a $40k system to U.S. Steel in Gary, Indiana, all over the phone and using a web-based meeting tool, they knew management system software was going to be an integral part of management systems going forward.

As Wayne's tenure with Q5 was a pivotal point in his auditing career and professional audit management development, he would be remiss if he didn't at least give a shout-out to the guys at Q5 for where they have taken the product in support of the internal HSEQ audit community. In fact, here is a recent review of the Q5 product, SMS. The examples in this profile are something you can also use and reference in the development of your own functional requirements for an HSEQ software product. If there's a product you're considering, do a web search for reviews on the product by real-world users. Alternatively, you can put your audit software requirements into an AI tool and see what you get. Great job, Q5 guys . . . good to see that you're still a highly rated and respected audit management product. Hope my early work with the original product development helped in bringing the Q5 audit technology to where it is today.

Comparing Two Integrated Quality and Safety Management Systems: QMS versus SMS

Do You Have Too Many Software Systems?

Many mid-sized to large aviation service providers have two software systems where one solution would suffice. These systems are:

- Safety management system (SMS); and
- *Quality management system (QMS).*

The logical leap would be to improve efficiencies and determine whether these systems can be merged. Another logical leap would be to use these existing systems to track other things, such as:

- Environmental issues
- Security
- HSE, OHSA, and so on

Is this the smartest choice? Maybe not. There are some considerations that we'll review.

The safety department uses the SMS data-management tools for

- hazard reporting;
- risk management;
- *managing safety policies and procedures;*
- *safety promotion activities;*
- *safety performance monitoring; and*
- *safety assurance.*

The quality department uses its QMS system for conducting audits, such as,

- internal audits;
- *tracking customer complaints and service issues; and*
- *supplier/vendor audits.*

In this article, we discuss the benefits of having one integrated quality and safety management system. We will also compare two QMS programs and offer feedback based on secondhand user accounts. These reports often come from frustrated users; however, we also share some good news.

About Q5 and Quality Management Systems

Before the ICAO SMS mandate in November 2006, IATA started the IOSA program to ensure participating airlines were audited in a consistent and standardized manner. This is a good program, yet there are some concerns about corruption and inconsistent application of standards across the globe.

Many IOSA and ISAGO auditing questions are based on evaluating an operator's SMS. These questions may initiate action on the part of management that would otherwise not be taken without such an oversight program. Management is participating in IATA with an expectation of financial benefits. Consequently, management will be more motivated to pass an IATA audit than a regulatory SMS audit. Do you disagree?

When an operator is not in jeopardy of losing their operating certificate, the lure of additional financial benefits will always be stronger than some lofty goal of "continuous improvement of the SMS." Sure, there may be an SMS requirement, but if I'm passing my SMS regulatory audits, why spend more money on making my SMS better? On the other hand, an IATA audit may make it easier and faster for the operator to conduct business in foreign countries without jumping through the foreign country's safety requirements.

In short, having an IATA certification smoothens the way for operating in different markets. This is a powerful motivator to improve SMS, or at least demonstrate that your company can pass an IATA audit.

IATA audits are made up of many checklists. Each checklist has many questions that should be objectively evaluated. If you have never seen an IOSA (or ISAGO) checklist, don't feel as if you are missing anything special, especially if you are already well-versed in ICAO's Document 9859 (Safety Management Manual).

IOSA and ISAGO checklists are not much fun to read. If an auditor or quality manager had to manage them manually without automated tools, they would go crazy, especially if they were doing this on a recurring basis.

IOSA audit management is where Q5 and other quality management solutions shine. For approximately $750 per month, five users can use the auditing tools to conduct audits and manage corrective actions arising from the IOSA audits.

Some Quality Software Programs Have Evolved

When I mention the "Q" auditing program, the star "*" refers to all QMS programs on the market. "*" is a wildcard character denoting "all." The most popular aviation auditing solutions on the market are Q5 and Q-Pulse.*

Q5 claims to also have SMS capabilities. Based on end-user accounts, don't expect much functionality or a complete safety system to manage your safety program. If your auditing team is considering a solution to manage quality audits and you also want to include your safety program, then we don't recommend Q5. Users are complaining of too much copying and pasting from one part of the program into another part of their system.

As I stated, Q5 claims to have integrated SMS functionality called Q5 SMS. They may have been premature in coming to market without managing expectations. The biggest complaint about Q5 that I've heard is that an airline with several hundred employees has no way to involve all employees in the safety process. Many time-consuming safety functions need to be duplicated, such as taking paper-based hazard reports and copying them into their risk-management system.

Unless Q5 evolves rapidly within the next few years, many more disenchanted users will move away to more complete integrated quality and safety management systems. If you are looking only for an auditing solution to track IATA audits, then this may be worth considering, yet $750 per month seems a bit steep just for auditing. There are other less-expensive auditing solutions with IATA checklists, such as the SMS Pro auditing system.

Better Integrated Quality and Safety Management Software

Q-Pulse started out as an auditing program and evolved nicely into an integrated quality and safety program. From the latest reports by safety and quality managers, Q-Pulse has very much the same functionality as SMS Pro. Conversely, SMS Pro started as an SMS and risk-management program and included audit capabilities in year two (circa 2009).

If you are considering an integrated safety and quality management system, you will not go wrong with Q-Pulse. Q-Pulse is considered to be a good auditing system. Q-Pulse workflows are unique to SMS Pro, but they both get the job done.

The best integrated QSMS solutions have offline auditing capabilities. Offline auditing allows quality managers to use iPads, iPhones, laptops, or Android devices to perform audits without Internet connectivity.

With offline auditing software, audit forms are still created and managed online but can be filled out either in online or offline mode. Q-Pulse claims to have offline auditing capabilities. SMS Pro's offline auditing tools were released in November 2015.

If offline auditing is important, you may wish to ascertain whether the system supports all modern web-enabled devices and not just one particular platform, such as iPad. Some operators needlessly lock themselves into one platform, and when hardware changes, the software is not so forgiving.

Final Thoughts on Integrated Quality and Safety Management Systems

The two top aviation SMS software products are Q-Pulse and SMS Pro. They are both truly integrated quality and safety management programs. Many wannabes have sprung up in hopes of making a quick buck. Many of these wannabes cater to other industries, such as automotive, chemical, and food industries.

For database providers that work across multiple industries, you may not be satisfied with the lack of qualified subject-matter experts on their staff. There are distinct benefits to working with database providers that only focus on one industry, such as SMS Pro. The system is more aligned with aviation industry requirements, and the workflows were developed by aviation safety professionals and not by professionals in the auto or oil and gas industries.

The aviation SMS software market is not about making a quick buck, but about providing great service to aviation service providers. To be effective, your SMS software provider must consider you as their partner and be willing to adapt their solution to suit your unique needs. SMS software providers that work across industries may have very flexible databases, but reports indicate that setup times can exceed three to six months, versus two weeks for industry-specific software, such as SMS Pro.

> *If you are only needing auditing tools, SMS Pro has an Audit Management System for just the quality departments. Otherwise, if you are looking for a complete, all-in-one SMS database that includes these same auditing tools, check out these short videos below:*

Reference https://aviationsafetyblog.asms-pro.com/blog/comparing-two-integrated-quality-and-safety-management-systems

Of course, as a previous cofounder and vice president of Q5 System, Wayne would be less than honest if he expressed nothing but a soft spot for a mobile audit technology that was making waves even as far back as 2001. And for those of you who want to gain an appreciation for the world of HSEQ auditing today, and the technology solutions that can be leveraged to make your auditing processes faster, easier, and more accurate, it's always good to remember those pioneers who have blazed a trail to where many of us in the auditing and auditing technology world find ourselves today. It's with that nod to technology for HSEQ auditing that we share this profile of the Q5 auditing technology, as profiled by the Government of Newfoundland and Labrador in their *Vision* magazine profile of 2006. It's now 2024. In some cases, technology has matured and come a long way. In other ways, some of the early trailblazers who saw the opportunity to leverage technology for HSEQ audit processes still make today's HSEQ technology solutions relevant, viable, and practical. In fact, as we look to the HSEQ technology audit world, some of the baseline technology applications that Q5 established in 2006 are still in use today. No small feat for a small technology company, with a vision for best-in-class HSEQ audit software from St. John's, Newfoundland.

INFORMATION TECHNOLOGY

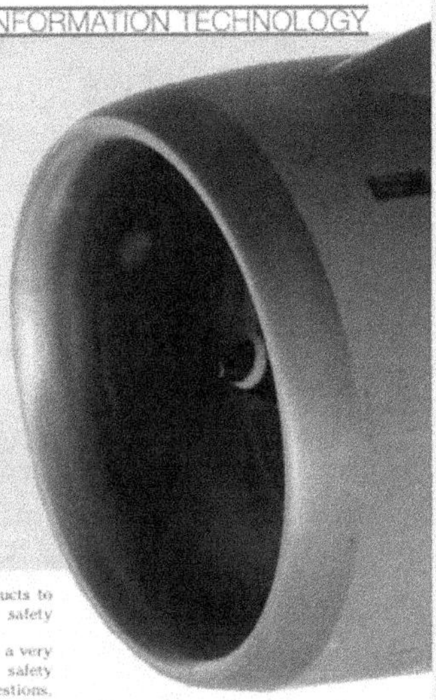

Q5 Systems Takes Flight in Airline Industry

If you don't know exactly where to find Q5 Systems in St. John's, you're likely to pass it by. There's no splashy sign out front and nothing prominent to hint of its status as an internationally-recognized developer of occupational health, safety, and security management solutions for some very big clients.

Well-established U.S. companies such as Liberty Mutual, Southwest Airlines and US Steel have implemented the Q5 solution. With a few exceptions, Q5 Systems is focused on export markets beyond Newfoundland and Labrador's backyard.

Q5 sells to companies across a number of industries where health and safety standards are crucial to a company's bottom line. Hence the software is applicable to virtually everyone. Construction, mining, insurance, air travel, food services, universities, even national parks are all customers. They use Q5's products to ensure compliance with safety standards and regulations.

Think of the Q5's software as a very sophisticated version of a safety checklist, one that asks questions, sends reminders, and prompts staff to get things done.

The company's technology solutions have a broad range of applications, but Q5 has spent the past year making a name for itself in the airline industry. In fact, 2005 was the year Q5 really took off - literally!

Q5 sells to companies across a number of industries where health and safety standards are crucial to a company's bottom line. Hence the software is applicable to virtually everyone. Construction, mining, insurance, air travel, food services, universities, even national parks are all customers.

The company signed an agreement with the International Air Transport Association (IATA) to implement a system for conducting operational safety audits of all of its 256 member airlines around the world.

The IATA's membership list is substantial and includes the biggest airlines you can think of, including Lufthansa, Air France, Air Canada, United Airlines, Australia's Quantas Air and many more.

"The contract is a milestone in our history," says John Lukins, one of three company founders who started Q5 in 1997. "If an international organization, like IATA, has adopted your software, and say it's the one they want to use, it really gives us huge credibility in the airline industry."

Over the next two years the software will be used to conduct operational safety audits on IATA's 265 airlines around the world.

"We pulled out all the stops to get the IATA contract because we knew if we could sell to IATA, it would be a breakthrough. Now we've got our foot in the door of almost every airline worldwide - actually we've got most of one leg in the door!" jokes Lukins.

"When someone like Air Canada or Air France comes along and asks what kind of software you use, the fact that we have the contract with IATA gives them some comfort that we might be the right solution for them as well."

www.gov.nl.ca

VISION Newfoundland and Labrador 25

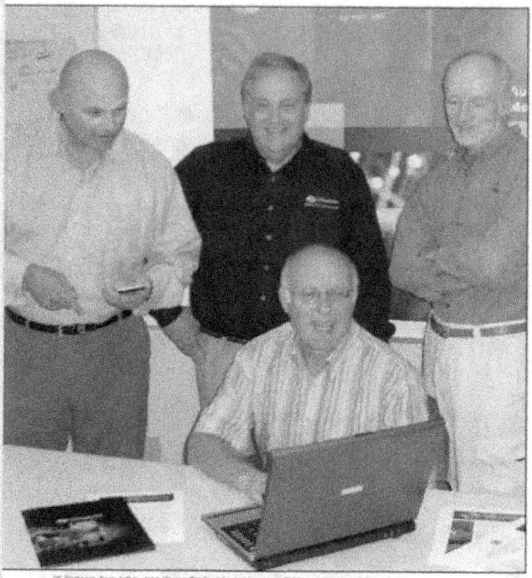

Q5 Partners, from left to right, Wayne Pardy, John Lukins, Larry Feltham (sitting), and Brian Dicks.

The roots of Q5 go back a few years, to the days when the three partners were still at Newfoundland Power: Lukins in IT, Wayne Pardy in safety and Brian Dicks in human resources. They saw potential in creating a safety audit software solution that wasn't available for over-the-counter purchase.

Lukins and the other company founders each had over 20 years seniority with Newfoundland Power, where they could have worked until retirement. Instead of playing it safe, they started Q5 with partner Larry Feltham. Working out of their basements for a couple of years, they built the company to a point where they now have international recognition.

They developed greater business and marketing acumen as clients of the Genesis Centre from 1999-2002. The Genesis Centre is Memorial University of Newfoundland's technology incubation centre and works with young technology-based companies to help them turn their good ideas into sound business ventures.

"It was a hard decision leaving a company you've been with for years, but this was an opportunity I just couldn't pass up, and I've had great fun. There hasn't been a day that I haven't enjoyed coming to work."

"It was a hard decision leaving a company you've been with for years, but this was an opportunity I just couldn't pass up, and I've had great fun. There hasn't been a day that I haven't enjoyed coming to work," says Lukins.

Over the past few years there have been some very good days for Q5.

Another milestone for the company came in 2004 when its management system was accredited by the International Organization for Standardization (known internationally as ISO).

"It's a rigorous process that we go through to ensure that anything that touches the customer has been quality assured, that everything has been tested and checked and there are no mistakes," says Lukins.

The ISO stamp of approval is prestigious and tells the world that Q5's products meet the highest standards of quality assurance. The company is the only audit software company globally to receive this designation.

The recognition gives Q5 certain bragging rights when it looks for potential customers. The ISO designation and the IATA contract all add up and it's as good as money in the bank.

And there's something else noteworthy on Q5's resume – the company's role in the cleanup of the World Trade Center after September 11, 2001. American insurance giant Liberty Mutual provided most of the insurance coverage during the trade center's cleanup. At the time, Liberty Mutual was Q5's largest client.

Liberty Mutual used Q5's safety audit software to monitor the safety practices of those involved in the cleanup. It was a pretty risky work environment and insurance company officials were on site at all times.

"We were standing by almost daily to make sure everything was working well," Lukins recalls. "Our system was at ground zero, monitoring workers safety and it was good to be involved. We knew it was high profile and we wanted to be successful.

"Even now when we go to visit customers, that's one of the implementations we discuss. It gives us a certain credibility."

As the company's credibility increases, so does its clientele.

"We build very strong relationships with our customers," says Lukins. "They are very happy with the Q5 product and the level of service we provide." •

26 VISION Newfoundland and Labrador www.gov.nl.ca

Government of Newfoundland and Labrador. Vision Business magazine. Fall, 2006. pp. 25–26

E-AUDITING: BEWARE PENCIL WHIPPING (OR DIGITAL SMARTPHONE OR TABLET WHIPPING)

Remember our profile on the cautions of pencil whipping? Well, just because you move to a technology-based approach to audit data capture doesn't mean the potential for "data whipping" automatically goes away. While accurate and timely data and information are necessary for management to make informed decisions, the old saying, "garbage in, garbage out (GIGO)," has as much relevance for paper-based data collection systems as it does for technology-based data collection systems. Don't just assume that because you have a process to capture data, the information is always accurate and valid.

Beware of pencil whipping or the more modern version, mobile technology whipping (completing a form, record, or document without having performed the implied work or without supporting data or evidence). Here are two examples for your reference to ensure that you have enough oversight in place to ensure this does not happen to you.

- **AUDIT PENCIL WHIPPING EXAMPLE #1** During an annual inspection program, we had to look at several substations in an operating area and examine things like key risk and safety barriers and processes needed to protect the public from the asset and to ensure asset integrity. Prior to completing our inspection, we pulled all the previous records that the individual responsible for completing those inspections had completed. In all the inspection records, there were no deficiencies noted. Everything was 100 percent perfect; however, when we did the very same inspection using the exact same form and checklist criteria, we found that about 25 percent of the items were, in fact, not in conformance with requirements and could not have degenerated so quickly from the last inspection. Long story short, the individual in question did not actually conduct an inspection "in situ" and instead completed it while sitting in his pick-up truck because, as was the perception, the paperwork had to be turned in. The emphasis was on the paperwork and getting it submitted in time—not the risk-based nature of the inspection focus or the consequences of not being disciplined in its completion. So, while it was important to actually do the inspection, the real point was to do it with accuracy and integrity to ensure that the asset was safe and that risks were identified and remediated.
- **AUDIT PENCIL WHIPPING EXAMPLE #2** Many organizations have some variation of behavior-based safety audits in use for their safety system. Simply stated, behavior-based safety is a data-rich process that continually focuses on workplace safety behavior, with the aim of reinforcing "safe" or acceptable behaviors and taking actions to correct at-risk behaviors which could eventually lead to accidents or injuries. On a large construction project, there was an HSE adviser who continually scored 100 percent on every safe work observation he conducted. In looking at the analysis of the behavioral observation data, we actually looked at the raw record of the observations.

One hundred percent compliance on each and every observation was, in the opinion of the authors, a red flag. No one is 100 percent perfect 100 percent of the time. Yet, over a period of several months, the aggregate behavioral audit score was consistently high, in large part because of the 100 percent compliance score of each and every behavioral observation audit this individual made. We decided to conduct a team-based audit with this individual, and when the exact same observation process was done with the team, audit scores dropped to around the 70 percent level. Again, long story short, investigation of the situation determined that the individual did not complete the observation audit in the field. He simply used the observation requirement as an opportunity to chat with the work crews (which, in and of itself, is not a bad idea); however, he never documented or discussed his field-based audit observations with the crews in question but completed the data observation card when he was back in the office.

What's the lesson here? Don't assume that when some slick software marketing tells you that their data-management system can solve all your problems and provide you with better and more accurate data, this claim will be automatic. Any software or data-management system will need to be implemented with diligence and discipline. And people will invariably still be involved in this activity. Auditing and surveillance of the way the software is being implemented and used will also need to be an important part of your implementation. Don't just assume that because you have a software solution with smartphone or tablet capabilities, the lack of paperwork and written records will automatically solve all your data-management problems. People can "whip" any type of audit data-management process—paper checklists or smartphone applications.

What is important is the integrity of the data and the discipline by which it is captured and entered in your audit management system software. A word of caution: Don't just accept that the next or best generation of audit software will raise your management system to the next level. Without discipline and oversight, the potential for the "garbage in—garbage out" scenario could exist for you as well.

One of the biggest challenges for any audit program is to ensure effective management, control, and distribution of the information and data generated by the audit. Several critically sensitive documents are generated as a result of each audit. These include (1) draft and final audit reports prepared by the audit team, which document the deficiencies or findings at the site or within the audited organization or system; (2) a plan generated by the audited entity, which defines the measures needed to correct the deficiencies; and (3) a report that continuously tracks the status of all proposed corrective actions for all audits. It is generally the responsibility of the corporate (or headquarters) HSEQ audit program manager to monitor and analyze the data and information generated by these audit reports and plans.

An HSEQ audit program manager must provide documented assurances to the corporation that the sites' corrective actions are being completed on time and are consistent with the findings of the audit teams. It has been stated many times by attorneys and regulators that one is better off not implementing an audit program if the organization cannot (or will not, for some reason) ensure that identified deficiencies are corrected in a timely fashion. In sum, organizations need to reach verifiable closure on all audit findings, especially high-risk audit findings.

A second critical documentation issue for the HSEQ audit program manager is determining whether audit reports and documents can be protected from discovery in a legal proceeding and, if not, deciding what should be done to minimize liabilities to the corporation posed by a potential release of these sensitive documents. This demands that audit program managers treat the management, retention, and destruction of records very seriously. Historically, this has been an arduous task since most programs have principally used paper-filing systems. In the past few years, automation has made some breakthroughs, particularly in the area of tracking audit reports and the status of corrective action plans (CAPs).

TRADITIONAL RESPONSES TO HSEQ AUDIT DOCUMENT MANAGEMENT

The HSEQ audit report documentation process can be quite complex and involved in many organizations. Typically, as a first step, the audit team develops a draft list of findings and a draft of an audit report. These receive extensive reviews by site HSEQ staff, line management, corporate HSEQ staff, and, in some cases, corporate legal staff. In some organizations, these reviews are conducted simultaneously, which accelerates the process, but at the risk of the audit team receiving conflicting comments.

In other organizations, corporate HSEQ affairs and legal staff must receive copies of the draft reports first (even draft findings sometimes), and comments must be incorporated before the site or line management receives their copies. This helps to protect the auditors and the organization, but the process often bogs down substantially, with the site potentially not receiving draft reports for several months. This is a stronger reality for more litigious jurisdictions than others, which might be a little more liberal.

In an organization with multiple sites, or multiple national and international sites, one can imagine how quickly the document management process can get out of control. At any given time, various document types for each site, in various stages of completion, are winding their way through the organization. As an example, take an organization with twenty sites, each on a two-year audit cycle. After six years, the organization will have developed 60 draft audit reports, 60 final audit reports, 60 draft CAPs, 60 final CAPs, as many as 480 quarterly status reports, and numerous other program documents. Is it any wonder that most HSEQ programs have challenges in meeting their established scheduling standards for report and CAP completion?

As a result of these challenges, many organizations have increased their reliance on IT solutions, including portable computers, such as tablets and laptops, in the field. Field use of computers now allows audit teams to develop the skeleton of a report prior to visiting a site. This can accelerate the report-generation process.

Organizations have also instituted automated audit-tracking systems. These systems rely on commercially available databases and HSEQ management systems. Using these systems, HSEQ audit program managers can monitor the progress of draft and final audit reports and periodically (usually quarterly) review the status of all outstanding corrective actions. Audit reports, where all corrective actions are completed, will be formally closed out, and the program manager will "red flag" those planned actions that are behind schedule. Leading-edge technologies have made this job much easier in many respects, but that technology is also not inexpensive and, in many instances, needs time and resources to custom program to meet organization-specific requirements or individual idiosyncrasies.

For periodic tracking to be effective, the audited entities must submit or self-enter a status report of some kind, which is usually entered into the database and then updated. In addition, the data are also reviewed to determine the progress the site has made toward completing the corrective actions by the original target date. In fact, timely completion of corrective actions is probably the most critical performance factor for the site that was audited, even more so than other factors, such as the number of deficiencies observed by the audit team. The reason is workload management and continued visibility and relevance of the actions in question.

Unfortunately, some audit systems in use are cumbersome and not easily maintained and updated. For example, audit reports are completed using a word-processing program, tracking data are maintained in another relational database, and performance charts are developed using a charting program like PowerPoint. Although many of these programs can be used relatively seamlessly, the links are often manual. That is, a clerk reenters the data from the audit report into a database and subsequently enters key elements from the database into the charting program. Not surprisingly, without a true champion, the databases, quarterly reporting, and tracking often fall by the wayside. That is why a "one shop stop" technology solution can incorporate all these technological challenges. But again, these technologies are not inexpensive. And finding the system which best meets all your defined functional requirements can be challenging.

THE ADVANTAGES OF INTEGRATED DATA-MANAGEMENT SYSTEMS

Integrated data-management systems can make the audit-tracking process much more manageable and effective. An integrated system allows groups of users to work together by sharing information across a local or global network. The information can include files created in the system or from other software packages, comments attached to those files, and a variety of other file formats and types of information.

Conceptually, integrated systems can be a very powerful tool for managing an audit program. If taken to its full potential, an auditing system could allow for a paperless audit documentation system, similar to the Q5 audit system we profiled earlier. Let us explore some of the possibilities.

Under the integrated-system scenario, findings from audits can be loaded directly onto the system network during the audit, allowing for real-time review of the audit reports by the site and other interested parties. This would allow designated reviewers to review a draft audit report the evening before the closing conference and to incorporate any proposed changes into the report prior to the meeting. The same could be done by the corporate HSEQ audit program manager. Then all comments could be incorporated, and the file replicated so that all recipients have the same version. In fact, where all relevant parties have access to the report findings, there may be no need for a written report, although a printed set of findings might be useful for the closing conference at the site.

Further, the CAP can be quite easily loaded onto the groupware system and keyed to the audit findings and report. Screens can be designed using user-defined fields so that for each audit, individual findings with their proposed corrective actions can be shown together. Real-time adjustments can be made here as well.

One of the more powerful ways to use integrated systems is in the continuous updating of CAPs. There would no longer be a need for formal, quarterly status reports. Updating can be done at the site level since actions are completed through direct input into the network as opposed to transmitting status reports by paper or email and then manually entering them into a database.

It might be prudent to exercise certain controls or security measures over the corrective-action updating process, because the corporation may not want to allow uncontrolled modification of the CAPs. That is, only certain individuals should be given authority to update the plans. Establishing read-only files for most users of the audit reports and CAPs would be an appropriate security measure. This is quite easy to accomplish with most systems.

Finally, this approach allows the audit program manager to easily develop and update the periodic tracking reports and distribute the reports directly and electronically to the interested parties. The audit program manager should decide in advance which characteristics are appropriate to analyze and display for his or her organization. Some companies will statistically analyze each plant's performance. Others will assess only a division's performance. Still others will "roll up" the data to show only overall corporate performance. These strategic views can help the audit program manager better understand the relative strengths and weaknesses of the organization's HSEQ program.

A practical example is from the software which one of the authors, Wayne Pardy, had an opportunity to help design and program. In the example in question, the software, Q5, was designed in order to be able to pre-program/pre-populate an audit report based on the following criteria:

1. Each audit question could include a range of "scoring" based on the response options available. Based on the answer selected from the audit, the system automatically scored the question based on the findings and evidence.
2. Each audit question could then couple be pre-programmed/pre-populated with a generic audit finding. For example, for any answer not in the affirmative, the system would be asked to pre-populate the narrative section of the report with the commentary, "The audit was unable to verify any objective evidence in support of confirming that the requirements of XXXXX was in place and functioning as required." This narrative was then "mapped" to the audit report if a "No" answer was selected for the audit requirement being asked.
3. Based on #2, the audit then generated a pre-populated/determined corrective action, such that if the exact same evidence was identified in five completely different audits, in five different locations, and all based on the exact same audit criteria, the audit action was consistent across all five audits.

EVALUATING AUDITING SOFTWARE SYSTEMS

Choosing an audit system from the numerous commercially available environmental auditing software systems is not easy. Some systems can be purchased outright for less than $1,000. Others, if purchased or licensed and used company-wide, might cost as much as $100,000 or significantly more for a corporate license. Yet, these more expensive systems are more flexible and usable throughout the corporation. That said, they typically require more administrative time to program, customize, and maintain.

To select from among the options offered, in general, potential purchasers should first develop program specifications and requirements and then evaluate the offerings against these specifications. For example, a buyer might want an audit program management system to meet some or all of the following requirements. That is, in a perfect world, the system should be able to

- operate on the company's hardware configuration and be accessed by laptop computers with remote communication capability;
- allow for widespread access to HSEQ regulatory databases, if available ("talk" to other applications);
- load and sort company-designed or commercial federal, provincial, and state compliance checklists;
- allow the easy updating of the checklists;
- load (at times remotely from the field) and search audit reports;
- produce tabular audit-findings reports;
- produce periodic reports of incomplete action items across all facilities;
- code and retrieve findings by class (e.g., air emissions, confined space, customer complaints), location, year, organization, and severity (e.g., low, medium, and high risk);
- calculate simple statistics (e.g., number of significant compliance issues in various locations) across all audits;
- produce graphics-oriented management reports using data across all audits; and
- provide selective data security.

Once the above design specifications are further refined, staff need to evaluate any offering against the following criteria:

- Is the program truly preexisting, or will the buyer be paying for its design or major modifications?
- Can the system readily meet the design specifications?
- Is the system flexible?
- Is it user-friendly? Is there mobility and/or a smartphone option?
- What types of reports can be generated?
- Are search capabilities broad enough?
- Is the documentation complete and clear?
- Can the system handle text (e.g., checklists) as well as numeric data?
- Will it have on-screen help?
- Can data be transferred among modules?
- Are presentation graphics available?
- Is updating or upgrading the program design easy or a major undertaking?

Possibly, an otherwise attractive system may not fulfill all these requirements in its current form. However, the question really is: Can the system be modified readily to take into account the needs of the company? If so, many of these software packages can add significantly to the auditor's tool set.

Note: The mention of any commercial product in this chapter is not an endorsement of that product.

REFERENCES

This chapter has been adapted from Lawrence B. Cahill and Raymond W. Kane. *Environmental Health and Safety Audits*, 9th Edition. Government Institutes, 2010. It has been updated for this edition.

Wayne Pardy and Terri Andrews. *Integrated Management Systems: Leading Strategies and Solutions*, 2nd Edition. Bernan Press, 2019.

https://aviationsafetyblog.asms-pro.com/blog/comparing-two-integrated-quality-and-safety-management-systems.

Government of Newfoundland and Labrador. *Vision Business magazine*. Fall, 2006. pp. 25–26.

Chapter 11

Managing and Critiquing an HSEQ Audit Program

Assuring regulatory compliance and operational conformance is a complex challenge for today's industrial manager. Shaping HSEQ audit programs to help meet this challenge is also no less a challenge. Programs must be well-thought-out and receive the understanding and support of senior managers.

This chapter is directed at those managers who will be given the complex task of developing or managing an HSEQ audit program within a large or demanding corporate structure. The chapter first presents an approach for developing a program, consisting of several recommended steps, beginning with a policy-setting and planning exercise and ending with the full implementation of the program. Using this as a starting point, the remainder of the chapter discusses a variety of management techniques that can be used to control, assess, and evaluate an ongoing audit program.

BEGINNING A PROGRAM

As one is immersed in the complex and pliable concept of HSEQ auditing, one can become overwhelmed with the choices that need to be made in setting up a comprehensive yet workable program. It is often useful to consider the opportunity one step at a time. The sections below outline a suggested step-by-step approach that could be used in creating a successful audit program.

1. Develop an HSEQ Audit Policy and Procedure

Successful HSEQ audit programs uniformly receive strong support from senior management. The explicit backing of the program by senior managers creates a supportive attitude throughout all levels of the organization. Thus, quite often the first step in any program is the development and distribution of a policy statement, signed by a senior corporate executive, describing and supporting the initiation of a formal HSEQ auditing program. This policy statement sets the tone of the program.

The policy statement should be supported by a set of program procedures, which is a natural follow-up to the policy. These procedures deal with key planning and structural issues. The statement should be responsive to the criteria selected by the organization, as appropriate. These criteria might include regulatory auditing requirements, industry best practices, ISO, EPA, or COR® auditing guidelines, and/or other internal or external HSEQ auditing mandates, requirements, or suggested opportunities.

The successful HSEQ audit program should also respond to any quality management principles established by the organization. Some that come to mind include the following:

- *Focus on Customers:* Define the customers of the program, both internal and external. They include corporate management, line management, HSEQ management, site staff and other employees. In some cases, clients, shareholders, or other external stakeholders are included as well. Make sure that key documents, such as the facility audit reports and third-party certifications, respond appropriately to those customers.
- *Look for Continual Improvement Opportunities:* The program should be evaluated annually to determine if it has met preestablished objectives. Moreover, a new set of objectives should be established each year, which should correspond to program improvements. It is especially important that line management perceives that the program is adding value each year and not simply becoming "pickier" with each subsequent audit. Meaningless, picky findings can cause credibility problems.
- *Remove Program Barriers to Audit Success:* Although it is difficult to remove the "performance-evaluation" flavor of an HSEQ audit completely, the program should focus on management systems and site procedures and performance. Depersonalizing the program can make it more credible at the site level.
- *Remove Staff Barriers to Audit Success:* The audit program can help facilities understand that HSEQ compliance is not simply the responsibility of HSEQ Managers or their staff. Line management has a clear role in achieving compliance. With line and staff organizations working together, more can be accomplished.
- *Don't Focus on Generalizations or Make Audit Scores the Prime Audit Objective:* Audit programs should be careful about incorporating broad, unachievable objectives, such as "Compliance will be improved." The audit

program is only part of that equation. One should also be careful not to put quotas on the number of audits that must be conducted each year, without some risk categorization of the sites being audited. And while some audits might be rated or scored, don't make this the focus. Yes, some audits are developed with a risk-based question ranking or scoring process. And if you must base your focus on higher risk issues or scores, that's OK. But don't be consumed by the audit "score" At the end of the day, the objective evidence will drive the scores and not the other way around. So, if a high or low "score" is supported by objective evidence, so be it.

- *Don't Focus on Mass Audits:* There is a common tendency for organizations to "count up" the number of findings on each audit and compare one site against another. This should be avoided since each site is different, and they are not generally comparable. One comparison that can be made is how a site performs on audits over time. Are deficiencies being corrected? Is the site performing better over time?
- *Make Sure Your Audit Team is Trained and Competent:* Most companies require that auditors must be formally trained prior to their first audit and that experienced auditors receive refresher training and periodic updates on relevant regulatory issues. This is a good practice and consistent with ISO 19011 and other industry HSEQ Auditor Certification expectations.

2. Set Up the Organization

The second step on the agenda is deciding how to organize the audit program. For larger, multidivision or multinational organizations, there are a variety of options, including

- a corporate audit function with full-time corporate auditors;
- a corporate audit function with full-time auditors supplemented by part-time auditors selected from other operating divisions or countries;
- a small corporate oversight group with the audit function delegated to the operating divisions;
- a small corporate oversight group with self-audits conducted by plant staff; and
- a small corporate oversight group with the use of external independent auditors.

Or any variation of the five points highlighted above, based on the business, organizational, and regulatory realities of the organization in question.

Even in smaller companies, similar organizational issues can arise. Beyond the choices listed above, the types of individuals who should serve as auditors must be selected (e.g., financial vs. engineers vs. legal counsel or other internal resources). It must also be decided how corporate counsel is to be involved in the audit, if at all. Further, should auditors be full-time, in a full-time rotation, or part-time, and who is to have ultimate responsibility and authority for running the program?

Unfortunately, there is no standard organizational solution for the management of an audit program. Each organization must investigate the strengths and weaknesses of the variety of options open to it and select accordingly. That said, the auditors have seldom, if ever, seen a representative of legal counsel on an HSEQ audit team, but they have been involved in audit report reviews. This can become more critical depending on how transparent the organization is with the distribution of its audit reports, sometimes impacted by its corporate and social-responsibility commitments.

3. Develop Tools

The third part of the program-planning process is the early development of the audit tools. Many of the tools and techniques commonly used in industry have been discussed elsewhere in this book. These include

- statement of the HSEQ audit policy;
- pre-visit and audit-evaluation questionnaires;
- site visit and opening/closing conference protocols;
- audit checklists and protocols; and
- formats for audit reports, corrective-action plans, and status reports, including leveraging available technologies.

Each of these tools should be developed in a standard and compatible way to ensure consistency within and among individual audits. If you have a Document Control department, they can assist you with the controlled development and content. Eventually, they can be included in an all-encompassing audit manual or other audit guidance document that will serve as a training device and as the audit working document.

4. Train Staff

The fourth step in the process is auditor training, a certain amount of which will be required early in the program. The extent and nature of the training will vary depending on the backgrounds of the individual auditors (e.g., corporate HSEQ staff versus any other internal staff or people resources). Additionally, the frequency of recurring training will vary depending on the organizational choice selected earlier. That is, the training of full-time auditors is pretty much a one-time effort, while the use of rotating or part-time auditors will require training on a regular basis.

Understandably, auditors must be trained technically to deal with very complex compliance-management requirements. But perhaps more importantly, they must also develop skills in conducting probing interviews with personnel having a wide variety of educational and employment backgrounds. Auditors must walk a fine line between being supportive of the facility, its management and staff in their management of HSEQ, and being assertive in their probing for areas of known or suspected noncompliance or nonconformance. This task requires both diplomacy and firmness.

A final point on training—and this is an area where outside help may be useful: HSEQ audit consultants or trainers can bring a large number of experiences to a training exercise and can provide the expertise for program start-up. These may be otherwise unavailable to the organization, depending on the existing experience or skill sets of those conducting the training.

5. Test the Program

With the organization, tools, and trained auditors in place, the fifth step is to test the program. Testing involves conducting one or more practice audits at select sites. In this light, the audit program manager may want to test the auditors' abilities to conduct an investigation commensurate with the potential liabilities associated with the range of organizational sites. Therefore, they may want to select one large, complex facility and one small, fairly risk-free facility (e.g., warehouse and distribution center) to audit. The intensity and duration of the investigations for these facilities should vary considerably; therefore, testing the audit method at each site would be a useful exercise. Having a facility manager at one of these facilities who is a willing and welcoming participant in having their site "test" audited would be a plus. These folks can also be champions of the HSEQ audit process going forward.

6. Set a Review Schedule

With the program fully tested, the sixth step is to set a schedule for reviewing all of the organization's sites. To provide some rationale for determining how often sites are to be audited, for how long, and by how many auditors, many companies rank sites based on risk-potential criteria, which would be a recommended advantage. For this exercise, use whatever your internal risk-ranking process and matrix is for consistency, or compliance risk. The resulting classifications are then used to determine the frequency and duration of the audit and the audit team's size. This type of exercise can be completed for all facilities to help ensure that audit resources are applied effectively and efficiently. Remember that this schedule might take place over a three- to five-year period, so some of these schedules can be rather detailed and complex.

7. Conduct Audits

With all preparatory tools in place and a schedule set for facility audits, the seventh step is to actually conduct the audit using the tools and timetable developed.

8. Implement the Full Program

The central purpose of an HSEQ audit program is to ensure continued compliance with regulatory requirements as well as operational and standard conformance to the organization and any other HSEQ commitments—say what you do, do what you say, and prove it. And just as important, prove that it's effective. Audits are (should) not one-time effort but must be conducted on a regular basis. And while *regular* can be subjective we again rely on our risk-ranking process for determining audit frequency.

As has been stated, where instances of noncompliance or nonconformance have been identified, these must be corrected within a reasonable length of time so that corporate vulnerability is not exacerbated. Thus, in implementing the full program, most companies have designed a follow-up mechanism to monitor subsequent corrections made to eliminate noncompliance and nonconformance. One approach has been to develop brief "exception reports" or "action-item reports" as a result of each and every audit. These reports are then entered into a database or spreadsheet, together with a program that produces periodic status reports on the completion of the action items. As corrective actions are taken at sites and progressed to closure, these are noted. In addition, semiannual or annual reports are generated that summarize key compliance-management statistics, such as items of noncompliance or nonconformance per facility type, type and cost of corrective measures, lag time between identification of noncompliance or nonconformance, and implementation of corrective action, and so forth. Management reviews are also a source for analysis of this audit data.

Others have provided some guidance on the risk-ranking of action items. A burned-out light bulb may not have the same demand or priority as a missing guard off a grinder. So, while findings are important, just as important are the risks to the organization of continuing to leave the finding open and uncorrected. Depending on the finding, some can place the organization at greater risk than others.

MANAGING A PROGRAM

Too often the value of a management technique, such as an HSEQ audit program, is lost to an organization because of incomplete or poor execution. This can happen even in cases where the program-planning exercise has been extremely successful. The management techniques discussed below can be useful in keeping a program on track. As we've heard one supervisor say to us, "We do best what we plan best."

Assessment Tools

Audit programs often are implemented without any prior consideration of how program success might be measured or determined. This is not good management practice. Truly successful programs will typically incorporate some type of monitoring and evaluation techniques. Most of these use the reduction over time of noncompliance and nonconformance items as a yardstick.

Sometimes compliance or conformance measures are formally incorporated into the performance standards of facilities and individual managers. Since community and customer complaints, violation notices, and fines are in fact measurable events, management can be held accountable. In some observed cases, facility managers have maintained graphs on their office walls depicting historical compliance or audit performance at the facility. These graphs can also depict trends in audit findings. Some find these pictorial displays more effective than narrative or numerical displays. Use whatever you find works best for you and your team.

Incorporating these techniques into the management system and evaluating managers based on successful execution will help to ensure that risks and liabilities are understood and handled appropriately. This practice establishes a clear message that HSEQ management is taken seriously at high levels within the organization.

Management Reports

Top management's role in assuring HSEQ compliance is crucial. Constructive HSEQ policies and procedures must be developed and communicated. Senior management must demonstrate a serious commitment to ensuring compliance with and conformance to all stated or identified requirements.

In addition to being involved in the setting of policies and procedures, senior management should also be apprised of the successes and failures that occur during program operation. In organizations where the reporting of audit results does not go beyond corporate HSEQ or facility managers, these managers have, in some cases, found themselves in a troubling situation. They may lack the institutional leverage needed to convince line managers—often peers—that expenditures for achieving HSEQ compliance should be budgeted on par with normal operating expenditures. "Why" might be a question asked? "We haven't had any real issues which would warrant these new expenditures." Like a lot of things in life, audit reports which are out of sight are often out of mind. And at the end of the day, the outcome of the audit process is not for the benefit of the auditor. It's for management and their management team, as these folks are, at the end of the day, the ones responsible and accountable for the HSEQ performance of their respective facilities.

One way to ensure management awareness and commitment is to design an audit program that formally requires reports be delivered to senior management. Some develop a standard distribution list for this or specify in the audit notification who will be a recipient of the final audit report. Precedence for this can be found in corporate safety programs in which summary safety statistics are routinely reported to levels as high as the Board of Directors. Audit results can (and should) be a part of this process.

A key to making the "reports-to-management" idea work is designing a report that provides useful information efficiently. Most senior executives are not in a position to read all audit reports, and even if they were, they would typically be unable to reach any strategic conclusions without some supporting trend or snapshot analyses. Moreover, many of them are pressed for time and want to quickly get to the point of any issue.

Typically, then, reports to management should be brief tabular and/or graphical presentations (PowerPoint, etc.), transmitting the maximum amount of information with the minimum number of pages. Assuming that these reports will probably be semiannual or annual, they might contain the following information:

- Number of audits completed in the quarter (by organizational unit or by suppliers audited).
- Highlights of risks or potential liabilities most affecting the organization (e.g., new or pending regulations).
- Trends in noncompliance or nonconformance items identified.
- Statistics on success rates in meeting action-item schedules.
- Specific instances in which audit program findings and recommendations have resulted in significant cost savings (e.g., major potential fines avoided or substitution of non-hazardous materials for hazardous materials, etc.).

Presenting this information in a concise, digestible format will aid HSEQ audit program managers in their efforts to establish and maintain corporate credibility for their programs.

HSEQ Audit Staff Management—Keeping Them Engaged

The role of an HSEQ auditor is a difficult one. Even under the auspices of a supportive program, much of what an auditor does involves evaluating the performance of the organization's operational staff. Constantly "dinging" facilities (and their management) in written audit reports can become a fatiguing exercise (although some people, for better or worse, seem born to it). This is often not perceived as a positive process on the part of the auditee. Also, in most situations, extensive travel is required. While this seems glamorous at first, regularly spending weeks on the road—locally, nationally, or internationally—can add to fatigue and can strain an individual's home and social life.

In order to maintain a motivating environment for auditors, the audit program manager should initiate some efforts to counter the downsides of auditing. These efforts could include:

- *Rotating staff:* Most companies rotate audit staff on a regular basis. This helps to keep auditors fresh and enthusiastic and also help to spread HSEQ awareness among a large group of individuals. Burnout is real. Try to structure your process as best you can to avoid it.
- *Establishing career-progression tracks:* Supplementing the need for rotation is the need to convince staff that the HSEQ auditing slot is a logical step in one's career and not a "dead end" or part of a "holding pattern." The goal is to create a sense of HSEQ awareness in the managers of the future.
- *Maintaining the technical edge:* Keeping up with HSEQ trends is an overwhelming task. It seems that every month significant HSEQ regulation is either proposed or promulgated. Audit staff need to do more than read the *regulations applicable to the scope of their audit* (a task to be reserved for strong hearts and sharp eyes) to keep abreast of developments. Participation in activities like regular seminars or workshops will maintain a cutting edge in staff, put auditors in a setting with auditors from other companies, and provide a perquisite that can enhance morale.

It's also very important to look for symptoms of burnout in your auditing staff, especially if you are in charge of a dedicated audit team. By way of a personal example, one of the authors was asked to be the HSEQ audit team lead for a major oil and gas company. A total of twenty-four supplier audits were scheduled and delivered over a relatively short, twelve-month period, due to being way behind on the schedule for the current and previous year. Aside from the differences which each auditee brought to the equation, after twenty-four instances of preparing audit notifications, scheduling and planning logistics, traveling to twenty-four different audit locations, coordinating the efforts of the audit team, and overseeing the audit and development and distribution of twenty-four different audit reports, the burnout factor was high.

After a year of this fast and frantic pace, it was time to look for a change of scenery. That said, the individual who then assumed the role remained in that position for ten-plus years, although the annual audit plan for suppliers was almost cut in half. So, consider "balance" for the annual audit plan. High performance is fine in terms of a targeted number of audits completed, but consider the potential for audit burnout. Too much of a good thing can be a bad thing. At least it was for this auditor!

Of course, managers can use many other traditional techniques to motivate staff (e.g., good salary increases for good performance), and these techniques should indeed be used. Over time, an audit program is only as strong as the quality, integrity, and professionalism of its people, and their ability to perform to a realistic performance level.

Quality Assurance

One of the key challenges with any program is to ensure it meets or exceeds its stated objectives. Exceeding those objectives can be challenging. Meeting those expectations can be more realistic from a planning and execution perspective. But many organizations like to set "stretch targets" for their operations. Assuring a quality program requires regular performance reviews. One way to accomplish this is to have an annual self-evaluation. The evaluation can be completed as part of the year-end planning and scheduling for next year's site visits, which is done by most companies. Thus, the planning exercise should be not only a look forward but a look backward as well.

- What have we accomplished?
- Did we meet our objectives?
- Where did we exceed our plan?
- Was the quality of our efforts as high as anticipated?
- Were the "customers" of our products pleased with the outcome?
- What changes can we make/will we make/did we make to improve our program?

In addition to self-evaluation, audit programs also benefit from occasional third-party evaluations. For a modest expenditure to an outside firm, an organization could conduct an audit of its audit program. This audit could include requesting that the third party observe an actual audit or review audit reports for substance, format, and language, or interviewing auditors and auditees for their feedback and experience.

Lastly, the audit program manager faces a very difficult quality-assurance challenge in order to keep current with changing HSEQ regulations or standards. Most programs use some form of audit checklist drawn from current standards and regulations. If no effort is made to keep these checklists updated, they will quickly be viewed as irrelevant or out of date, jeopardizing the program's viability. As part of the HSEQ audit program, some mechanism for regulatory or standard updating must be chosen and put into practice.

Maintaining Awareness

It is frequently surprising how much selling is a part of a job—any job. You might not like having to sell yourself, but we all need to do it. And we all do it, to different levels of success (or failure). We all must sell ideas, approaches, plans, strategies, and the like to our bosses, our peers, and even our staff. Strong-arming goes only so far. Running a successful audit program is no different. Senior management and line managers must be convinced of its value. And perhaps most importantly, facility managers, through the audit program, must understand the HSEQ consequences of their actions. They are where "the rubber meets the road." Techniques companies have used to make this happen include posting important notices and procedures in the workspaces of unit operators.

Too often emergency-response procedures, spill procedures, and HSEQ targets are found as blueprints on the shelves or bulletin boards in facilities but not in the operating environment where they would be the most useful. Also, regular training and orientation of both new and seasoned employees is an important awareness technique for management. This should include not simply classroom exercises but practice drills for spills and upsets. Finally, publicizing good HSEQ practices in the way strong safety performance has traditionally been rewarded in some organizations can help improve the visibility and credibility of the HSEQ audit program.

CONCLUSION

This chapter has been designed to assist company managers and staff in developing and running audit programs to monitor compliance and management system conformance at their facility sites—be it one site or fifty. It is our hope that the concepts and approaches presented herein will guide the development of efficient and effective programs that will minimize both the liability exposure of corporate managers and the exposure of the public at large.

REFERENCES

The points of a successful HSEQ audit program and related quality management principles have been taken and modified from Mary Walton, *The Deming Management Method,* Putnam Publishing Group, 1986.

This chapter has been adapted from Lawrence B. Cahill and Raymond W. Kane. *Environmental Health and Safety Audits*, 9th Edition. Government Institutes, 2010. It has been updated for this edition.

Wayne Pardy and Terri Andrews. *Integrated Management Systems: Leading Strategies and Solutions*, 2nd Edition. Bernan Press, 2019.

Chapter 12

Conducting an HSEQ Audit

INTRODUCTION

The core of any audit program lies in the actual completion of individual facility audits. Like the phrase "location, location, location" is key to real estate, "execution, execution, execution" is key to HSEQ auditing. Audits must be conducted efficiently, consistently, and comprehensively by competent auditors who must elicit the cooperation of plant managers and staff. This can be a tall order for uniquely complex facilities whose basic day-to-day operations fully tax on-site staff resources.

But a key word of advice before you start: Many criticisms of HSEQ audits in general is that they have no relationship to other key performance indicators of a facility—in other words, there's no "cause and effect" relationship between the outcome of an audit or the improvement of a facility's customer service, incident or injury experience, or environmental performance. So just remember to keep in mind that when you're developing your audit, you need to be very, very clear on what those objectives are and what you hope the audit program will bring to your overall HSEQ management system.

Consider this perspective from famed safety author Dan Petersen when we spoke about the issue of audits and regulatory compliance:

> ***Audits predict results in safety.*** *Petersen once backed the use of audits, but he said correlational studies between audit results and injury records in large companies show very little predictive value. That is because audits "tend to measure regulatory compliance as much as they do the effectiveness of the safety program."*
>
> *For example, said Petersen, most audits start with paperwork. "Paperwork doesn't necessarily dictate what the actions have been. There's a little slippage there," he noted. "Also, the more paperwork you require people to do, the less*

they're out there talking with their people and working on improving their behavior." Nor do the parts of audits that focus on physical conditions prove very helpful, he added, except to ensure regulatory compliance.

Can audits be a good measure of safety effectiveness? Yes, says Petersen, if the audit interviews employees about their perceptions of the safety program. This leads back, he said, to asking employees not only "what is wrong, but how to fix it. That gets back to involvement."

Regulatory compliance ensures safety results. *Being in compliance with OSHA and ensuring you have a safe workplace, Petersen stresses, are "totally different things." Compliance with OSHA, he said, "demonstrates to the hourly workers that their safety is important to management, but it certainly doesn't ensure" that a company will have a safe workplace.*

Petersen said injury statistics bear him out. Over the last twenty-five years since OSHA was founded, he said, the physical layouts of factories and other workplaces are "safer than we've ever had before." Fatalities have been reduced. But there is no "significant change" in either minor or lost-time injuries, and lost days are "50 percent worse than they were 25 years ago."

He said Heinrich's maxim that the vast majority of accidents are caused by unsafe acts provides a clue to the problem with OSHA. "If we concentrate on the 10 percent [of accidents that are due to] unsafe conditions and we have a law that fixes the 10 percent, how much improvement do you think we can get?"

Little wonder, then, that Petersen opposes the movement toward standardizing safety programs embodied in California's SB 198 and OSHA's guidelines for safety management, now being examined as a possible standard. Petersen said he finds it "difficult, if not upsetting" to find the country going in that direction "when the research clearly says, 'That isn't it.'"

Asked whether we need OSHA, Petersen said the issue is debatable. "I think OSHA has been, and probably is, good in making the worst companies better. I don't think it's been good in making the good companies better."

So, with that in mind, let's go forward. And keep in mind that equipment and facilities don't have an opinion, they don't talk back, and they don't agree or disagree with you.

Accordingly, this and the following chapter discuss the detailed steps and procedures typically undertaken in the course of an HSEQ audit. It should be noted, however, that every facility is different, and this chapter can only address those elements of an audit common to most facilities and programs. That is, some of the material presented here may not be applicable to certain programs; conversely, some HSEQ compliance issues of concern to a reader's operations may not be included here.

The next chapter will provide insights and perspectives into the conduct of an HSEQ audit from the "typical" facility viewpoint. The following key questions will be addressed:

- How should I prepare for the audit?
- What records and documentation should I review?
- What part of the facility should I inspect, and what compliance issues are key?
- Whom should I interview, and how should I do it?
- How do I communicate my findings to the site?
- What should be done after the audit is completed?

There are three major phases to an HSEQ audit: (1) preaudit activities, (2) on-site activities, and (3) post-audit activities. Because of the distinct procedural differences in each of these phases, the remainder of this chapter addresses each separately.

PREAUDIT ACTIVITIES

Several key activities should be completed before an audit team arrives on-site:

- Team selection and formation
- Completion and review of the preaudit questionnaire
- Review of relevant regulations and other facility HSEQ requirement and commitments
- Audit-scope definition and establishment of team responsibilities
- Review of audit protocols
- Development of a detailed agenda

Taken together these tasks are often compiled in what is commonly referred to as the "audit plan." This stage of the process should not be underestimated. Many an audit has failed due to inadequate preparation—especially where an organization has relied on part-time auditors from other divisions or facilities. These are typically very busy people who quite often begin preparation for the audit when they climb aboard the plane. This is too late and often results in peculiar behaviors such as "herding," where the team members follow the team leader around all day because they have not been assigned individual tasks or protocols (very inefficient). Take the time to prepare. Not only is it professionally essential but it will yield substantial rewards. A detailed discussion of the preaudit activities is presented below.

Team Selection and Formation

The HSEQ audit program manager selects the audit team leader, and together they typically select the remainder of the team members. Team members should have complementary and overlapping skills, if at all possible. Auditors should be prepared for any circumstance in the field. Auditors can become ill, especially overseas, or otherwise indisposed. Individual or family emergencies sometimes come up. One is sometimes asked to pitch in and cover areas that a member of the team is not addressing. Thought should also be given to teaming up relatively inexperienced auditors with suitable mentors; not every audit should get the "A" team, or the experienced auditor pool will never expand.

It is helpful to have one or more auditors on the team from the same state or province as, but independent of, the site. This aids in conducting an independent review of any applicable state or provincial regulatory applicability.

SAMPLE PREAUDIT CHECKLIST

Audit Background

Site Name:
Site Location:
Audit type:
Audit dates:
Team Leader:
Team Members:

Team Leader Only

No.	*Pre-Audit Planning Activity*	*Done Yes/No*
	Define the audit objectives, scope, and schedule	
	Form the audit team	
	Contact site six weeks in advance to discuss the audit. Address the following:	
	Audit objectives, scope, and schedule	
	Scheduling of site manager for opening/closing conferences	
	Identification of any current regulatory challenges or issues	
	Completion of preaudit questionnaire/information, including a list of documents to be provided prior to the audit and those documents that should be available during the audit	
	Team room availability	
	Phone availability	
	Site internet access and/or Wi-Fi or corporate network availability	
	Printer availability	
	Audiovisual equipment availability (e.g., computer projectors)	
	On-site lunch availability (optional)	
	Site contact name(s) and phone/fax numbers	
	Directions to the site	
	Ground transportation needs	

No.	Pre-Audit Planning Activity	Done Yes/No
	Hotel recommendations	
	Dress code and personal protective equipment (PPE) requirements	
	Send preaudit questionnaire to site	
	Assign areas of review to team members	
	Distribute completed preaudit questionnaire and previous audit report to team members	
	Develop detailed audit agenda, including timing for opening/ closing conferences	
	Distribute audit agenda to site staff and team members	
	Develop/tailor opening conference presentation	
	Hold preaudit team meeting. Address the following:	
	Areas of responsibility	
	Report-writing responsibility and expectations	
	Need for laptop computer(s) or other technologies	
	Review of completed preaudit questionnaire and previous audit report	
	Dress code and PPE requirements	
	Arrival time and means of transportation	
	Departure time and means of transportation	
	Site contact name(s) and phone/fax numbers	
	Hotel name, location, and phone/fax numbers	
	Site and hotel directions	

All Team Members (Including Team Leader)

No.	Pre-Audit Planning Activity	Done Yes/No
	Determine audit scope, objectives, and schedule	
	Identify individual areas of review	
	Participate in the preaudit team meeting	
	Assure the above items are covered by the team leader in the meeting	
	Review applicable preaudit information, including:	
	Complete preaudit questionnaire or equivalent	
	Company auditing standards and guidelines	
	Applicable local, national, or federal regulations	
	Applicable local site permits	
	Previous audit report	
	Applicable audit protocols	
	Applicable policies, standards, and guidelines	
	Obtain local weather forecast	
	Research country norms and customs (if applicable)	
	Bring language dictionary (if applicable)	
	Determine/comply with Passport, Visa, and Vaccination requirements (if applicable)	
	Determine electrical applicable requirements (if applicable)	

Many companies today assign "subject-matter experts" to their audit teams when particularly complex issues at the audited facility require in-depth, technical HSEQ knowledge. These staff members may not be the most experienced auditors, but their technical knowledge of a regulatory compliance or ISO conformance area is often essential to the success of the audit. Technical subject-matter experts are increasingly being included on audit teams for areas like security, environmental management, OHS management, transportation, sustainability, and process-safety management, to name a few. Or they could be in the technical engineering disciplines such as electrical, mechanical, or structural.

Some companies assign the HSEQ coordinator from the next site to be audited to the audit team. This gives them a good idea of the process and helps them better prepare for the upcoming visit. These individuals, sometimes referred to as "guest auditors," do not typically have audit assignments, but in some cases, they may assist another audit team member.

One should also consider language when creating an audit team. Even in North America, this issue can come into play. Having an auditor who can speak French on an audit in Quebec, or an auditor who can speak Spanish on an audit in Mexico, can be very advantageous. For better or worse, cultural issues should be considered, at least to some extent. Cultural diversity on audit teams can be a wonderful asset when auditing a wide geographic and culturally diverse area.

Finally, once the audit team is selected, there should be a team meeting prior to the audit. This can be handled in a variety of ways. A face-to-face meeting is preferred but not always possible. A videoconference on a web-based platform like Zoom or Teams is an acceptable substitute and is, in fact, becoming more and more common, especially in remote auditing processes. The team may also schedule a meeting for the evening before the audit. This approach should be used sparingly because it might be too late at that point to make any last-minute adjustments. There is always the risk that one or more auditors' flights will be late, and the meeting will never take place. If you've flown lately, you'll understand.

Completion and Review of the Preaudit Questionnaire

The purpose of the preaudit questionnaire is twofold. First, it enables the audit team to familiarize itself with the general HSEQ-related activities and operations before they arrive on-site. Second, it serves as a timely alert to the facility manager so that they may better prepare themselves and their staff for the audit.

An important element of a good preaudit questionnaire should be its brevity. Normally, fifteen to twenty-five pages is sufficient. Of course, audit scope and facility complexity will be in play here, but this is a good rule of thumb. The preaudit questionnaire should ask only for general information about the facility. Its primary purpose is to make the audit team sufficiently aware of facility HSEQ activities so that relevant regulations and operational requirements can be obtained and reviewed.

Several important points about preaudit questionnaires are worth mentioning. If the audit team wants the questionnaire completed, the team should ensure that it is simple and straightforward. For example, the questionnaire should not require the site to provide reams of performance data that can be reviewed better when the audit team arrives on-site. It should focus only on the facility's operational activities and the related HSEQ impacts so that the questionnaire can serve as a screening tool for the auditors. Questions on compliance should be avoided. For example, "Is your facility submitting monitoring reports as required by your air permit?" is a wasted question because it is the auditors' job to verify this, not the facility staff's.

Make sure the questionnaire is distributed to the site well in advance; two to four weeks prior to the audit is typical. Most importantly, each member of the team must review the questionnaire prior to the on-site activities. There is nothing more inconsiderate than requiring the site to complete a questionnaire, then not having it reviewed by the team in advance of the audit. Courtesy is always in vogue.

A useful part of a preaudit questionnaire is often a list of typical records and documents that the audit team intends to review during the audit. This allows the staff at the facility to be better prepared and to compile these records ahead of time so that they are available to the audit team.

It has become a more common for many organizations to request several of these key documents during the preaudit phase to allow time for the auditors to review them prior to the audit if they have the time and opportunity. The advantage of this approach is that the auditors gain insight into the specific audit criteria they will be verifying once on-site. Taking the time to read through a respiratory-protection program or vendor pre-qualification documents prior to the audit allows the on-site audit time to be spent more efficiently. It is best to request only documents that contain specific requirements that will not usually be listed in audit checklists or protocols. Requesting detailed records prior to the audit is typically not done as these records are best reviewed during the on-site audit phase.

Review of Relevant Regulations

Numerous regulatory requirements are administered by federal, state, provincial, and local authorities. Once the preaudit questionnaire has been returned to the audit team, a thorough review of the relevant regulations affecting the facility should be undertaken. Several methods can be used to obtain the regulations. Directly contacting regulatory agencies and asking for copies of the regulations is an appropriate technique. Or checking tier online websites. These are all free to anyone.

Computerized regulatory database systems are available that provide fast retrieval of applicable regulations through the use of keywords. These products have become quite cost-effective in the past few years. Most provide regulatory information on CDs, websites or the "cloud" or other internet sources, or the same information can be loaded onto a company's intranet. Auditors often bring the CDs into the field or can access web-based data. Internationally, teams can access country regulations through books, the Internet, local consultants, embassies, and, to a limited extent, computerized regulatory database systems. Simply because an audit is international does not mean that regulatory data gathering should be ignored. In almost all cases, at least limited regulatory information is available. Suffice it to say that audit teams must have some access to national and local regulations during the course of the audit. Protocols and checklists only go so far.

Definition of Audit Scope and Establishment of Team Responsibilities

An important preaudit activity is clearly defining the audit scope and audit team responsibilities. It is not necessary that all areas be audited during the site visit if it is felt that time would be better spent concentrating on a few compliance areas that represent a higher exposure.

Once the team decides on the areas that will be the subject of the audit, each team member should be given a specific assignment and responsibility to serve as the auditor for that audit scope area. The auditor can then fully prepare to start their portions of the audit efficiently once the team arrives on-site. In some cases, it may be appropriate to have two members of the team audit the more complex compliance areas. This should be decided by the team before the audit commences.

Development of a Detailed Audit Agenda or Plan

The success of the on-site audit will depend largely on how well the audit team has prepared itself and the facility staff. A good technique is to develop a daily agenda that describes the activities planned for each day of the audit. The agenda allows the facility manager to alert key facility staff of when they will be required to talk with the auditors and, generally, about the audit topics that will be covered.

Review of Audit Protocols

Audit protocols are typically used with some discretion. More experienced auditors will often use the checklists as reference documents, reviewing them in detail each morning and evening, to assure themselves that they are not overlooking any aspect of compliance. These auditors sometimes develop one-page reminder sheets that cover the major compliance categories for each area. Other, perhaps less-experienced, auditors will use the checklists verbatim during the course of the inspections and interviews.

The advantages of the first approach are increased flexibility for the auditor and their ability to interview staff without the intimidating presence of a checklist. Although these advantages are typically lost in the more rigorous second approach, its use is less likely to result in the auditor's overlooking noncompliance items. And generally speaking, findings will be based on great measure on how well the auditee is meeting the intent of the requirements detailed in the checklist guidance.

Some organizations have decided to utilize the commercial, computerized audit protocols available in the marketplace. These are excellent tools, both comprehensive and current. However, one should be wary of their use in the field. Teams required to answer every protocol question in order to generate a report may find that protocol completion can interfere with the conduct of the audit. The team will often spend too much time behind the computer screen, or looking for interpretations of the protocol, and not enough reviewing records, observing the facility and its activities, or otherwise verifying compliance and conformance.

Regardless of the protocol techniques selected, the auditor should familiarize themselves thoroughly with the protocol prior to the audit. If the auditor chooses the first approach (i.e., using the protocols as reference tools), they probably should develop the one-page summary sheets prior to the site visit. It is also important to include compliance items on the protocols that reflect local (e.g., city, county, province, country) regulatory requirements.

Arrange Logistics

Logistics is not a trivial concern on HSEQ audits. The team leader must discuss these items with the site staff well in advance of the audit. It is not fun to stay at a hotel located ninety minutes from the plant site because there is a major league baseball game or Rolling Stones concert in town and nearby hotels are sold out. Also, the team should take advantage of the Internet whenever possible as the list of available travel web sites is virtually unlimited. Utilizing the resources at hand will help to ensure that the team arrives on time, prepared, and rested. Many audit programs include a scheduled preaudit conference call between the facility staff and the audit team during the week prior to the audit to discuss the logistical issues noted above. This call, while usually brief, can sometimes identify last-minute conflicts and issues with the facility that could impact the audit schedule.

In summary, and as mentioned previously, all or most of the above preaudit activities are often documented in an "audit plan," which serves as a summary of all the key planning activities that have taken place. It is a good management tool to ensure that all parties involved in the audit are on the same page and all people participating in the audit are prepared.

SAMPLE ITINERARY FOR AN AUDIT

Day 1 – Monday a.m.

The audit team meets with the host facility manager and environmental manager to make introductions and review the purpose of the audit. They refine schedules for interviews, tours, and special requirements.

The environmental coordinator makes a brief presentation to the audit team, highlighting major features of the facility.

There is a general tour of the facility to provide the audit team with an orientation of the overall facility. This is a brief "ride through" of key areas in the facility.

Day 1 – Monday p.m.

The team conducts a detailed audit of *XXXXXXXXXXXX* compliance. They physically inspect discharge points, treatment facilities, monitoring records, and other related data. Conduct interviews with key facility staff.

The team conducts a detailed audit of *XXXXXXXXX* compliance. They physically inspect XXXXXXXXXXXXXXX. Review XXXXXXXX records, inspection records, permits, and licenses. Conduct interviews with key facility staff.

The team meets at the end of the day, without the site HSEQ staff, to discuss interim findings and general observations.

Day 2 – Tuesday a.m.

The audit team briefs the site HSEQ staff on interim findings, and they plan the daily agenda.

Conduct audit of *XXXXXXXXXXX* compliance. They physically inspect hazardous waste generation points (e.g., shops, process areas, storage yards, warehouses). Inspect manifests, waste analysis records, permits, groundwater monitoring, and inspection plans/schedules. Conduct interviews with key facility staff. (Depending on facility size and hazardous waste activities, this audit could take a full day or more.)

Day 2 – Tuesday p.m.

Conduct audit of *XXXXXXXXXXXX* compliance. They physically inspect hazardous waste chemical storage areas and warehouses. Review spill contingency plans, spill reporting procedures, and incident reports. Conduct interviews with key staff.

Conduct audit of *XXXXXXXXXXXX* compliance. They physically inspect oil storage areas, tank farms, and drum storage areas. Review oil spill contingency plans and spill reports. Conduct interviews with key staff.
The team meets at the end of the day, without the site HSEQ staff, to discuss interim findings and general observations.

Day 3 – Wednesday a.m.
The audit team briefs the site HSEQ staff on interim findings, and they plan the daily agenda.
The team conducts an audit of XXXXXXXXXX compliance. They physically inspect areas where transformers/capacitors are maintained and conduct interviews with key staff.
The team conducts an audit of XXXXXXXXXXXX. They physically inspect XXXXXXXX storage areas. They review records of XXXXXXXXXX and disposal records. They conduct interviews with key staff.

Day 3 – Wednesday p.m.
The team conducts an audit of XXXXXXXX compliance. They physically inspect XXXX facilities and XXXXXXX facilities. They review records of quality monitoring and system inspection records. They conduct interviews with key staff.
The team conducts an audit of XXXXXXXX. Physically inspect areas of the facility with XXXXXXX. Inspect handling/disposal procedures. Review records of disposal of XXXXXXX. Conduct interviews with key staff.
The team meets at the end of the day, without the site HSEQ staff, to discuss interim findings and general observations.

Day 4 – Thursday a.m.
The audit team briefs the site HSEQ staff on interim findings, and they plan the daily agenda.
The team conducts a general inspection of areas just outside facility boundaries, especially residential areas. They look for potential nuisance problems (i.e., emissions, noise, odor).
The team continues audits as before.

Day 4 – Thursday p.m.
This period is reserved to conduct audits of any special areas that are uncovered once the team is on-site. It is a period to review the previous days' activities. Additional data or information needs are identified, and any unfinished items are completed. Perhaps a second visit to an area on site is needed, or some discussion on the applicability of certain regulations is required. This period is also used by the audit team to develop a preliminary list of audit findings for any information briefing to key staff.

Day 5 – Friday a.m.
The audit team gives an informal briefing to key HSEQ staff on preliminary findings of the audit. The purpose of this briefing is to alert the staff to any significant problems found so that corrective actions may be initiated. The meeting is also used to verify the validity of the findings with site HSEQ management prior to meeting with the facility manager.
The audit team conducts a formal closing briefing for the facility manager.
The audit team departs the facility.

On-Site Activities

On-site activities during an HSEQ audit will include the following primary functions:

- Opening conference
- Orientation tour or tour of some aspect of the process related facility
- Overview of HSEQ management systems and the organization
- Records/documentation review
- Staff interviews
- Physical inspection of facilities
- Daily reviews
- Closing conference
- Development of the audit report

Not all of the above activities relate, strictly speaking, to auditing. Be aware that the three principal auditing verification tasks—records reviews, interviews, and facility inspections—represent only approximately 50 percent of the time spent in the field on an audit. So, a five-day audit involves about two and a half days of actual auditing. This takes many first-time auditors by surprise.

OPENING CONFERENCE

Each audit should begin with an opening conference or meeting involving the audit team and site operational and HSEQ management. This meeting, while it might begin with a welcome by the facility manager, is the responsibility of the audit team leader, who sets the agenda and keeps it running on time. One of the most important things to remember about the opening conference is to arrive on time. The audit will not proceed smoothly if the audit team is late and the site's management team must waste time waiting for them to arrive. Late arrivals occur more than one might imagine.

Orientation Tour

After the opening conference, the audit team is usually taken on a facility or site orientation tour, which may be preceded by a facility safety orientation presentation. This allows the team to gain an appreciation of the relative complexity of the site and its operations. Some tips for completing this tour are as follows:

- Give the site escort a time limit for the tour (usually about one hour) and, for subsequent scheduling purposes, assume you will run over by fifteen minutes. Tell the escort what you would like to see. Use the preaudit questionnaire to help focus the exercise.

- If you need to request a vehicle to observe remote areas, do so. Generally, you will be able to return to most facility areas later, but for remote areas this may not be the case. Make careful initial observations in these situations.
- Be careful not to spend too much time in the process or manufacturing areas. Auditors generally find these areas personally fascinating, but detailed observation of manufacturing does not always provide substantial HSEQ compliance or performance information, except regarding topics such as personal protective equipment (PPE), machine guarding, and the like. The alternative to this is if the scope is on quality and customer service and the quality of the product being manufactured.
- If the audit, because of the size of the site, requires a large team (more than four), split the team in two and request two escorts. Organize the orientations based on relative areas of interest among the two audit sub-teams.
- Take notes when on the tour, but other than for remote areas, do not get into too much detail. Doing so will slow down the process. Try to note areas you would like the team to revisit.
- Bring a one-page plot plan or site map with you to help with the site orientation.
- If feasible, do not retrace your steps so that you see as much of the facility in as short a time as possible. That is, try not to return to the office on the same route you left.
- Try to have the team or teams stay together as much as possible. There will be a tendency for team members to wander off. Not only does this slow down the process, but the escort often makes significant comments during the tour, which some team members might not hear.
- Arrive at the facility early on the first day of the audit and attempt to drive along the site boundary to obtain a different perspective. This may help during the orientation tour.

Overview of Management Systems and the Organization

After the orientation tour, it is often helpful to have the team sit down with the site HSEQ manager (and his or her staff) to discuss how HSEQ at the site is managed. Topics to consider include organizational structure, roles and responsibilities, management systems and procedures, and the like. This discussion will help the audit team better understand how things actually get done at the site. And since the questions (and answers) will generally be relevant to all the auditors, this will avoid having the site staff answer the same question multiple times.

Records/Documentation Review

As noted earlier, a good audit protocol will provide the auditor with instructions on the records, files, and reports they should request during the audit. More importantly, it should help the auditor understand what he or she should be looking for when the documentation is reviewed. Normally, records should be reviewed just before interviews are conducted and facilities inspected. However, often it is useful to review documentation at the same time an interview is being conducted or an operation is being inspected. This will depend on the area being audited and the individual style of the auditors. As a general rule, however, auditors should spend their initial efforts reviewing the records and files associated with the specific area to gain a better understanding of the key issues at the facility.

One of the important things to remember when reviewing documentation is that many requirements are contained within the records. The auditor will need to scan these documents, looking specifically for applicable terms, conditions, or requirements, and then verify that these requirements are being met.

When appropriate, auditors should obtain copies of relevant documentation uncovered during the audit when doing so can aid them in evaluating the compliance status of the facility. Also, it is useful as reference material when writing the audit report at the conclusion of the audit.

During the course of the audit, a file of working papers or field notes will be developed. It is not uncommon for an audit team to leave the facility with a thick file of records, reports, or other documentation. However, the rule of thumb is to make copies only of those materials that the audit team needs to perform a complete and thorough evaluation of the facility's status. Finally, be careful about leaving the site in possession of documents that you have yet to review. This may mean that you have not completed your review, and it will be difficult to conduct a follow-up verification of apparent deficiencies once back in your office.

The following listed items provide some helpful guidance on developing an effective document-review strategy:

- *Obtain what you can ahead of time, within reason.* By way of example, requesting a copy of the site's written confined-space entry procedure is prudent and reasonable.
- *Review records first.* Many auditable requirements (e.g., inspections, maintenance procedures) are found in the documents.
- *Do not get overwhelmed with the task at hand.* There can typically be thousands of pages of records. Start with strategic documents in each of the compliance areas (e.g., written programs and procedures), and see where that leads you.

- *Ask for quiet time if you need it.* Nobody wants to be watched while reading. When a site person is hovering next to you, concentrating becomes difficult.
- *Develop a list of verifiable requirements.* These are items such as training and inspections. You will want to ensure they are being completed at the site and are consistent with the stated operational requirements.

Remember, reviewing records is a critical, if tedious, audit task. Do it completely but do it efficiently.

Interviews with Facility Staff

Proper interviewing during an HSEQ audit is perhaps the single most important aspect of the audit process. Yet, too often, a lack of attention to the subtleties of interviewing results in less-than-optimal results. There are a number of interviewing skills and techniques that, if followed, can enhance the outcome of the audit.

Schedule Interviews Ahead of Time (If Possible)

Popping in on busy managers or fab shop supervisors is a sure way to cause ill feelings and poor audit results. An interview should be scheduled well ahead of time so that the person being interviewed is prepared and ready for the auditor. If possible, the interviewee should be told ahead of time about the purpose of the audit, the general types of questions that will be asked, and the types of documentation the auditor will want to review. This is not intended to be a "gottcha" exercise. Often the interviewee will suggest that someone else in the shop be available for the interview because the auditor's questions can be better answered by that person, or that other person can give additional context in the answer. This is to be encouraged because the whole purpose of the interview is to obtain the best evidence available, relative to the status of the facility. If at all possible, at least a one-day advance notice should be given to all interviewees.

However, there are exceptions to this rule of notification. In some instances, the auditor might simply want to walk the shop floor and ask operators or technicians a few questions, such as

- What would you do in case of an emergency or a spill?
- Do you attend any safety meetings?
- What PPE is required in the various areas?
- Do you use an inspection and text plan when you fabricate your client's product?

You should receive permission first to conduct these "casual" interviews, especially in union shops, but they should be part of your audit process. Do not be too concerned about the unannounced nature of the interviews; everyone at the site will be on high alert, as you can be assured that they will have been notified of your presence well in advance.

Conduct Interviews in the Workspaces

Conducting interviews in the workspace of the interviewee serves several purposes. First of all, the person being interviewed is more relaxed and less defensive than he might be if summoned to the plant manager's office or another similar location for the interview. Second, some key records and files are often maintained in the workspace, if not already on the network, and will be more readily available to the auditor. Third, the auditor has an opportunity to observe firsthand actual workplace conditions, the attitudes of plant staff, and other subtleties that would not be observable in the facility manager's office or a conference room.

The one disadvantage to conducting interviews in the workplace is that distractions and interruptions likely will occur. The interviewee will face phone calls, emails, employees with problems, and other similar distractions. Also, it is often noisy in many workplaces and difficult to communicate.

The auditor should make it clear to the interviewee that he would like their attention and would appreciate some uninterrupted time. An appropriate opening statement might be something like:

> Hello, Mr. Smith, I know you have a tight schedule, as I do. If you could put your telephone or cell calls on hold and minimize interruptions from your staff, I know I can be finished with these questions in short order and let you get back to work.

Be Sensitive to the Interviewee's Nervousness and Defensiveness

This may seem obvious, but often it is not perceived by auditors. There is a normal negative reaction associated with an audit of any kind, regardless of the auditor's plea that "I'm only here to help you." That might not have been their previous experience. The auditor must continue to reassure the interviewees that the purpose of the audit is to uncover the areas that need more attention, resources, staff training, and the like to comply with the law and/or corporate expectations. It is not an audit of the interviewees or individuals but rather an evaluation of the systems and related controls needed to help them do their jobs better and more efficiently. Of course, people are essentially at the heart of all systems, as all systems were created by people (Artificial Intelligence aside).

Some people will view the auditor as a threat to their job security or credibility. The auditor should be sensitive to this and ask questions in a constructive, respectful, and unemotional manner. If an interviewee becomes overly negative, sarcastic, or uncooperative, it is better to suggest terminating the interview at that point and discuss the problem with the team's site host. Most people who are interviewed are nervous to begin with and become more so if they sense their responses to the auditor's questions are not the *correct* ones. Sometimes, they will dig a hole for themselves as they grope for what they perceive to be the right answer. When the interviewee is struggling, the auditor should change the subject rather than probe more deeply. Either move on to other audit questions or perhaps curtail the audit temporarily and talk about some other topic to relax the interviewee.

Avoid Closed-ended Yes/No Responses to Questions

Questions asked during an audit should focus on getting the interviewee to open up and discuss compliance issues. That is, ask open-ended questions. Avoid closed-ended questions that give the person an easy yes-or-no response. "Do you inspect the customer property storage facility every thirty days as the contract requires?" may result in a simple "yes" because the interviewee assumes that is what he is supposed to do. He may not even be aware of any requirement to inspect customer property storage facilities. "Tell me about your procedures to ensure your customer property is protected while under the facilities custody" is a more open-ended question, which will reveal much more about the interviewee's knowledge of customer property requirements.

Be Open to Follow-Up Interviews with Other Staff

You may start with one interview with a facility staff member, then find that you end up interviewing three individuals to get the information you need. "I don't handle that part; Bill Jones does" is a common response during interviews. An auditor needs to keep probing for the knowledgeable staff that may be able to answer the questions at hand. Individuals at the plant may have been transferred to another job at the facility and be no longer handling tank inspections or overhead crane inspections, for example. Should you find some discrepancies in inspection records for these areas from two years before, seek out the individuals who conducted the inspections at that time, if possible, and try to get your questions answered. In some, albeit very, very rare cases, attempting to contact retired staff or individuals who have left the facility is acceptable if they can provide useful information to the auditor.

In summary, if these suggestions are followed, auditors will obtain more precise information about the conditions at the facility. Interviewing is a personal, interactive process. Each auditor will have his or her unique style and attitude. As an aid, a list of recommendations that all auditors should review before conducting interviews is provided here:

- Call interviewees and schedule the exact time and place of interviews at least a few hours ahead of time.
- Upon meeting interviewees, introduce yourself and explain who you are, where you are from, and why you are auditing the facility.
- First, relax interviewees and get them to explain who they are and their roles and responsibilities.
- Do not become captive to your checklist so that effective communication is hampered.
- Ask open-ended questions; avoid questions that require only a "yes" or "no" answer.
- Do not ask questions about compliance items that can be better evaluated by physical inspection or documentation review at a later stage of the audit.
- Do not preach to interviewees or intimidate them with your knowledge of the standards or regulations. Do not quote or cite regulations unless this information is requested, and you think it will help the interviewing process.
- Ask interviewees about previous audits/inspections relative to the compliance area you are auditing. This is a good place to start.
- Solicit input from interviewees about how the audit should be conducted for maximum effectiveness. Make them a part of the audit process, not the subject of it.
- Be careful not to tell or order interviewees to do anything during the interview. Remember that you are there to obtain information and identify problems, not to solve them during the audit. That will come later.
- When appropriate, and if it helps the interview to proceed more effectively, make general comments that are instructional in nature as long as they are not construed to be directives from the auditor.
- At the time that noncompliance items are being identified, do not make interviewees uncomfortable with your reaction. Continue to assure them that the audit is not intended to be a personal inquisition but a process to identify problems typically found at facilities.
- Be empathetic as you talk to interviewees, but do not cross the line and become too sympathetic to their problems. The interviews could last longer than they need to.
- Be quick to distinguish the "hostile interviewee" who does not want to cooperate from the "nervous interviewee" who is simply uptight about being questioned. And address this quickly and firmly, and then move on.

CLOSING CONFERENCE

A closing conference should (must) take place at the facility being audited before the audit team leaves the site. This is typically a formal meeting and involves the facility manager or other members of the site management team, who may not have been involved in the audit or interview process after the opening conference. Some thoughts on preparing for and conducting the closing conference are provided below.

Preparing for the Closing Conference

1. Determine the time, place, and invitees as soon as possible so that all parties are given proper notice.
2. Organize findings by compliance or conformance areas (e.g., air, wastewater, hazardous waste, confined space, hearing conservation, customer property, quality of products), and prepare a brief handout for people attending the meeting.
3. Plan the meeting to be relatively brief (less than one hour) and focus only on key finding and problems. Leave the nitty-gritty details to the audit report but don't have any surprises in the final report which weren't broached in the closing meeting.
4. Organize findings by type: (a) regulatory, (b) company policy or ISO Standard, and (c) company guideline or good management practice.
5. Organize findings by priority and importance (some use minor, major, or significant, others use risk based on high, medium and low), depending on degree of risk, health impact, customer impact, or other similar criteria.
6. Focus findings on the root causes of the finding or problems, not the symptoms.
7. Rehearse the closing conference with other audit team members and challenge each other to ensure that the findings are valid and "backupable."

Conducting the Closing Conference

1. Introduce the audit team and state the objectives of the audit and the format for the meeting.
2. Express appreciation to facility management for their cooperation and assistance.
3. Try to avoid using specific names of facility staff when presenting negative findings but try and specify individuals' names when presenting commendable findings.

4. Avoid confrontation during the meeting with any member of the facility staff who may disagree with your findings.
5. Avoid comparisons to another facility's performance unless it is helpful to make a point.
6. Resist requests to "reaudit" an area before the audit team departs the site so that findings can be left out of the audit report.
7. Discuss the follow-up requirements for the draft and final reports, the corrective-action plan, and periodic status reports.

If care is taken to prepare adequately for the closing conference, there should be little cause for concern. The conference principally entails the communication of factual findings that have been fully verified and previously communicated to site HSEQ staff.

REFERENCES

Dan Petersen. *Why Safety is a People Problem.* https://www.ehstoday.com/archive/article/21907885/dan-petersen-why-safety-is-a-people-problem.

This chapter has been adapted from Lawrence B. Cahill and Raymond W. Kane. *Environmental Health and Safety Audits*, 9th Edition. Government Institutes, 2010. It has been updated for this edition.

Wayne Pardy and Terri Andrews. *Integrated Management Systems: Leading Strategies and Solutions*, 2nd Edition. Bernan Press, 2019.

Chapter 13

Conducting Effective Opening and Closing Meeting and Conferences

Though it be honest, it is never good to bring bad news.

—William Shakespeare, 1564–1616

This chapter discusses a variety of issues that often arise during the preparation and conduct of opening and closing conferences. If these issues are dealt with professionally and appropriately, the audit will have a greater potential for success.

OPENING CONFERENCES

The opening conference, not surprisingly, occurs at the very beginning of the audit. It typically involves the full audit team, the site manager, the site HSEQ manager, and selected site staff. The basic intent is to provide face-to-face introductions, establish the audit objectives, set the agenda for the audit, and discuss, in a preliminary fashion, issues raised by a review of preaudit information. A meeting quite often has two phases: a first, shorter phase involving the plant or site manager, followed by a longer issue discussion phase during which the site manager may or may not be present.

The opening conference sets the tone for the entire audit. It can be stressful and is filled with potential "land mines" for the audit team. If the following six recommendations are kept in mind by the audit team, many of the mines can be avoided.

1. Take Charge of the Meeting

This may seem to be a simple point, but it is often lost on the audit team leader. The opening conference or meeting should be orchestrated by the audit team, not by facility or local management. This can be especially difficult with a domineering or aggressive facility manager who is several positions higher than the audit team leader in the organizational hierarchy.

Certainly, the facility manager will most often want to welcome the team, make general introductions, and provide an overview of the site's history and operations. But after this is accomplished, the HSEQ audit team leader should take over, based on an agenda that has been discussed previously with facility management. This is not to say that site staff do not have a major contribution to make during the meeting—they do indeed. However, the audit team will be on-site only for a short while and will have quite an ambitious agenda; therefore, any substantial deflections can jeopardize meeting the objectives of the audit. One must keep the audit on track at all times and at all phases of the audit.

2. Be Organized

Once the HSEQ audit team leader assumes responsibility for the flow of the meeting, they should conduct it in an organized fashion. A predeveloped series of slides and/or handouts works well to keep things moving and to ensure that all audits, regardless of the makeup of the team, are conducted consistently. A somewhat formal method is especially useful when discussing the audit objectives, approach, results, and follow-up. Quite often, organizations develop the handouts as part of the audit program guidance document so that they are generally available to all auditors. A list of topics that should be covered in the opening conference includes the following:

- Audit objectives and scope
- Audit "flow," including follow-up and closure
- Identification of key interview candidates and availability (including obtaining relevant organization charts)
- A summary review of the operations at the facility (including obtaining plot plans)
- Identification of important site activities occurring during the week
- A review of the preaudit information
- Scheduling of the daily and closing conferences
- Identification of the audit team workroom and phone/cell phone protocol
- Identification of site work hours and visitor safety and security protocols
- Identification of computer/printer support
- Discussion of the site escort protocol for visitors and PPE requirements

A couple of points here must be kept in mind. The meeting should be crisp and to the point. The HSEQ audit team's questions and inquiries should clearly reflect that they have done their homework—that the preaudit information has been read and digested well in advance of the audit. There is no greater insult to the facility staff than the failure of one or more audit team members to review (in detail) the preaudit information that the facility staff so painstakingly prepared.

And finally, remember that not all questions will be answered in full during the opening meeting. Do not involve ten or so people in a protracted discussion of an issue that can be resolved much more easily and quickly in a follow-up, one-on-one discussion.

3. Discuss Logistics

One of the biggest challenges during the audit week is managing the logistics of the effort, especially if the audit is not conducted as a remote audit. During the opening conference, the preset agenda should be modified as appropriate, and the actual names of interview candidates and escorts should be placed in the "time blocks" of the agenda.

Notwithstanding this noble objective, one can be assured that within a relatively short time after the formal initiation of the audit, a change to the agenda will need to be made. A new interview candidate will be identified, another will be called away for a day, or a surprise regulatory-agency inspection will occur, justifiably deflecting the attention of the site staff.

The audit team needs to be responsive to the various incidents that might require schedule changes; flexibility and common courtesy are paramount. Several techniques are useful in this regard. First, the audit team should leave some open time near the end of the audit agenda. This can be used to accommodate needed changes. This time never seems to go to waste.

Second, the auditor should address areas in parallel, not in series. In other words, if an individual audit team member is responsible for several areas, such as wastewater, PCBs and spills, confined space, lockout, tagout, and machine guarding, some work on each of these areas should begin early in the process, even if it is simply to review paperwork and schedule interviews. This accomplishes two things: it allows for better time management, minimizing the chance that an area will not be addressed at all if completely left to the morning of the last day, and it also avoids the issue of having the key site staff member take a holiday on the last day of the audit, unbeknownst to the auditor.

And third, do not think of the audit as taking place only from 8:00 a.m. to 5:00 p.m. each day. Conflicts in scheduling can sometimes be remedied through breakfast and dinner meetings. After all, what else is there to do far from home in a hotel two miles from the facility in a remote town? Audits in Chicago or Toronto offer more after-hours distractions.

4. Find Out What's Happening at the Site

Far too often, audit teams miss opportunities to observe important activities that might occur during the week of the audit. Examples include incident-related issues like

- a spill drill;
- a load out of a customer product;
- start-up of a boiler;
- monthly wastewater or stormwater sampling;
- weekly or quarterly inspections; and
- a confined-space entry.

There is no better verification technique than actually watching to see if something is done consistently with written procedures. These activities should be observed whenever possible.

5. Schedule Additional Conferences

Most mature audit programs include not only opening and closing conferences but also daily audit team and site HSEQ staff meetings. During the opening conference, a tentative time should be set for the closing conference and the daily meetings with the site.

The daily meetings do take time away from the actual audit, but they are crucial in maintaining adequate communication. These meetings allow participants to review findings to date, resolve any misunderstandings early on, and revise the audit agenda as needed. Based on numerous observations, the daily meetings with site staff appear to work better last thing in the afternoon as opposed to first thing in the morning. That way, there is an incentive to keep the meeting brief and to the point. On the other hand, morning meetings occur when people are fresh and not fatigued by the day. People on both sides of the table are often more articulate and patient. The morning meeting also allows the audit team to have some time alone the evening before to prepare and compare notes. Either approach is acceptable.

6. Address Important Topics

Certain special topics should be addressed during the opening conference. If they are ignored, misunderstandings can arise. These topics are as follows:

- There will be findings (no site is perfect). Site staff need to be told that an audit will result in findings, no matter how well managed the site. Stated another way, audit findings in and of themselves are not necessarily reflective of poor management, which has more to do with the number of significant or repeat findings.

- Audits require verification. Acceptable audit methods require verification; hearsay evidence is generally not sufficient. This implies that when a site employee claims, for example, that all staff members have received appropriate training, the auditor typically will not, or cannot, take that statement at face value; audit records will have to be reviewed. However, unless site staff are made aware of the need for verification, any given individual could be insulted if the auditor seemingly does not believe his or her statements.
- All areas must be covered. Simply because the completed preaudit questionnaire stated, for example, that there were no underground storage tanks, permitted confined spaces, or customer-owned equipment at the site, that does not mean the audit team can ignore those areas. The person completing the questionnaire might not have considered a septic tank serving the maintenance shop as an "underground storage tank" or a five-foot construction trench as a confined space, or he might not have known that fluorescent light fixtures sometimes have PCB-containing ballasts. These issues can be important and cannot be ignored.
- How will "fixed" findings be handled? It is quite likely that some identified deficiencies will be remedied during the course of the audit. The audit team needs to inform the site staff about how these are to be handled in the report. Site staff typically will request that the fixed findings not be included in the report; however, most audit programs do include them but indicate that they were remedied during the audit. This approach is generally preferred because the findings, as trivial as they might be to the site staff, could sometimes be symptoms of a much larger site issue or even a corporate-wide issue. The larger issues could be lost if the symptoms are not included in the report.
- How will "significant" issues be handled? The audit team may, on occasion, identify a truly significant issue (e.g., an uncontrolled PCB spill, operation without a permit). The team should not wait until the end of the audit before raising these issues with facility management. Facility management should be told that it will be made immediately aware of any significant issue uncovered and that the audit may be halted temporarily until a plan of action is implemented.

As can be gathered from the above comments, the "bottom line" for opening conferences is free and open communication.

CLOSING CONFERENCES

The closing conference is the final on-site activity of the audit process. It typically involves the full audit team, the site manager, the site HSEQ manager, and selected site staff; the participant makeup is thus pretty much identical to the opening conference. The basic intent of the meeting is for the audit team to report back to the site on the findings of the audit. The meeting should be crisp and to the point; a goal of one hour (not including the inevitable questions and comments) is usually appropriate.

More often than not, a final working meeting with site HSEQ staff directly precedes the closing conference. At this meeting, most, if not all, of the differing points of view can be (hopefully) resolved. It is not unlike the daily meetings discussed previously.

The closing conference can be a stressful meeting, especially if the audit team is working right up to the last minute to produce a typed, formal list of findings or a draft report, as many audit teams are directed to do. Keeping the following closing conference points in mind can help to reduce, but not eliminate, the stress.

1. Take Charge of the Meeting

Having the audit team take control of the closing conference is an even more important issue than it is for the opening conference, so the point is worth repeating. The same issues discussed with respect to the opening conference apply here as well. The team leader should establish an agenda, there should be an allowance for significant input by facility staff, and the team should respect the position of the facility manager without being overly deferential.

Further, the correct message must be communicated to facility management, and this can only be done if (1) the team leader is in charge, and (2) the facility manager is present. If, in fact, the facility manager is unavoidably absent, the team leader should find some way to communicate the findings to him or her separately, whether by phone or face-to-face at a different time and/or location. This direct communication is essential because no matter how well-intentioned the site HSEQ staff is in relaying the information, there will always be filtering or screening of the findings when transmitted secondhand.

2. Be Organized

The audit team must certainly be organized for the closing conference; most often, time with the facility manager, in particular, is limited. It would not hurt to review once again the audit objectives, scope, approach, report format, and follow-up requirements. Although much of this information was transmitted in the opening conference, a second review helps when additional site staff are attending the closing conference; moreover, the staff who attended the opening conference, for better or worse, will not have retained all of the information in the days that have transpired since.

A proposed agenda for the meeting might be

- general reintroduction;
- statement of objectives, scope, and approach;
- overall summary of the audit, highlighting particularly commendable items and significant deficiencies;
- review of findings by individual area;
- discussion of the audit report format and schedule; and
- discussion of the corrective-action report format and schedule and next steps.

An organizational issue that audit team leaders face entails who should present the findings for the individual finding areas. The audit team leader could make all the presentations themselves, or each auditor could discuss their own subject-matter areas. In most cases, it is advisable to have the individual team members present their own findings, even if their presentation skills are not quite as good as the team leader's. Using summary slides, a good support tool even for experienced presenters, should be considered.

Having individual auditors present their own material is advantageous for several reasons. If they know that at the end of the audit they will be standing before a demanding audience and defending their findings, they are more likely to take care with the accuracy and precision of each. They are also the individuals who directly observed the deficiency and should be better able to respond to questions. Lastly, each of these closing conferences is an opportunity to improve presentation skills and, ultimately, to groom future lead auditors.

3. Be Appreciative but Do Not Bury the Message

It is very difficult to stand up in front of ten to twenty people, who might also be fellow employees and colleagues, and go into detail about all the things they are doing wrong. Thus, more often than not, closing conferences begin with a speech by the audit team leader thanking virtually everyone on the site for their help with the audit and praising participants for their cooperation and extensive knowledge and expertise. This courteous behavior is certainly appreciated by the facility staff, but if the praise becomes too effusive, site management can misinterpret what is being said. Or it may be perceived as "sugar coating." Managers will focus on the recognized expertise of their staff and assume the deficiencies or findings are trivial, administrative shortcomings, whether or not this is true. Auditors should not overdo the thanks and acknowledgments; they should be courteous but straight and to the point.

4. Set Priorities

On audits where there are numerous findings, some prioritization is in order. Many programs distinguish between regulatory, company policy, and good management practice (GMP) findings, or risk-based findings. Each of these finding types is often classified by the level of significance as well. In the closing conference, a similar organizational structure is needed. The facility manager should know before leaving the meeting whether there are any so-called showstopper findings. These significant findings should be addressed either at the very beginning or the very end of the meeting—preferably at the beginning.

5. Minimize Praise for "Acceptable" Performance

In school, scoring a 97 out of a possible 100 will get you a grade of A+. In regulatory compliance or conformance verification, it could get you a major fine or jail time. People often forget this important distinction. Therefore, audit team leaders need to stress that enforcement agencies expect 100 percent compliance with HSEQ rules and regulations. This is a little different from being perfect. Sites should not receive effusive praise for being "mostly" in compliance. This philosophy is quite consistent with total-quality-management principles of continuous improvement, no-defects production, and Six Sigma quality control.

By way of an example, sometimes scored audits can achieve a 100 percent score. This may be supported by evidence and facts, or it might be that the auditor was lazy, inexperienced, or simply did not perform all the work necessary to conduct a thorough audit and gave some "benefit of the doubt." A personal observation of the authors—regardless of the scope or complexity (or simplicity) of an audit, is to review audit scores of 100 percent. Nothing may be amiss. But then again, it is better to check (read between the lines on what "amiss" may mean).

6. Respond Professionally to Challenges

Each audit team aims to resolve all conflicts with facility staff prior to the closing conference. This is done mostly in the daily meetings and at the final preparatory meeting with site HSEQ staff. However, it is possible that controversies will arise during the closing conference.

The most important thing to remember in the closing conference is that the audit team should respond professionally to any challenge of its findings, if for no other reason than the facility staff might be correct in their assertions or opinions. Sometimes auditors get it wrong, and these "errors" have to be handled quite delicately, with professionalism and courtesy.

7. Focus on Root Causes but Avoid Evaluations of Staff Performance

A general trend in auditing today is to get behind symptoms and identify the root causes of the problems. This quite often results in a focus on management and organizational systems. The advantage of this approach is that focusing on root causes will more likely result in long-term fixes rather than Band-Aid solutions.

For example, a label could be missing from a drum containing hazardous waste. If this is reported as a finding, the site's response will most probably be to stick a label on the drum and be done with it. Yet, the audit team focusing on root causes will attempt to identify not only the what but also the why of the problem (e.g., why was the label missing?), and there could be half a dozen reasons. Focusing on these whys—such as lack of training, no ownership of the drum, poor labels, and so forth—should result in more appropriate corrective actions.

Yet, as valuable a tool as root-cause analysis can be, it can also more directly identify an individual's or group's lack of performance as the core of the problem—a much more difficult point to raise in the closing conference, which should be handled with great care. The old adage "Praise in public, admonish in private" should apply. If the audit team indeed has a sense that there is a chronic performance problem, the team might want to (1) make absolutely sure this is the case (e.g., maybe the individual did not receive the required or appropriate training), and (2) deal with it outside the public arena of the closing conference. Try very, very, very hard not to embarrass any auditee in front of their management team or their peers. This is embarrassing and unprofessional.

8. Understand How to Handle Repeat Findings

Every audit program should have a policy on how to handle findings that arise repeatedly from audit to audit. Many organizations will escalate the significance of the finding simply because it has not been corrected since the last audit. There is also the issue of how these findings are handled in audit reports. Some programs will specifically identify them as repeat findings, while others prohibit this practice due to concern about the potential liabilities stemming from apparent "willful and knowing" noncompliance or nonconformance. Should the audit discover any repeat findings, the audit team leader should be ready to address these issues during the closing conference in a manner consistent with corporate policy.

9. Avoid Comparisons

Whether they ask the question or not, facility managers are always curious about how their operations measure up against others in the organization. Responding to this question in the closing conference is generally a no-win proposition for the audit team leader. If the team leader states that the facility is exceptional by comparison, then any message of significance is lost on the site management. Also, "about-average" or "lower-quartile" responses are almost never taken at face value without challenges.

Some programs do require the audit team to score the audit, and this is done in a variety of ways for a variety of reasons. Occasionally, a point scale is used, such as the following example:

- In compliance or meets requirements (4.0 points)
- Generally, in compliance and mostly meets requirements (3.0 points)
- Needs improvement (2.0 points)
- Substantially out of compliance and conformance (1.0 points)
- No evidence of compliance or conformance (0 points)

Even this more simplified scoring can create disputes and arguments, however, given the competitive nature of most organizations.

Notwithstanding the above policies for scoring some companies, it is best for the audit team not to provide comparative judgments when, in fact, facilities cannot be evaluated fairly against one another. Different facilities handle different materials, use different technologies, are of varying ages, have different customer requirements, make different customer products, and are located in different physical and regulatory settings. Also, different auditors and their experience and skill sets might be a factor in different audit scores with similar objective evidence, or lack of the same. You can interpret this as you see fit.

10. Avoid Guarantees or Absolutes

The facility manager may also want the audit to identify any and all problems so that if a regulatory-agency inspection were to occur within a short time after the audit, there would be no surprises. The audit team leader should never make this guarantee. An audit, especially a systems HSEQ audit, is a spot check of the facility's operations using statistical and/or representative sampling techniques. That is, it occurs over a limited period, with a limited scope, and not all records are necessarily reviewed. It is quite possible that an agency inspector could subsequently review a certain compliance area in considerably greater depth. The inspector could, therefore, come across a compliance problem not identified by the audit team.

11. Leave Some Form of Written Findings (If You Can)

It would be remarkable to observe the look on the site HSEQ manager's face when told by the audit team leader during the closing conference that the team will leave no written record of the findings with the site. It is usually a look of bewilderment and disappointment, and one can sense that the momentum built up during the week of the audit is in jeopardy of being lost.

Some believe that providing a verbal debriefing alone should indeed be sufficient feedback to the site during the audit. After all, the site staff is hearing the essence of the message. These same people would prefer that any written report, be it a draft list of findings or a draft report, receive an independent (legal) review before even a limited distribution to the site and others.

There are at least two problems with this approach. First, momentum can be lost as the site waits anywhere from two weeks to two months for the draft report. The lack of on-site written documentation lessens the likelihood of quick or immediate responses. One could argue that the liability stemming from not addressing an issue in a timely fashion while awaiting the draft report is greater than that associated with leaving a draft list of findings with the site, which may need legal "massaging" later. In point of fact, the audit team leader should stress that if there are to be changes of significance between the draft list of findings and the draft or final report, site staff will be alerted prior to the distribution of the report. This is common courtesy.

Second, there can quite often be a major difference between the spoken and written word, especially with the interpretation of the words spoken or unspoken. Time and again, people will agree with what an auditor says in a closing conference; yet once they see these words in written form, they will disagree with both form and substance. This is because there are communication filters between the observation, verbalization of the observation, and documentation of the observation. Misinterpretations caused by these filters should be resolved face-to-face in the closing conference, not via "e-mail missiles."

12. Discuss the Next Steps

It is important for the audit team leader to close the meeting with a precise discussion of the next steps in the process. These steps relate principally to any follow-up work required of the audit team and to the schedule and distribution of the draft and final reports, and of the corrective-action plan. The team leader should explain that much is expected of the site in the final phase of the audit process. The site really determines the success of the audit by its dedication to correcting identified deficiencies in a timely manner. If all participants leave the meeting agreeing about the importance of this commitment, the audit has been a success.

13. Solicit Site Feedback

Many companies require that audit teams solicit formal feedback from the site on the value of the audit. This is often done via a questionnaire. A model questionnaire is provided in appendix K. Some thoughts on this process: First, it is appropriate and valuable to solicit feedback formally. Second, the completed questionnaire should be returned not to the team leader but to the audit program manager. And third, care should be taken not to misinterpret the results. A high-scoring result could mean an excellent audit, or it could mean that the team was too lenient. Conversely, a low-scoring result could mean a poorly performing team or a site that was not pleased with the justifiable rigor applied to evaluating its HSEQ performance.

REFERENCES

This chapter has been adapted from Lawrence B. Cahill and Raymond W. Kane. *Environmental Health and Safety Audits*, 9th Edition. Government Institutes, 2010. It has been updated for this edition.

Wayne Pardy and Terri Andrews. *Integrated Management Systems: Leading Strategies and Solutions*, 2nd Edition. Bernan Press, 2019.

Chapter 14

Drafting and Writing Quality HSEQ Audit Reports

Much has been written on developing effective HSEQ audit reports. Unfortunately, authoring a chapter on how to write effective audit reports is a bit like giving a speech on how to be an effective speaker. Nothing but perfection will be tolerated.

Notwithstanding this heartfelt reservation, this chapter examines a variety of issues that need to be considered when developing an audit report. These issues never quite seem to go away, no matter how many reports are written or how often the frustrated audit team leader refers an auditor to the audit report requirements. In the audit report, the audit team presents its findings with respect to the compliance status of the facility. As such, it is the key document of the audit program. The audit report should be a working, supportive document that will assist the facility staff in attaining and maintaining compliance.

Assuring that an audit report is accurate, precise, thorough, and helpful to facility staff is a considerable challenge. It requires proper preparation during the audit, deliberate efforts in the week following the audit, and a consistent follow-up program. This chapter discusses each of these equally important phases.

FIELD PREPARATION

Preparing well in the field is vital to developing a useful audit report. In most cases, a return trip to the site to gather overlooked information is infeasible. Follow-up phone calls are about the only avenue open to the auditor, and the information gathered from these remote efforts is not sufficiently verified.

Yet, an auditor can do several things to help ensure that sufficient data has been obtained to write the report without following up with the site later.

Keep the Customer in Mind

One of the key tenets of quality management, "keeping the customer in mind," is often forgotten in the heat of an audit battle. Audit reports should be written principally for facility management specifically and those responsible for correcting deficiencies. Yes, there are of course other customers. Senior management should have a sense of whether it has a problem facility on its hands after reading the executive summary. And there should indeed be an executive summary, for quite often that is all some reviewers will read.

However, the body of the report, the findings, must be written so that the reader both understands the nature of the problem and can readily envision corrective action. Thus, when the team leader reviews the report, they should put their "facility hat" on and ask, for every finding, "do I understand the problem well enough to know how to fix it?" If the answer is "yes," then the auditor has done the job of serving the customer.

Look for Underlying Causes

Root-cause analysis is a value-added effort and should not be ignored for efficiency's sake. For example, the lack of secondary containment at a hazardous waste storage facility might be due to

- an untrained site manager who is unaware of the requirements;
- the permitted use of a temporary location while a permanent one is being built;
- a disapproved capital improvement request by division management; and
- a general uncaring attitude on the part of site management.

The recommended corrective action will vary depending on which of the above is the underlying cause. In a case where site staff are not trained in the applicable requirements, simply constructing a dike or berm will not likely avoid the possibility of additional problems (e.g., wall penetrations) arising in the future.

Organize Daily

An individual auditor can produce hundreds of pages of field notes during the course of on-site work. How these field notes are recorded should be left to the personal preferences of each auditor. Some will use bound journals, some loose papers, and others loose-leaf or spiral-bound notebooks. Others may use a tablet or a smartphone or send themselves emails. Regardless of the technique used, it is imperative that the auditor take some time daily to organize their thoughts and findings. Otherwise, they will probably be unable to decipher their own work when it comes time to write the report. Daily organizing of the working papers or notes also allows the auditor to determine whether any particular area has been overlooked. This organization of tasks may require allocating some time each evening in a hotel room, but this will be time well spent.

Pinpoint the Bottom Line of Interviews

An auditor might interview scores of people during the on-site effort. Interviewing is probably the most important of the field activities. During an interview, an auditor is typically very busy—especially when, as is often the case, conducting the interview alone. The auditor will be referring to the protocols, company policies or procedures, asking questions, hopefully listening to the answers, and taking notes (hopefully good notes). Too often, auditors are thinking about what the next question should be, as opposed to truly listening to the answer. The auditor should not be intimidated by "dead airtime" during the course of the interview and should take some time to allow their notes to catch up with the conversation. You can even indicate to the interviewee that your pause is so that you can capture their feedback accurately.

Quite often, auditors question whether a small tape recorder or a voice recorder on a smartphone might help in documenting interviews. In general, this is not an effective or recommended approach. Interviewees quickly "clam up" when a recorder is present. If, however, the auditor later wishes to make notes to themselves on the tape recorder or smartphone as a way to document findings, this would be acceptable. It's not a crime scene.

Probably the most important thing an auditor can do is pinpoint the "bottom line" of the interview immediately following the interview itself. In other words, interviews should be scheduled so that time is available after the session to summarize their results quickly. The benefits of this effort will be realized later when the auditor attempts to write the report using field notes.

Another effective technique is to summarize the results of the interview at the end with the interviewee, that is, to repeat back to the individual one's perception of the key findings resulting from the conversation. The auditor will often learn that the recap has lost something in translation, and this gives the interviewee a final opportunity to clarify any misunderstandings.

Develop an Annotated Outline

The auditor should begin to develop an annotated outline of their sections of the report on the very first day. This will help in preparing for the debriefing and will serve as a check to ensure that all areas the auditor is responsible for are covered adequately. This effort will also aid in organizing field notes properly, as discussed above.

Challenge Each Other

In most cases, the audit team will be required to debrief site management as a way of concluding the fieldwork. It can almost be guaranteed that the audit team's findings will be challenged in this meeting. Therefore, it is important that the team members challenge each other's findings (respectfully) throughout the fieldwork in preparation for the debriefing. This often proves a valuable exercise and will result in more precise findings and in double-checking sources of information. Each team member should be aware of the benefits of this internal challenge and not immediately become defensive if another team member questions a finding. It's not about you as the auditor. It's about the evidence. And it's about the final product of the audit for the auditee.

Develop a Consistent Debriefing Approach

The debriefing is a vital part of the entire process. It informs facility staff of significant findings and clears up any misunderstandings held by the audit team. If the debriefing is structured properly, it can also provide the basis for the audit report. One good way to ensure that proper findings are eventually developed is to use a four-step process in communicating findings to site staff and management. Each finding should be communicated

1. when first observed;
2. during a daily meeting with site staff;
3. during a preclosing conference with site staff; and
4. during the closing conference with site management.

If the auditing team strictly adheres to this process, the closing conference should (hopefully) not be a contentious exercise.

REPORT PREPARATION

Having properly done everything in the field, the auditor is now prepared to undertake what many consider the most difficult part of the process: writing the report. The audit report typically includes a discussion of the audit process, an overview of the facility, an executive summary, and a presentation of findings and recommendations. The report addresses both regulatory and procedural findings. A regulatory deficiency is one involving an applicable regulatory obligation. A process or procedural deficiency is one involving internal requirements or good management practices, such as internal policies or procedures or any other standards such as ISO 9001, and so on. Findings are often classified as significant, major, or minor, or some make no reference to the priority of the finding at all. Still others base them on risk and categorize them as high, medium, or low. Where a finding is corrected prior to the departure of the audit team, the report will typically contain the finding but will indicate it as corrected. After all, the process needs to recognize all efforts of the auditee.

Audit team members will write those sections of the report that relate to the areas reviewed. The audit team leader is responsible for assigning other sections of the report (e.g., introduction, facility overview, and executive summary) to themselves or other team members. Based on past experience, team members would do well to adhere to the following guidance.

Organize for Monitoring

Many reports the authors have seen are rambling narratives in which it is difficult to sort background information from the findings. This does little to help the facility or allow for later tracking of corrective actions. The audit report should be organized so that the findings are broken down, listed, and codified. It is normally best to list only findings that are deficiencies. It makes little sense to codify a finding that requires no corrective action. If positive findings are listed, there will be a numbering gap in the sequencing of corrective actions, which can confuse those responsible for managing the close-out process. Save the positive findings and commendable items for the executive summary. Some use a Positive Finding section in their report template.

Some assign each finding of each report a two-field numerical code, which includes the year of the audit and the number of the finding. When coupled with a code for the plant that was audited, this allows for computerized tracking of the closure of all findings. This closure step is critical to the success of a program. In independent reviews of audit programs, problems with the management of the follow-up and closure system for findings are among the most commonly observed deficiencies.

Start Early

The auditor always returns to their office with good intentions. The first order of business is to complete the audit report. However, most people who have been away from the office for an extended period will spend the first couple of days back returning phone calls, reading emails, and catching up with the latest office politics. It is crucial that the auditor not let these distractions prevent them from completing the report in a timely fashion. To paraphrase Yogi Berra in this regard, "The more you procrastinate, the more you'll put it off." Procrastination builds on itself. The law of recency applies here. Start the report while events are still fresh in your mind.

As an auditor, you do not want to be in the position of committing to write a report in the field as you undertake yet another audit. Nor do you want to be back at your office with several reports due to team leaders. You can become quite confused in trying to recall exactly what you observed at any given site, especially if there is any ambiguity in your written notes.

Several approaches may help the auditor quickly complete the report. Developing an annotated outline before one leaves the facility is a technique that works well. One of the more interesting approaches is the increasing use of laptops or tablet computers in the field. In some cases, draft reports are basically completed before the team leaves the site. The laptops or tablets are also helpful in developing very impressive debriefing packages.

In summary, however, each auditor must do what works best for them. For many of us, simply taking an hour to organize our notes for one finding area and writing the first paragraph is enough to get us going. If we continue to struggle, reviewing a previous audit report should be a source of ideas on how to approach the material. And while we won't get into the area of Artificial Intelligence (AI) for this book, the advances in AI will, in our opinion, one day have the potential to revolutionize audit report writing. And while there may be ethical questions ahead in using AI for audit report writing, that day is quickly coming, we predict.

Establish a Report Format

Regardless of the report format chosen, it should be adhered to consistently so that subsequent audit reports are prepared in the same manner. This allows common elements of reports among different facilities to be compared. It also allows for easier assessment of how a specific facility is improving its compliance status over time via a comparison of findings in one report to those in subsequent audit reports.

The audit report should typically contain the same information each time. Generally speaking, section 1.0 is a brief executive summary written for upper management that highlights the key findings and recommendations of the audit report and any especially commendable items. Section 2.0 stipulates the who, what, where, and when information to familiarize the reader with the administrative aspects of the audit. Section 3.0 provides a general background on the facility.

Section 4.0, "Audit Findings and Recommendations," should be written with respect to noncompliance or nonconformance items as a first priority. Many companies take the viewpoint that the audit report should be an exception report; that is, the report should *only* document those items found to be deficient. Conditions found in compliance or in conformance with stated requirements are not documented, and an individual section begins with a phrase along the lines of "The facility was found to be generally in compliance and conformance to the requirements with the following exceptions . . ." Other companies take the view that all observations, both good and bad, should be documented.

The exception report approach appears to be the most prevalent form of documentation of audit findings by companies with audit programs.

Recommendations typically stipulate the auditor's suggestions on actions needed to come into compliance or conformance with stated requirements. These may range from simple administrative suggestions to recommendations for a capital improvement project (e.g., facility or plant upgrade). The recommendations may also focus on the need for additional investigation or further analysis before a final solution is chosen to correct the condition observed.

A significant issue of concern to companies with audit programs is the liability created when recommendations documented in an audit report are not implemented. The guidance that can be given is to document only recommendations that are known to be implementable by the facility. If there is some doubt that the audit's recommendations will be carried out (due to lack of resources, staffing, or funds), then it would be better to recommend that facility management come up with its own action plan to address the problems. In these cases, the auditors should focus on the what and not the how in the recommendation.

Specifying a responsible party and a time limit or date for a recommendation is more often left to the site's corrective-action plan. The concern about including a recommendation that cannot be implemented in an audit report is a valid one. Audit report writers should be sensitive to the positions in which they are potentially putting facility managers when they pose their recommendations.

Supporting data, such as tables of analytical data, copies of notices of violations, plot plans, schematics, and photographs, are sometimes included as attachments to the report to provide relevant backup information. There is great variability among audit programs regarding the inclusion of this material in a report. Photographs are excluded from many audit reports because they are considered to be potentially damaging and provide only a snapshot in time of the facility.

The benefits of including supplementary materials in a report should be weighed against the impact the material might have on the reader of the report. A picture may be worth a thousand words, but it might also be worth a thousand words to an attorney in the event the report is used as evidence in a legal case. A simple rule of thumb is to include only supplementary information that is absolutely needed to convey the point to the reader. If the point can be made clearly and completely in the body of the report, the use of supplementary material to support the finding should be discouraged. You're not writing the great American novel.

Pay Attention to Repeat Findings

The handling of findings that remain uncorrected from the previous audit is quite a challenge for most programs. Many auditors will argue, rightfully, that labeling them as "repeat" findings in the audit report creates added liabilities for the organization. Yet, for senior managers, it is important to know if documented problems are being corrected or if they are slipping through the cracks. Some would say that not knowing whether problems are being fixed is an even greater liability than documenting repeat findings.

Some organizations have a specific and proactive policy regarding repeat findings. The policy calls for auditors to pay particular attention to problems identified in the previous audit that have not been corrected. In classifying these findings, auditors are asked to consider assigning them a higher risk priority than would otherwise be the case.

Be Careful of Good Management Practices or Opportunities for Improvement (OFI)

Most audit programs classify findings into one of three types: regulatory, company policy or procedure, standard or good management practice (GMP), which some call opportunities for improvement (OFI). GMP/OFIs are sometimes also called good engineering practices or observations. Difficulty often arises in crafting effective GMP/OFI findings.

Hour-long discussions (or, more precisely, arguments) have occurred between the audit team and site management over the validity of a single GMP/OFI finding. The discussion usually centers on the justification for it. Auditor statements like "That's the way we do it at our site" or "We will accept nothing less than best-practice procedures" usually raise the hair on the back of the facility manager's neck.

There is a place for GMP/OFI findings in an audit report. Regulations or company policies or procedures do not always address all practices that might pose a risk to the organization. However, there needs to be solid justification for each GMP/OFI finding.

One way to develop that justification is to frame GMP/OFI findings in the same way as suggested above for repeat findings. What is the situation? What is the requirement? Too often, GMP/OFI findings begin with phrases such as "The site should . . ." or "The site needs to . . ." These are not findings; they are really "soft" recommendations. This is the trap that many auditors fall into, crafting GMP/OFI findings as recommendations with no supporting justification.

Set Priorities

Not all findings are created equal. Some are more important than others, and some left uncorrected present greater risk to the facility than others, although all need to be addressed. Thus, it is usually helpful to categorize findings by significance. Some companies do this by bringing the most important findings forward into the executive summary. In other cases, individual findings are classified by level of significance. The following three-tiered classification process, as follows, can be helpful:

1. *Significant:* A problem categorized as significant requires immediate action. It poses, or has a high likelihood of posing, a direct and immediate threat to human health or safety, the environment, or customer service. Some administrative issues can be categorized as significant. For example, failure to ensure that hazardous waste is destined for a permitted facility, failure to report when required, and failure to meet a compliance schedule are all significant deficiencies.
2. *Major:* A problem categorized as major requires action, but not necessarily immediate action. This category of deficiencies usually results in a notice of violation from regulatory agencies. Major deficiencies may pose a future threat to human health or safety, the environment, or the customer. Immediate threats, however, must be categorized as significant.
3. *Minor:* Minor deficiencies are mostly administrative in nature. They may involve temporary or occasional instances of noncompliance or nonconformance, and customers are seldom impacted.

An alternative to prioritizing audit findings can be similar to the following:

- Level I—highest-priority action required: This applies to findings that could result in substantial risk to the environment, the public, employees, stockholders, customers, the company, or its reputation or in criminal or civil liability for witting violations.
- Level II—priority action required: Findings included here do not meet the criteria for Level I but are more than isolated or occasional situations. They should not continue beyond the short term.
- Level III—action required: Findings in this category may be administrative in nature or involve isolated or occasional situations.

No matter what approach is used; however, there should be some way to establish priorities among findings and to highlight those items that are truly in need of immediate attention. Whatever your risk-based approach is, having a risk-based approach always rationalizes which items need priority attention, and why.

Be Clear and Concise

Generating a good audit report should not be an attempt to write the great American novel. Reports should not include gripping, suspenseful, or emotional stories. Findings should be written in a simple and straightforward manner based solely on observations, tests, and interviews. Use of general or vague statements will do little to help the reader understand the magnitude and nature of the issues found during the audit. Best put, the writer should put himself/herself in the facility manager's place and ask, "If I were to read this report, would I know the exact nature of the problem, and would I know how to resolve it?" Again, the auditor needs to be precise and accurate about underlying causes.

The importance of writing clear and precise audit reports and findings has been discussed at length in classic auditing texts. Here, the intent is to reinforce the importance of the topic and to suggest an approach to writing findings that can help achieve a quality product.

The use of indefinite adjectives should be discouraged or minimized in audit reports. "Very," "some," "significant," "small," "high," and the like are often found throughout audit reports, and their meaning and intent are wrongly left to the interpretation of the reader. One tip is to spend the time counting items when it is appropriate. For example, it is often a good idea to count drums at hazardous waste accumulation areas. Then, when it is reported that five drums were stored past the ninety-day deadline, the auditor can state whether it is five of ten or five of two hundred. There is a difference.

The auditor should not attempt to prove a point using sensational language or hyperbole in an audit report. Words such as "dangerous," "negligent," "willful," "criminal," and the like are often overstatements and imprecise, and they can lead to misinterpretation by the reader. They are subjective.

The auditor should also use proper English and avoid slang and excessive use of acronyms. The average length of sentences, according to writing experts, should range from fifteen to eighteen words; that is, short, crisp sentences make the technical information more easily digestible for the reader. Where acronyms are necessary, they should be spelled out the first time they are used, or the auditor should include a table of definitions or acronyms in the report.

Deemphasize Numbers

Quality management principles suggest that numerical quotas should be eliminated. In the context of an audit report, this suggests that one has to be very careful about how the number of findings is handled within the facility. It seems that no matter what is said or done, line managers and others have a tendency to add up the findings and compare. Perhaps this is just human nature, but this is neither a meaningful nor constructive exercise and should be discouraged by senior management.

It is nearly impossible to make effective performance evaluations solely by keeping track of the number of findings. First, individual facility situations differ greatly due to a variety of factors.

Second, audit teams differ in composition and makeup. One can send two different audit teams to the same location and have them audit something as straightforward as an accumulation point, and they will return with a wide variance in the number, priority, and type of findings.

Finally, as audit programs have evolved over the past few years, there has been a movement toward evaluating management systems. This has resulted in the "rolling up" of individual compliance findings into an overall system finding. This makes quantitative comparisons over time even more difficult.

In summary, using the number of audit findings as a measure of performance is fraught with problems. As an alternative, some companies have asked audit teams to classify the site overall. An example ranking system, based in part on a scheme sometimes used by financial auditors, might be to classify the site as follows:

- Good
- Meets most requirements
- Needs improvement
- Unacceptable

This approach is more compelling, although each of the classifications would have to be defined.

Use Evidence in the Discussion of Findings

During the course of the audit, evidence will be obtained using one of three methods: inquiry, observation, and testing, including document reviews. Inquiry gathers evidence through interviews; observation, not surprisingly, gathers it through visual inspection; and testing does so through means such as running an emergency-response drill or physical sampling, including document sampling (records, etc.). When writing findings in the audit report, the method of discovery should be clear from the language used. For example, where appropriate, phrases such as “it was observed” or “it was reported” should be used. This phrasing gives more meaning to the auditor’s findings.

The auditor should be very careful to avoid outright conjecture, that is, conclusions deduced by guesswork. This is a common pitfall in auditing. There should be at least one solid piece of evidence for each finding and probably two pieces of evidence for each significant finding. Speculation on the part of a maintenance supervisor that there might have been a fifty-gallon spill of perchloroethylene last month is not sufficient evidence. The supervisor may have been reprimanded recently and possibly wants to damage the reputation of the plant manager. When the auditor runs into this kind of situation, they should try to find corroborative evidence. This could include independent confirmation by another facility staff member, a spill report, or regulatory-agency correspondence. Where no confirmation can be made, the auditor should raise this issue at the debriefing. Usually, the issue will be resolved in one way or another in this forum.

REPORT FOLLOW-UP

With the report now finished, one could assume that the process is complete. It is not. Audit follow-up is a crucial part of the entire process. Without adequate follow-up, the system is likely to fail. One should pay special attention to the following items in particular.

Assure Legal Review of Reports where Required

Some companies manage their audit programs through their legal departments, due to concerns about protecting the confidentiality of the findings, especially where occupational health and safety or environmental management is concerned. Whether or not the audits are done under these mechanisms for protection, it is most prudent to have a lawyer review the draft audit report. The lawyer can help to ensure that legal references in the report are correctly stated and applied. More importantly, the lawyer can make suggestions regarding the wording and tone of the report from a legal point of view. It is a good rule of thumb to assume that the audit report may be discoverable in a subsequent legal proceeding against the company. Review of the draft report by the lawyer may be very helpful if he or she is required to defend the company in litigation.

Limit Distribution of the Report

The draft report should be sent to the facility and HSEQ managers for review within two weeks of the audit. That two weeks is a suggested target, but in our experience, it's a prudent target. A time limit should be stipulated for responses so that any disagreements can be resolved quickly. The facility staff should have no longer than a week to respond. Upon review, a final report should be issued. The final report should be distributed to upper management, as well as to the facility manager and his immediate supervisor.

Producing more copies of the audit report than needed, as stated above, should be discouraged. These extra copies tend to find their way to people who do not necessarily have a need to know. Many companies number the copies so that distribution can be controlled, and people can be held accountable for their copies of the report. Many companies have adopted a policy of destroying draft copies once a final report has been issued. Final reports are kept either indefinitely or until the next audit report is issued for that site. Some require that the auditors' notes and working papers be destroyed after the audit report has been issued. Others require their maintenance. Obviously, it is a good idea to develop a formal records-retention policy covering audit reports and associated documents and papers. If your facility is managed according to the documented information requirements (control of documents and records) of something like ISO 9001, you will perhaps have very good guidance here.

Accept No Mistakes

Not much needs to be said here. Audit reports should be mistake-free. The smallest typographical error should not be allowed, not even in a draft report. In fact, in the audit business, much like in the consulting business, there is really no such thing as a draft report. If it is to be sent to the client or customer, it can be considered final, no matter if words like "draft" or "preliminary" are used. Based on experience, we think it is better to take the heat for a report being a day or two late than for it being sloppy. People will remember a report with all the typos for ten years and will forget the perfect report within a month.

Every report should undergo a third-party review by someone not on the audit team. Also, do not rely solely on computer-software spell-checkers to eliminate all typos; they will not. Context for all words is very important. A human must conduct the final check.

Remove Barriers to Efficiency

Auditors must be given the tools to develop a high-quality report. This includes a sample audit report to be used as a guide. Many companies have also developed a separate audit report writing guide, which typically includes a discussion of the writing process, pitfalls to avoid, and a sample report with sample findings.

Develop Action Plans

Approaches to follow-up actions on audit findings vary among organizations. Still, this is viewed as one of the key factors of a successful audit program. Each audit report typically results in an action-item table generated by the facility, which lists each finding, the associated recommended remedial action, the responsible party, and the expected date of completion. Tracking can be accomplished by technology reports, follow-up phone calls to facility management, or by expedited follow-up audits.

Action-item tables are quite often entered into a computer database or something like Excel spreadsheets, and quarterly tracking reports are generated to monitor progress. Responsibility for this monitoring usually rests with the audit program leader, who may delegate it to audit team leaders for particular facilities. The option of whether to give facility staff the ability to revise information on the database or spreadsheet is handled in a variety of ways. In some cases, the system is secured with password protection, preventing entry by anyone but an auditor.

Regardless of which method is used, the audit process is not complete unless some formal measures are instituted to ensure that each of the audit findings and recommendations has been addressed by the facility staff. Clearly, some recommendations made in an audit report may involve large capital expenditures that cannot be made immediately. In this case, including the item in a subsequent year's capital-expenditure plan is an appropriate step, as long as this action does not implicitly condone continuing noncompliance or nonconformance. Corrective actions do not necessarily have to take place immediately. As long as the facility management has a reasonable schedule for completion and is tracking the status of corrective measures, it can demonstrate a good-faith effort to operate in a responsible manner.

More recently, companies have established firm deadlines for the completion of any and all action items. These have ranged from 120 days to six months, to one year. Should any action item require longer than the established deadline, a senior executive must formally sign off on the exception. In the experience of the authors, some organizations have made it a policy that they will never extend the timeline for the completion of an action. In their opinion, this "creep" has the potential to keep pushing actions out longer and longer. They pick a target due date and stick with it. If it continues to be late or past due, so be it. That's what their action status reports will profile.

Train the Auditors

Train, train, and retrain! All auditors should receive formal training before they embark on their first audit. A good part of this training should deal with report writing or, at a minimum, the writing of individual findings. Receiving on-the-job training in how to write findings at an inopportune time (e.g., on a Thursday night at 11:00 p.m.) for someone's first audit is no fun. Unfortunately, though, this happens too often.

Preparing a quality audit report is a difficult task. It takes time, effort, discipline, and lucidity. But the effort is well worth it. The report is the decision-making document for the HSEQ audit program.

REFERENCES

This chapter has been adapted from Lawrence B. Cahill and Raymond W. Kane. *Environmental Health and Safety Audits*, 9th Edition. Government Institutes, 2010. It has been updated for this edition.

Wayne Pardy and Terri Andrews. *Integrated Management Systems: Leading Strategies and Solutions*, 2nd Edition. Bernan Press, 2019.

Chapter 15

Planning to Achieve High-Quality HSEQ Audits

Twenty Tips for Success

It is one thing to show a man that he is in error, and another to put him in the possession of the truth.

—John Locke, 1632–1704

DEVELOP AND MAINTAIN A "LIVING" AGENDA THROUGHOUT THE AUDIT

Audits consist of records, reviews, interviews, and physical observations sandwiched between an opening and closing conference. Generally, records are reviewed right after the opening meeting and facility orientation tour. If the team is tasked with developing a draft report or draft set of findings while on-site, they usually need time specifically to prepare these findings. This occurs just before the closing conference and sometimes late at night. Auditors should develop an agenda that allows for this logical approach. This agenda should be sent to the site ahead of time so that appropriate interviews and location visits can be scheduled. The agenda should be adjusted constantly during the audit, depending on what the audit team is finding and any changes in the daily work schedules of the site staff.

Leave an open slot in the agenda just before you are scheduled to prepare the findings. This time will never go to waste. There will be additional people to interview, records to review, and locations to visit to further verify your findings.

YOU WILL NEVER FINISH, SO MANAGE YOUR TIME WISELY

We have never been on an audit where the team managed to review every single HSEQ document or interview all site staff involved in HSEQ management or compliance—if for no other reason than that there is simply not enough time on an audit to cover over a dozen areas using a census-type approach. Moreover, audit sampling (statistical or otherwise) is a time-honored approach that allows one to capture the salient issues on the relevant topics. This sampling of records or interview candidates does not mean that the audit is incomplete, just that audit teams need to use their time wisely, spending more time on higher-priority issues. So, use your "living agenda" to continuously set your priorities.

Remember, it is better to address all areas to some extent than to ignore one or two areas entirely. Thus, the audit agenda should be structured so that each team member conducts his or her assessments in parallel, not in series. For example, if one team member is tasked with reviewing customer service, security, environmental management, or safety procedures, they should do some initial review of each area on the first day of the audit and not leave one area for the last day. By reviewing each of the areas upfront, time priorities can be established based on the relative risks identified. The auditor will not be caught in the uncomfortable position of not leaving enough time for one or more full compliance areas. This parallel approach will also help to identify whether any key site individuals might not be available later in the week. Their interviews can then be moved up.

KEEP A BALANCE BETWEEN RECORDS REVIEW, INTERVIEWS, AND OBSERVATION

The audit team leader is always challenged by the different tendencies of individual team members. Some auditors are bored or intimidated by paperwork and ready to undertake the physical audit almost immediately. Some people are more comfortable with field-level activities than office-based tasks. This can be very risky, even where the auditor has encyclopedic knowledge of regulations and company policies, procedures, or standards. Many requirements are found in site permits and licenses; ignoring these before you interview and observe activities can be perilous. Review records first.

On the other hand, some auditors can be intimidated by the interview process or inspecting the physical facility itself. These auditors will pore over records until they have them virtually memorized. The team leader needs to push these individuals into the field to ensure an adequate verification process.

As with most things in life, balance is the key. Try to avoid your own tendencies to focus on one or two of the three core audit activities.

"THINGS" WILL HAPPEN ON THE AUDIT, SO BE FLEXIBLE

Have you ever had an auditor become unavailable in the middle of an audit because they got a "come home now" call from their spouse or been called back to the office? Has there ever been a surprise agency inspection during an audit in which you participated? Has your otherwise reliable laptop gone on the fritz, or you can't get a secure Wi-Fi connection as you were preparing the draft report? If you audit long enough, any or all of these things will happen to you, and more.

Be flexible and have a contingency plan for unexpected occurrences. If you are participating in an audit team because of your fall protection expertise, do not be surprised if you are asked to help out with confined-space entry, especially if you finish early. That's why organizations develop audit protocols—to help guide the auditor through a compliance and/or systems review.

An agency inspection or other outside activity (e.g., Regulatory inspection by US OSHA or Transport Canada, or an ISO 9001 surveillance or re-registration audit) might also take place during the week. Some adept scheduling or scoping changes can minimize the impact of these distractions. It is generally not appropriate to postpone or cancel the audit once the team is on-site, especially if a significant expense was involved in getting the audit team on site.

If you rely on information technology, always have some kind of backup for your laptop or tablet, presentation device, or printer, especially overseas. Check ahead of time to see if the facility has compatible computer capabilities. Typed draft reports are impressive; having the facility staff stand around a computer screen because you do not have the correct printer driver is not. One option is to write findings neatly on a preprinted digital form as they are developed. These digital forms can be inserted into the report if time allows, but they can also be used as presentation handouts if technology fails.

If you intend to develop a formal draft report for the closing conference, as many organizations do, schedule the audit so that the report can be printed and copied the night before. Giving yourself two hours on a Friday morning to accomplish the final editing, printing, and copying of the report or handout materials is flirting with catastrophe. A late night on Thursday can decrease the team's anxiety considerably. It is also usually better to work through the final stages at the facility and have a late dinner as opposed to having dinner and then working on the report. A lot of momentum and energy can be lost after dinner.

And be careful about designing a program approach that ensures the team will work until 2:00 a.m. the night before the closing conference. Aside from those individuals who relish the pain of a late night, audit team members typically do not find it a morale booster, and it does not have to be an integral part of each audit.

ALWAYS BE ON TIME, EVEN WHEN THE FACILITY STAFF ARE NOT

Always, always be on time during audits. On the other hand, the audit team may find that facility staff are not always available for prescheduled interviews. This can happen because of normal day-to-day interruptions. Remember, facility staff still have to perform their normal job duties during the audit. Unless the lateness or no-show problem becomes chronic, the audit team should "grin and bear it." As the saying goes, "Half of life is just showing up."

REMEMBER SITE STAFF WILL ALWAYS CONSIDER AUDITS A PERFORMANCE EVALUATION

As much as we kid about the saying, "We're from corporate, and we're here to help you," second- or third-party audits are generally intended to be a supportive exercise. Yet, there is no way to completely avoid the facility staff's feeling that their personal performance is being evaluated. While you can tell them not to take it personally, guess what—many invariably take it personally. That is probably because it is true, especially on management-systems audits. Auditors should never forget this and should therefore strive to be empathetic (to understand, be aware of, and be sensitive to the feelings, thoughts, and experiences of another) without becoming sympathetic (feeling loyalty or tending to favor or support). That's why it's important to focus your efforts on the objective evidence—not individuals.

REMEMBER THAT DESPITE THE EXISTENCE OF GOVERNMENTAL REGULATIONS AND COMPANY POLICIES, PROCEDURE OR ISO STANDARDS, CONSIDERABLE JUDGMENT IS STILL REQUIRED

Isn't it comforting to know that the corporation has prepared audit protocols for us that define precisely the government regulations and company and

ISO procedures and standards against which we will audit? It takes all the guesswork out of the review, right? No, of course it doesn't. Probably a good 25 percent of all findings in an audit have very little to do with requirements definitively prescribed in protocols. Even where requirements are provided, sometimes the specific facility applicability is complex. One also has to be cognizant of the fact that even detailed regulatory protocols only serve as a guide because they can never be completely up to date. As a consequence, auditors should always receive some sort of training prior to that first audit. This will help immeasurably in their learning to apply practical interpretations to complicated situations.

REMEMBER THAT EVERY COUNTRY, STATE, PROVINCE, AND REGION IS DIFFERENT

Audit teams need to reflect the differences in local requirements on every audit. Yet, the lack of an independent review of country, state, province, and regional differences and realities is one of the most common deficiencies observed in audit programs. Auditors, then, are often expected to conduct an independent review of the local realities of their audit scope.

The challenge of undertaking an adequate regulatory review is magnified with overseas audits. Even national-level regulations are difficult to obtain and often require extensive translation. Some of the commercial databases have recognized this problem and compiled HSEQ regulations for a number of developed countries.

LEARN AND APPLY THE AUDIT PROTOCOLS, BUT DO NOT FORGET TO USE YOUR COMMON SENSE AND NATURAL CURIOSITY

It is comforting for most auditors to have access to an extensive set of audit protocols. It is literally impossible to have total recall of all regulatory requirements and company policies, procedures, or standards on any given audit, even where the auditor might be responsible for only one area (e.g., procurement). The protocols will guide the review, but they do not replace common sense and natural curiosity. Asking naive, open-ended questions that are not in the protocol can result in some remarkable answers. Don't be uncharacteristically intentionally "stupid" but do ask questions which, to you, might seem stupid. Examples include, where does this drain lead to and how do you know? What if this vessel were to rupture? Why doesn't your boiler need a permit? What if the HSEQ coordinator is not on-site when an incident occurs? What happens if you lose your customer's property? Auditors should let their natural instincts guide them in their interviews.

TRY TO OBSERVE THINGS AS THEY HAPPEN

Verification is, to varying extents, what auditing is all about, but audit teams do not always accomplish this effectively. This can be a special challenge overseas. Different cultures have different value systems, and individuals may react in surprising ways to requests for verification. It may seem perfectly logical in North America to request training records to verify the statement by the site HSEQ coordinator that staff have been trained properly. This same request could be considered an insult in other cultures.

To maximize the verification process, auditors should attempt to observe key activities as they occur. These activities could include spill drills, wastewater and air-emissions sampling, routine inspections, chemical loading and unloading, and waste pickups by contractors. It is one thing to read in the standard operating procedures how these activities are to be conducted (e.g., "There will always be a company person attending all loading and unloading of hazardous chemicals or wastes"); it is quite another to actually observe them in practice.

Auditors should review both the design and implementation or operation of physical and management systems. Many an emergency-response plan has met the regulatory requirements, but because of a lack of training or drills, the plan is ineffectual when implemented during a real emergency. It is common to observe in an audit situation perfectly acceptable secondary-containment system designs have been compromised by poor operating practices (e.g., valves kept in the open position, containers stored on or outside the dike wall, breaches in the containment wall created to allow fork trucks to enter the area). The engineer had the right design in mind originally, but the operators, because of other demands, have negated the system's effectiveness. The bottom line for the auditor is to make sure that all plans and procedures created in response to regulatory and company requirements are actually practiced in the field. Test the systems.

OBSERVE ANCILLARY OPERATIONS (IF POSSIBLE)

On too many audits, the auditors fall into the trap of spending most of their time with the HSEQ coordinator and, to a lesser extent, line managers and operators. Not only should more time be spent with line operations, but the team should also increase its efforts in reviewing ancillary operations such as maintenance, site purchasing, document control, and on-site contractors, especially if you're auditing to any of these requirements in the respective ISO Standards we've been referencing.

For example, maintenance, which is usually assessed for its safety compliance (e.g., machine guarding, confined-space entry), also handles numerous hazardous chemicals including oils, degreasers, and chlorinated fluorocarbons used in the air-conditioning system. Some of these machines might also support of a customer-related process or service. Maintenance is often overlooked when audit teams are making these determinations.

Site purchasing can also pose quite a challenge to facility auditing. A classic component of any audit of management systems is to ensure that there is a procedure in place for purchasing to notify the site HSEQ staff when new chemicals arrive on-site. If there is proper notification, safety data sheet (SDS) books and systems can be updated, regulatory threshold determinations can be made, and the chemicals can be added to any regulatory reports, if and when required. The auditors should also determine if quantities of chemicals can possibly arrive on-site without going through on-site purchasing. At times, a business unit can acquire materials through central or divisional purchasing, thereby bypassing on-site purchasing. These potential channels of acquisition must be explored in audits.

OBSERVE, ARTICULATE, AND WRITE—IN THAT ORDER

Auditing is a process that, hopefully, results in clearly articulated findings. Some auditors forget that an effective process begins and ends with an observation in the field that must then be presented orally in the closing conference and then written into the report.

When auditors do not take detailed notes about what they have observed, they often find themselves in serious trouble. Trust us—we've learned this the hard way. Reporting in the closing conference that there "were some hazardous waste drums without labels" or that "several safety data sheets were missing from the maintenance shop book" reflects improper investigation and is not helpful to the site in determining the appropriate response. Auditors must clearly define what they observe in the field and translate it precisely and accurately in the closing conference and audit report. Clear definitions come from meticulous note-taking.

REMEMBER THAT WRITING IS THE HARDEST PART; DEVELOPING "BULLETPROOF" FINDINGS IS AN ELUSIVE GOAL

Findings are verified statements of fact. Auditors should leave conjecture, speculation, hearsay, and editorializing for other endeavors. Sounds simple enough, right? This is, of course, easier said than done. Developing unassailable findings is the most difficult part of the entire process, especially as audit programs move more toward management-systems reviews. How does one communicate that an organization is not very effective in achieving its goals? Not easily. Nonetheless, each auditor should strive to develop findings that, when challenged, will withstand intense scrutiny from the site. Appropriate evidence gathering and verification will provide the foundation upon which an auditor can build an effective case.

WRITE THE FINDINGS AS YOU GO

Experienced auditors find that it is one thing to communicate a finding verbally in a closing conference and quite another to communicate it in a draft report. Many times, when the site reads the written findings for the first time a few weeks after the audit, the response is, "But that's not what you said in the meeting." Accordingly, many audit programs aim to prepare and distribute a draft report for the closing conference. This considerable amount of extra on-site work is generally worth the effort as the site can respond to the actual report that will be distributed to management.

This approach means that the audit team must prepare written findings as they go in order to avoid pulling an all-nighter the night before the closing conference. This also adds discipline to the audit process and means that the audit team leader will not have to rely on team members preparing audit findings once they have returned to their respective offices, a risky proposition at best. Most companies use standard forms or templates to compile individual findings as well as laptop or tablet computers and report templates to expedite the process.

PREPARE WELL FOR THE OPENING AND CLOSING CONFERENCES

Opening and closing conferences are key to establishing audit team credibility. As they are the main interface between site management and the audit team, the team is often judged by its performance in these forums. Good presentation skills and communicating technically correct information are integral to success. The conferences work better when auditors use standard presentation tools developed by the corporate audit group. Auditors should also listen attentively to questions and respond directly. If they do not know the answer, they should admit it and commit to gathering the information needed to respond.

MAKE SURE THE FACILITY HEARS THE REAL STORY IN THE CLOSING CONFERENCE

There will be a tendency to soften the findings in a closing conference. The environment can be very intimidating, in part because the audit team leader is reporting findings to the facility manager, who might be several positions higher in the organizational hierarchy. As a consequence, many closing conferences begin with high, subjective praise for the facility staff and operations. While this approach is fine, if warranted, the facility manager must also hear any significant issues clearly. This means that the audit team leader should separate these issues from the rest and communicate them with emphasis. It is best to highlight these priority issues together as a group early in the closing conference. By waiting until the end to wrap up the high-priority issues, one runs the risk that the facility manager will have been called out of the meeting and may miss the importance of the message.

PLAN TO BE DONE WHEN YOU DEPART

The audit team should minimize the number of issues requiring future analysis. The facility staff will want to be assured that in the closing conference they are hearing what will appear in the final report. Although the audit team should make no guarantees in this regard, the team should be close to 100 percent finished before leaving the site. If findings surface later, it is common courtesy for the audit team leader to communicate those to the site HSEQ staff or facility management prior to their appearance in the draft or final reports.

ENJOY YOURSELF

HSEQ auditing is hard work but personally and professionally rewarding. There is always something new to learn in an audit, no matter how many you have done. Take advantage of the trip; experience the local audit city or town, whether it is the U.S. Midwest, Atlantic Canada, or Asia-Pacific. You might never return to that location again.

REFERENCES

This chapter has been adapted from Lawrence B. Cahill and Raymond W. Kane. *Environmental Health and Safety Audits*, 9th Edition. Government Institutes, 2010. It has been updated for this edition.

Wayne Pardy and Terri Andrews. *Integrated Management Systems: Leading Strategies and Solutions*, 2nd Edition. Bernan Press, 2019.

Chapter 16

HSEQ Audit Guidance

On-Site Activities

A certain amount of opposition is a great help to a man. Kites rise against, not with, the wind

—John Neal, 1793–1876

Every HSEQ audit typically consists of three phases: preaudit preparation, on-site activities, and post-audit report-writing and follow-up. During the on-site phase, trained and experienced professionals are expected to conduct rigorous evaluations of the audited site's HSEQ practices. In most cases, this expectation is met. Independent observation of numerous audits suggests that on-site activities typically represent the strongest aspect of the HSEQ audit.

Nonetheless, on-site audit activities frequently fall short of the ideal. Problems are especially likely to arise when companies do not utilize full-time auditors but instead borrow HSEQ professionals from other parts of the organization. "On-loan" personnel will be restricted by the amount of time their management determines they can be made available. With such sporadic involvement in the auditing process, it is sometimes difficult for them to maintain the sharp edge needed for an effective audit.

The guidance presented here is intended to help those who conduct HSEQ audits by allowing them to learn from the experiences of others.

KEY ON-SITE ACTIVITIES

The on-site audit process tends to be a complex (and intense) undertaking for both auditors and facility personnel. It typically consists of the following activities:

- Opening conference with facility management.
- Site orientation tour.
- Review of site HSEQ management systems and related processes.
- Records review.
- Interviews with personnel.
- Field observations.
- Daily meetings with facility staff.
- Daily audit team meetings.
- Preparation of audit findings and recommendations.
- Preparation of the preliminary draft report.
- Preclosing conference discussion with the audit team.
- Closing conference with the plant manager.

When these activities are not performed well, any number of problems can arise. Given the complexity of the on-site process, it would be difficult to achieve a perfect audit—although that of course is the goal.

COMMON ON-SITE PROBLEMS—AND HOW TO COPE WITH THEM

Discussed below are some of the scenarios of on-site HSEQ audit problems that can be encountered most frequently:

- Poor time management (for both the audit team and facility management).
- Inadequate sampling and verification.
- Poor balance among record reviews, interviews, and observations.
- Disorganized records review.
- Poor interviewing techniques.
- Poor communication of findings.
- Poorly structured closing conferences.

Watch out for these pitfalls and put plans in place to avoid them.

Poor Time Management

Failure to Understand How Much Time Is Actually Available

In general, typically only about 50 percent of an auditor's on-site time is spent on "core" audit activities (records review, interviews, and field observations). The remainder is taken up by meetings, orientation tours, preparation for the closing conference, and the like. So, when you are told that you will be involved in a four-day HSEQ audit, remember that you will typically have only two days to verify HSEQ compliance and conformance requirements.

Clearly, time management is critical. Mistakes made early in the week can result in a miserable night before the closing conference. Too many audits end with auditors attempting to craft eloquent and accurate findings at 2:00 a.m. It cannot be done. Or if able to be done, many times it is not done well.

Tips for avoiding the problem: Develop your own personal, detailed agenda for the on-site audit. Review your progress against the agenda daily and make adjustments accordingly. Allow for contingency time at the end of the audit, should things not go exactly as planned. Trust us. Things invariably do not go as planned.

Poorly Designed Audit Agendas

Developing an agenda in advance of the audit helps ensure that all scope topics are covered sufficiently. But remember that the agenda must be a living document. Most agendas require change—often beginning early on as a result of opening conference discussions.

Be aware of agenda "red flags." For example, if (as an audit team member) you receive an agenda from the team leader that presupposes the team will be writing audit findings or a draft report until midnight on the evening before the closing conference, question that approach. Audits typically are very intense exercises, but there is no reason they should be designed to be "hell on earth." Such an approach just reduces the available auditor pool very quickly and can generate a perception that the process "doesn't pay you enough" for the effort required.

Tips for avoiding the problem: Review the overall audit agenda carefully. Get a good understanding from the team leader of how he or she intends to manage the last full day.

Team leaders should clearly define in advance when field audit activities must be completed and then hold firmly to that deadline. For example, team members might be told that all field verification must be completed by Thursday at 1:00 p.m. The remainder of the time on-site can then be used to write up findings and conduct a closing conference on Friday morning.

This schedule may not prevent Thursday evening from becoming a test of patience, but it works better than simply allowing audit team members to continue conducting field-verification activities until 6:00 p.m. That approach almost mandates a very late evening.

Failure to Focus Full Attention on the Audit

Time-management problems often arise because auditors fail to focus fully on the audit activities at hand. How does this happen? Most often, it is because auditors become sidetracked from their on-site activities by a perceived need to respond to other job responsibilities via cell phone calls, voice mail, and email. These intrusions are very disruptive to the flow of the audit, and they can become a chronic problem. When the first question an audit team member asks site staff is, "Where can I set up my computer so that I can access my e-mail?" anticipate problems ahead.

Tips for avoiding the problem: Establish a policy that audit team members will use cell phones and access email and voice mail *only* during lunch or other suitable breaks. High-speed Internet connections and Wi-Fi are available in most hotels these days; non-audit-related communications can be made quite easily in the mornings and evenings.

Failure to Schedule Time Needed to Produce On-Site Deliverables

Audits vary widely regarding the output expected from the team at the conclusion of on-site activities. In some cases, it is simply a verbal debriefing. In others, it is a draft set of findings. In still others, it is a complete draft report. Sometimes the technology you may be leveraging will determine which approach you'll follow. When there is inadequate communication regarding on-site output expectations, time-management problems almost always arise—usually accompanied by unpleasant verbal exchanges ("You should have told me you wanted a complete set of findings by Thursday close of business!"). In addition, when all findings write-up activities are left for later, there is a tendency to let them slide. Reports may be issued months after the audit—or not at all. This is unprofessional at best, unacceptable at worst.

Tips for avoiding the problem: Auditors should set aside time to develop a draft set of findings (if not a draft report) while still on-site. Do not be afraid to schedule an extra half day on-site in order to ensure that you have time to prepare at least a draft set of findings prior to leaving. You will have to spend time on this step anyway; you might as well do it while the audit is fresh in your mind. A solid knowledge of the audit report format will help make the process more efficient.

Inadequate Sampling and Verification

HSEQ auditors must be thorough in their field activities. This is true whether the activity is a review of paperwork or a physical inspection of facility infrastructure or equipment. But being thorough does not necessarily mean that the auditor must review hundreds of records. HSEQ auditors commonly use sampling when a large number of items need to be reviewed. Formal statistical sampling procedures can provide a means for identifying the number of items that must be reviewed in order to gain reasonable confidence that your results are representative. You must beware of the pitfalls involved in sampling and verification, however.

Improper Sample Size

Auditors often struggle to determine the proper level of sampling. On the one hand, it would be a mistake to draw conclusions based on a sample of one. On the other hand, the auditor can spend so much time reviewing records on a particular issue that other audit areas are compromised.

Tips for avoiding the problem: Not all sampling must be statistically representative. As with everything, there is a balance. In general, the "rule of threes" applies. Thus, for example, at least three instances of noncompliance or nonconformance should exist before the auditor can draw the conclusion that there is a finding. This is not a hard-and-fast rule, simply an audit guideline. Another rule commonly used in HSEQ audits is to sample 10 percent of the population. This applies generally to larger populations. Currently, there is no specific guidance from any standard-setting organization on whether statistically representative sampling must be used on audits, although certain audit organizations may have prescriptive guidance or requirements here. So, use your judgment.

Remember that auditors can never really "finish." There is always another record to review or another person to interview. Keep in mind that you are not doing a census. Do not spend too much time on any one topical area at the expense of others. Balance is crucial. It is a snapshot, not an ongoing commentary.

Lack of Auditor Independence in Verification Activities

When reviewing records, interviewing staff members, or observing physical activities, the auditor must decide not only how many, but which ones, to review. Too often, the audit site's staff may make the decision about who should be interviewed or which documents should be reviewed. Although this can offer the path of least resistance for the auditor, it compromises the independence of the audit and will likely bias the results.

Tips for avoiding the problem: When determining who should be interviewed or what documents should be reviewed, the auditor—not site personnel—should decide. As an example of how to proceed, the auditor might ask for a list of employees who have received hazardous waste training, fall protection training, or training in ISO 9001. In order to verify the adequacy of the training, the auditor can then randomly select from this list people to interview and training records to review. Proceeding this way ensures a more independent approach to verification.

Lack of Field Verification

The old adage "Say what you do, do what you say" is highly relevant to HSEQ audits. Added to that saying is the caveat, "prove it and/or demonstrate that it's effective." Too often, auditors review site procedures and plans for relevancy and completeness but fail to verify whether such procedures and plans are actually being implemented as claimed. Field verification is a critical step in the audit process.

Tips for avoiding the problem: Auditors should look for opportunities to field-verify plans and procedures. In the case of HSEQ audits, excellent areas for verification include

- new construction or demolition;
- emergency-response drills;
- inspections and sampling;
- loading and unloading;
- materials handling and transfer;
- process and equipment start-ups or shutdowns; and
- waste packing and pickup.

Remember, substantial field verification should be undertaken during an HSEQ audit.

Here's a recent practical example. The audit scope required that on an annual basis the facility conduct a "comprehensive risk assessment" of all their processes. The result was to be a record of that risk assessment which was then intended to inform facility staff of the risks and hazards associated with their work. At the time of the audit, the HSE staff presented the record for the last comprehensive risk assessment which they had completed, including when it was completed and who was involved. All in all, it was a very good process and document for what had been accomplished. The only issue was that it was not as "comprehensive" as it should have been. They forgot to include a very important aspect of their operation—the garage area. A field visit to the garage confirmed this, and interviews with the mechanic confirmed it as well.

So, while they had what they believed to be a comprehensive risk assessment for the facility, omitting the very important risk-based issues in the garage meant that it was not in fact comprehensive and that they needed to include the scope of the work performed in the garage as well. The evidence was clear, and there was no pushback. Action was needed to ensure the garage was included in the comprehensive risk assessment going forward.

Poor Balance among Records Review, Interviews, and Observations

Although the on-site HSEQ audit phase typically includes a wide range of tasks, three activities form the "core" of every on-site audit: records review, interviews, and field observations. All auditors have a tendency to gravitate toward their activity comfort zone. For some, it is records review. For others, it is field observations. For a few, it is interviews. This tendency can lead auditors to spend the majority of their time on only one of the core activities, at the expense of the others. The result is an unbalanced approach to auditing.

Tips for avoiding the problem: Auditors should keep track of how much time they spend on each of the three core audit activities. In general, the "rule of thirds" should apply. That is, an auditor should spend roughly one-third of his or her time on each of the three core audit activities.

Disorganized Records Review

HSEQ requirements can potentially generate tons of paper and thousands of electronic records. Deciding how to approach a review of these records can be a daunting task—and one that trips up many auditors. Auditors should recognize that although records are critical to demonstrating compliance, they are not the whole story. Spending a majority of your time on records review compromises the efficacy of the audit.

Tips for avoiding the problem: Reviewing records is not a random undertaking. There should be a method to the review. Following the steps listed below will make for a more efficient and effective records review process:

1. Obtain what records you can ahead of time (within reason).
2. Make records review your first on-site activity. Many auditable requirements can be found in the documents.
3. Do not get overwhelmed; stay organized.
4. Start with "strategic" documents, such as written programs or procedures.
5. Ask for quiet time if you need it. Nobody wants to be watched while reading.
6. While reviewing records, develop a list of requirements to verify later through interviews or observations.

Poor Interviewing Techniques

Proper (and while "proper" can be subjective, we will use the word "proper") interviewing is perhaps one of the single most important elements of the on-site HSEQ audit process—and one of the most challenging for many auditors. During the audit, you may need to interview people with a wide range of roles and responsibilities, including site management, site staff, line management, site HSEQ management, and unit supervisors or operators. Unfortunately, auditors often do not recognize that they must modify their style depending on the person being interviewed. Remember . . . it's not about you. Skilled interviewers will be sensitive to individuals' nervousness and different personalities, while still obtaining responses that enable them to accurately evaluate past and current HSEQ operating practices.

In many cases, auditors fail to verify interviewees' statements through records review and physical observation. "Trust but verify" is the mantra. This verification step should be used routinely in auditing, and site staff should understand that it is not meant as a challenge to their truthfulness. It's simply one of the steps you have to take as an auditor to ensure a professional outcome for your audit efforts.

Tips for avoiding the problem: The following steps can help you conduct more effective interviews:

- Always introduce yourself. You never know what interviewees may have heard about "the auditors."
- Explain what you are doing. Be succinct.
- Try to put interviewees at ease and relieve their stress. Ask them about their jobs.
- Ask open-ended questions ("Tell me about . . . ," not "Do you . . .").
- Do not be captive to your checklist. Share the checklist with the interviewee and use it as a guide—not the "bible."
- Ask about previous audits the interviewees may have experienced. What were their impressions?
- Wait for the interviewee to answer. Do not get impatient—some people actually need time to think before they speak.
- Demonstrate that you are listening. The interviewee should be doing the great majority of the talking.
- Keep the discussion on track. It is acceptable to talk about fishing for a while—but only for a while.
- Restate key findings at the end of the interview. See if the interviewee agrees with them.
- Avoid taking excessive notes during the interview. Extensive note-taking can be very intimidating.
- Keep names of interviewees confidential. Explain that individuals' names do not appear in the audit report.
- Do interviews one-on-one if possible. This is more relaxing for the interviewee.

- Distinguish between inquiry and observation. Do not ask a lot of questions about things you can see for yourself.
- Follow up on leads from interviews. This helps identify root causes.

When you have an auditor who spends more time talking about their experiences and "war stories" than they do listening to the auditee, you're in for a problem. Ok . . . your trip to Japan sounds very interesting, but keep it for lunch or a break. Don't do the auditee the discourtesy of regaling them with the boring details of your vacation or travel experiences (yes . . . this has actually happened!).

Poor Finding Communication

Full, accurate, and timely communication of findings is crucial to a successful audit. Too often, however, auditors wait until the closing conference to communicate their findings to site management and staff. This is a very risky approach for at least two reasons. First, your findings could come as a total surprise to facility personnel and others on the audit team (never a good thing). Second, your findings might actually be in error (this can happen if you have failed to get staff feedback that would allow you to track issues down completely). Obviously, either of these outcomes is undesirable.

Tips for avoiding the problem: Auditors should communicate their findings to facility personnel in a four-stage process:

1. When first observed (even if you are not totally convinced yet that you indeed have a finding).
2. At the daily conference (to get feedback and calibration from site staff).
3. At the preclosing conference or meeting with the audit team (to get confirmation and agreement).
4. At the closing conference (to ensure that the facility manager receives the message firsthand).

When you use this four-step process, your audit team may actually be able to achieve an unusual (but highly desirable) outcome—a boring closing conference.

Poorly Structured Closing Conferences

The closing conference is the final on-site HSEQ audit activity. It typically involves the full audit team, the facility manager, the site HSEQ staff, and selected facility staff—typically the same people who were in attendance for the opening meeting, if they are still around and can make it. The basic objective of the meeting is for the audit team to report back to the facility on the findings of the audit.

The closing conference can be a stressful meeting, especially if the audit team is working right up to the last minute to produce a typed formal list of findings or a draft report. A mishandled closing conference can jeopardize an otherwise excellent audit effort. Issues to watch out for include

- unsubstantiated findings;
- "surprise" findings that have not been discussed previously;
- disagreement on a finding or its priority;
- an unengaged audience that is unwilling to discuss the merits of the findings until the draft report has been issued; and
- breakdown of computers, projection equipment, or copiers.

Tips for avoiding the problem: For any on-site HSEQ audit closing conference, the following guidelines apply:

- Take charge of the closing conference.
- Be organized and professional.
- Be appreciative, but do not bury or "sugarcoat" the message.
- Highlight the highest-priority and repeat findings.
- Minimize praise for "acceptable" performance.
- Respond professionally to challenges.
- Focus on root causes and management system risks or opportunities.
- Avoid evaluations of staff performance.
- Leave written findings behind, if technically able.

During the closing conference itself, remember to do the following:

- Outline the meeting's agenda and explain how long the meeting will last.
- Review the audit's scope and objectives.
- Start your remarks on a positive note.
- Thank everyone for their cooperation.
- Communicate your findings objectively and specifically.
- Discuss follow-up requirements.

Remember that leading an effective closing conference is quite a challenge. It is analogous to visiting a friend's home and criticizing their housekeeping as you leave.

THE TOP THREE THINGS TO REMEMBER

If all else fails, remember the following rules, which are applicable to the on-site phase of any HSEQ audit:

1. It is a pressure cooker.
2. Focus is critical.
3. Be done when you leave.

REFERENCES

This chapter has been adapted from Lawrence B. Cahill and Raymond W. Kane. *Environmental Health and Safety Audits*, 9th Edition. Government Institutes, 2010. It has been updated for this edition.

Wayne Pardy and Terri Andrews. *Integrated Management Systems: Leading Strategies and Solutions*, 2nd Edition. Bernan Press, 2019.

Chapter 17

HSEQ Audit Report Guidance

Ensuring that an audit report is accurate, precise, thorough, and helpful to facility staff is a considerable challenge. Audit findings must be written so that the reader can both understand the nature of the problems identified and readily envision the necessary corrective actions. In some cases, HSEQ audit reports do not accomplish these critical objectives. There are a number of reasons for this, not the least of which is that effective, logical, and concise writing is becoming less and less of a skill these days, and AI will perhaps one day take this over as well. But we digress.

Every HSEQ audit consists of three phases: preaudit preparation, on-site activities, and post-audit report-writing. In this chapter, we address audit report-writing. For most HSEQ auditors, the main report-development responsibility involves writing up findings based on their observations. The guidance contained in this chapter focuses strictly on that task. The discussion begins by describing the components of a proper audit finding. It then covers the most common problems encountered in HSEQ audit report writing.

AUDIT FINDING COMPONENTS

Every HSEQ audit finding should contain the following key components:

- Statement of observation
- Statement of requirement
- Citation or reference
- Finding type
- Finding level
- Recommendation (corrective action/preventive action)

Statement of Observation

This is a brief factual statement summarizing a deficiency that the auditor has observed. The statement should be descriptive enough so that the reader can easily verify the deficiency. A statement of observation should also be limited to what the auditor knows (e.g., "the site could not demonstrate that inspections were being conducted" rather than "the facility was not conducting inspections"). It is inappropriate to include speculation or conjecture (e.g., "if this condition is allowed to continue, then . . ."). Simply put, a statement of observation should be "just the facts." Remember the Dragnet show, for those of you old enough to remember. For those of you younger, Google it with an emphasis on what Joe Friday said. Finally, note that a statement of observation is written as a complete sentence, not as a phrase or fragment. Don't be lazy.

Statement of Requirement

Each observation must have a specific basis—a requirement with respect to which the auditor has identified a deficiency. In many instances, the requirement is a regulation promulgated by a government entity, a clause of a specific standard, or an organizational policy or procedure. It might even be good management practice. The auditor should paraphrase or quote the relevant requirement in the audit finding. This will help site staff understand precisely what is needed to remedy the identified deficiency. No guesswork will be involved.

Note that the order in which the observation and requirement statements are placed in the written audit finding is not particularly important. It is important that every finding contains both an observation and a requirement.

Citation or Regulatory Reference

Each audit finding based on a specific rule (such as a regulatory mandate or company requirement) or specific nonmandatory provision (such as a company guideline) must include a citation to the applicable rule or provision. The citation should be as complete as possible. It is not sufficient simply to say "company policy" or refer to a regulatory agency, such as the U.S. Environmental Protection Agency or Transport Canada.

Obtaining the precise citation for an audit finding can take some effort. Most auditors do not have HSEQ regulations or corporate standards committed to memory. It is important to plan in advance how you will obtain access to the necessary citation sources while you are working on-site. This should be left for the audit team to verify later in the audit during the evidence verification process.

Finding Type

Each audit finding should be classified by type. There are four categories: regulatory findings, policy findings, guidance/observation findings, and commendations. These audit-finding types are discussed in more detail below.

Regulatory Findings

Regulatory findings relate to mandatory requirements contained in federal, provincial, state, regional, or local laws, ordinances, and regulations. This type of finding can also cover nonmandatory industry guidance provisions adopted as regulations by government agencies (such as National Fire Protection Association codes). In addition, regulatory findings are used to address the elements of regulatory-required plans or procedures, such as fall protection, confined-space entry written programs, and spill-prevention control and countermeasure plans.

In some instances, the audit site or its parent company may have built additional elements into regulatory-required plans or procedures that go beyond the specific regulatory mandates. Some do this to address multi-facility operations in many different regulatory environments. When this is the case, these additional elements become a de facto part of the applicable regulatory requirement. Deficiencies with respect to these elements should be covered in regulatory findings.

Policy and Procedure Findings

Policy and procedure findings relate to the mandatory provisions of applicable corporate policies and procedures. Also included in this category are site-specific mandatory policies, procedures, standards, and rules, if they are applicable in the audit scope.

Guidance/Observation Findings

Guidance/observation findings related to the nonmandatory provisions of applicable corporate or site-specific policies, standards, and guidelines. This category can include observations made by the audit team for which there are no specific corporate or site guidelines. Auditors should have substantial and compelling justification for any guidance/observation findings related to the nonmandatory provisions.

Commendations

Commendations should be limited to truly exemplary practices and programs, particularly those worthy of adoption by other facilities. Simply being in full compliance or conformance with applicable requirements is not in and of itself exemplary, although it is desirable.

For any given audit, the number of commendable findings will typically be quite limited. A general guide is to include no more than three to five commendations in an audit report unless absolutely warranted. It is perfectly acceptable to prepare an audit report with no commendable findings. Unjustified praise is manipulative and misleading.

Commendable findings do not require either a statement of requirement or a recommendation for action.

Finding Level

Audit findings are sometimes classified into priority levels. Although not specifically required by every organization, assigning levels, especially levels based on risk, can help the audit site establish priorities for action. Auditors should recognize, however, that unless there is very clear guidance and definitions on finding levels, considerable judgment may be involved in assigning priority levels.

In addition, it should be remembered that the facility must address all audit findings, regardless of priority level. Assigning lower priority to some findings does not imply that the site can ignore the deficiency or assume it is unimportant.

Recommendation (Corrective Action/Preventive Action)

For each finding, the auditor should consider developing a recommendation outlining how the site can address the identified deficiency. Recommendations (also known as corrective actions/preventive actions, or CAPAs) should include both immediate and long-term actions where appropriate. Some would suggest this is not the role of an auditor, but your experience as an auditor might be beneficial here to the auditee for a number of reasons.

No, you are not a consultant, but you can also provide some context for the auditee to be able to develop the best action plan they can. Just as some auditees might be immature in their response, so too might some auditors. It's not a punishment exercise. It's a learning and opportunity to improve exercise.

Auditors should not be too prescriptive in their recommendations if they do make any. They must allow facility managers the flexibility to develop their own responses or corrective actions. They need "skin in the game" as they will be ultimately responsible for the implementation and continued execution. Auditor recommendations should focus on the what (e.g., provide appropriate secondary containment for the oil storage tank) and not the how (e.g., build a concrete wall three feet high) of addressing deficiencies.

Audit "Findings Forms" or Templates

The discussion above makes audit report-writing sound simple enough. Yet, auditors continue to find the task challenging, and many HSEQ audit reports continue to fall short. In response to this problem, some companies now require auditors to use "findings forms" or technology, digital-based templates, in an attempt to force rigor into the process. This approach has proven helpful in many cases.

Using a form, however, cannot fully resolve some issues with writing audit reports. The following sections discuss a number of key problems that continue to arise in HSEQ audit reports.

COMMON PROBLEMS IN WRITING AUDIT FINDINGS—AND HOW TO AVOID THEM

All HSEQ auditors, without exception, struggle with writing effective findings. In fact, as a society, we're struggling with writing generally. Over the years, the same problems seem to surface on a regular basis, largely regardless of compliance or conformance area. The sections below describe the writing-related problems most frequently encountered in HSEQ audit reports and offer some suggestions for avoiding them.

Vague Observation Statements

Observations must be clear statements of fact that accurately and specifically describe deficiencies identified by the auditor. Vague statements such as "the fall protection program needs improvement" or "protection of customer owned property is inadequate" are not helpful to the audited site's personnel or management.

Some will argue that "general" statements are preferable because they avoid creating liability for the facility being audited. This argument simply does not hold up. Vague statements cannot clearly explain and delineate deficiencies. Without such clear articulation, facility personnel may not understand the nature of the deficiency and will thus be much less likely to take the corrective action needed to address it. This, in and of itself, increases an organization's potential liability.

It is not sufficient merely to identify specific deficiencies at the closing conference without including them in the written audit report. Such an approach makes it likely that the specifics will never be communicated to the facility manager or business owner, or to the next team that performs an audit at the site. Be clear, direct, and specific in communicating audit findings. The overriding goal of HSEQ audits should be to find and fix deficiencies and risks and address any identified opportunities for improvement.

No Statement of Requirement

Some auditors believe that statements of requirement are not necessary in audit findings and think it is adequate simply to cite the applicable rule or provision. In many cases, however, a citation is not enough. Rules often contain subtleties that can complicate both audit findings and corrective actions.

For example, it is common to see findings state that certain regulatory reports at the audit site have not been signed by "a responsible corporate official." A statement of requirement will explain who at the site meets (or could meet) the definition of "responsible corporate official," thus offering useful guidance to facility managers. By providing statements of requirement, auditors add rigor and value to the audit report.

Lack of Citations or Applicable Regulatory References

This is a chronic problem in HSEQ audit reports and often leads to inappropriate findings. In too many cases, a "finding" with no citation has proved to be nothing more than the auditor's faulty recollection of a policy provision or standard. Regulatory, policy, and guidance/observation findings must all be backed up with applicable citations in the audit report. Otherwise, the site risks having auditors set ad hoc policies in the field.

Overly Stringent Priority Classifications

The findings-level classification system was established to help set priorities and identify high-risk situations. However, a review of many HSEQ audit reports suggests that the level system is occasionally abused by auditors who are out to prove a point. Auditors should not classify all regulatory findings as Level I or high priority. This classification should be used only when the "highest priority" definition is actually met. Level I or high priority should be used for findings of truly significant deficiencies that "could result in substantial risk."

Other Challenges and Pitfalls

The preceding sections discuss the most common problems observed in HSEQ audit report findings. Resolving these problems will go a long way toward improving the audit process and product. Many additional challenges and pitfalls are involved in developing proper audit findings, but space constraints preclude the full discussion of every potential difficulty.

REFERENCES

This chapter has been adapted from Lawrence B. Cahill and Raymond W. Kane. *Environmental Health and Safety Audits*, 9th Edition. Government Institutes, 2010. It has been updated for this edition.

Wayne Pardy and Terri Andrews. *Integrated Management Systems: Leading Strategies and Solutions*, 2nd Edition. Bernan Press, 2019.

Chapter 18

Integrated HSEQ Management System Auditing

EXPLORING YOUR INTEGRATED AUDITING OPPORTUNITIES

While some may consider the total integration of safety, quality, environmental management, and operational integrity to be too large in scope to integrate 100 percent, or all at the same time, there are a couple of areas where it not only makes sense but which can also serve as a springboard to rationalize the practice of further management system integration, if developed and managed effectively. Those two areas include internal HSEQ auditing and the associated process of the management review. Of course, there are considerations of auditor competency if looking at a single auditor or the option of an integrated audit team, but we'll profile some recent success in this area based on real-world applications.

Why have different processes, systems, and approaches to internal auditing or management review? What is the point of having two or three separate audit functions (of the health and safety, quality, and/or environmental disciplines)? With the guidance of ISO 19011, Guidelines for Auditing Management Systems, and the common management system structure established in Annex L, the opportunity for integrated HSEQ audits is almost too good to pass up. In consideration of the valuable time of the top-management team and the need to take a 60,000-foot view of the overall performance of the organization, why have two or three different types of management review when an integrated program will remove any perceived discipline silos and allow top management to look at the critical management system processes collectively?

We thought we'd profile the basis for integrated HSEQ auditing and HSEQ management review to give you an example of how you can put a similar process in place. In fact, we've gone so far as to provide an example of an integrated HSEQ audit program procedure and an outline of the specific inputs and outputs required of an integrated HSEQ Management Review. If you are considering an integrated HSEQ audit or management review approach, consider this information as the logic for moving forward with your integrated HSEQ audit or management review process. These two approaches can be customized for any business, large or small.

The first place to start is to define what the purpose of your integrated HSEQ audit process will be. To that point, we offer the following as the basis for any procedure you might write, as it outlines the who, what, and why of the procedure:

- Purpose (What is this procedure intended to accomplish?).
- Scope (To which aspect of your operations does this procedure apply?).
- Responsibilities (so important—who does what?).
- Procedure itself (exactly what is expected to be done).

Here is some suggested text for an integrated HSEQ auditing procedure which you might consider in customizing your own:

SAMPLE CONTENT FOR AND INTERNAL AUDIT PROCEDURE

1. **Purpose:** The purpose of this procedure is to define the process and methods for conducting internal HSEQ management system audits to determine conformance to our defined HSEQ management system requirements, regulatory requirements, and the requirements of (state any additional audit criteria).
2. **Scope:** This procedure applies to all internal HSEQ audits conducted by ABC Company. The audit protocols and practices described in this procedure also apply to supplier audits conducted by ABC Company.
3. **Responsibility:** Process Owner—The HSEQ manager, or designate, is the process owner of the internal HSEQ auditing procedure and bears overall responsibility for the audit process, including
   - implementing and managing all internal HSEQ audit activities;
   - establishing the audit schedule;
   - assigning auditors and audit teams;
   - communicating audit results to responsible managers;
   - presenting audit findings and trends in a management review; and
   - ensuring that the effectiveness of the audit program is regularly evaluated. *Note: As the HSEQ manager is the process owner for internal auditing, he or she may not audit the process.

PRESIDENT (OR OTHER TOP-MANAGEMENT REPRESENTATIVE)

- review the status of all completed HSEQ audits during the Management Review;
- support the aims and objectives of the internal HSEQ audit procedure and associated processes; and
- ensure managers participate in any scheduled internal HSEQ audits and take ownership of any resulting actions to support them to conclusion.

MANAGERS AND SUPERVISORS

- review the status of all completed HSEQ audits during the Management Review;
- support the aims and objectives of the internal HSEQ audit procedures and ensure staff understand the importance of participating in any internal audit processes;
- review any HSEQ audit reports sent to their attention;
- support the time required for any of their staff involved in an internal HSEQ audit, whether as an auditee or auditor;
- ensure an audit response and audit action plan, if required, is developed, documented, and communicated to the HSEQ manager; and
- take responsibility to ensure that those actions are completed as documented.

Internal Auditors and Audit Leads are responsible for

- preparing audit checklists and plans;
- notifying auditees;
- assigning audit team responsibilities;
- participating in audits;
- chairing opening and closing meetings; and
- preparing and approving audit reports; internal auditors participate in any scheduled internal HSEQ audit for which they have been identified as an audit resource.

EMPLOYEES AND STAFF

All employees are responsible for participating in HSEQ audit activities as appropriate and for cooperating with any internal auditor.

Procedure—General—ABC Company shall

- plan, establish, implement, and maintain an internal HSEQ audit program, including the frequency, methods, responsibilities, planning requirements, and reporting, which shall take into consideration the importance of the processes concerned, changes affecting our organization, and the results of previous HSEQ audits;
- define the audit criteria and scope for each HSEQ audit;
- select competent auditors and conduct HSEQ audits to ensure objectivity and impartiality in the audit process;
- ensure the results of HSEQ audits are reported to relevant management;
- take appropriate actions without undue delay; and
- retain records as evidence of the implementation of the HSEQ audit program and its audit results.

AUDIT INITIATION

Internal HSEQ audits may be initiated for any or all of the following reasons:

- To determine the effectiveness of the implemented HSEQ Management System in meeting the specified HSEQ objectives.
- To determine if ABC Company is meeting the required statutory and regulatory requirements.
- To provide an opportunity to improve our HSEQ Management System.
- To verify the HSEQ Management System continues to meet specified requirements and is being implemented when significant changes have been made in functional areas; for example, reorganization and procedural revisions.
- When the performance of the products/services is at risk, or is suspected to be at risk due to nonconformities.
- When it is necessary to verify that the required corrective actions have been taken and have been effective.

FREQUENCY OF AUDITS

Audit frequency shall be determined based on a review, assessment, or consideration of any of the following criteria:

- Risk associated with audited activities.
- Organizational changes.
- Process requirements or concerns.
- Customer feedback.

- Frequency and type of nonconformances reported.
- Opportunities for improvement.
- Results of previous audits.

INTERNAL HSEQ AUDITOR QUALIFICATIONS AND TRAINING

Internal auditors are considered qualified to participate in an HSEQ internal audit as part of an internal audit team when they have completed a recognized internal auditor-training course or equivalent. Auditor competence is based on a combination of qualification (training), experience, and required personal attributes. Internal HSEQ auditor training can be by an external course or seminar provided by a qualified institution or in-house training provided by a qualified consultant/trainer. If training is provided in-house, the trainer must have documented qualifications as a Lead Auditor.

Internal auditors shall be

- non-biased or prejudiced in relation to the area being audited and not directly responsible for the work being audited; and
- responsible for and capable of performing a detailed audit and producing the subsequent audit report. Internal HSEQ audits may also be conducted by a third party on behalf of ABC Company.

AUDIT PLANNING, SCHEDULING, AND PREPARING FOR AUDITS

The Lead Auditor, or designate, shall be responsible for planning, preparing, conducting, and reporting the audit in accordance with the requirements of this procedure. All internal HSEQ audits shall be scheduled and recorded in the ABC Company management system software, with records of all completed audits maintained in the ABC Company management system software as well. The Lead Auditor, or designate, shall ensure an audit plan is prepared for the audit. For a scheduled internal HSEQ audit, an audit notification shall be sent to the manager responsible for the area being audited and to the auditee(s) via email.

Audit notifications identify

- the date and time of the audit;
- the purpose and scope of the audit;
- where and when audit activities and interviews will take place;

- distribution of the audit report; and
- details of opening and closing meetings.

OPENING MEETING

- Prior to starting the audit, an opening meeting shall be planned and conducted with the auditee using the internal audit opening meeting agenda form. The purpose and agenda of the opening meeting shall be to
- review the scope and the objectives of the audit;
- provide a short summary of the methods and procedures to be used in conducting the audit;
- establish the official communication links between the audit team and the auditee;
- confirm that the resources and facilities needed by the audit team are available;
- agree on the distribution of the audit report; and
- clarify any unclear details of the audit plan.

CONDUCTING THE AUDIT

The auditor(s) shall conduct the audit in accordance with the audit scope, their training, and this procedure. Audits will include interviews, records review, and observation of operational processes.

The management of the area being audited shall ensure a contact is made available to assist the auditor(s), and that required personnel are present during the audit. Prepared checklists, procedures, and other relevant documents shall be used by the auditor(s) to verify the suitability of the documented procedures and/or work instructions, as well as their effective implementation. The audit checklist, procedures, or notes used during the audit to record findings shall be retained. These documents are not included in the audit report but shall be maintained as part of the official record of the audit. Findings shall be recorded on an ongoing basis during the audit.

CLOSING MEETING

Upon completion of the audit, a closing meeting shall be held to communicate a summary of the findings to the management of the area audited and obtain agreement, based on the objective evidence identified, of any nonconformances found. The Lead Auditor shall present and review the findings from the obtained evidence at the closing meeting and shall clarify any issues identified and discussed in the closing meeting.

Reporting Audit Results

A formal audit report shall be prepared as soon as possible after the completion of the audit but shall be completed and emailed to the respective manager of the area or process audited no later than two weeks after the closing meeting.

When a nonconformity or opportunity for improvement is noted, it shall be brought to the attention of, and discussed with, the responsible manager. Upon completion of the audit, each noted nonconformity or opportunity for improvement is initiated in the action tracking log.

Managers are required to ensure the successful completion of the assigned actions within their area of responsibility. The responsible manager shall ensure that corrective actions are taken to investigate the root cause of significant or recurring nonconformances and that action is taken without undue delay.

AUDIT ACTION PLAN

Managers with responsibility for the area audited shall ensure that action plans are developed to address identified nonconformances or opportunities for improvement. Proposed action plans shall meet the SMART action acronym:

- ***Specific*:** Actions should be simplistically written and clearly define what you are going to do.
- ***Measurable:*** Actions should be measurable so that you have tangible evidence that you have accomplished the action.
- ***Attainable*:** Actions should be attainable; they should stretch you slightly so you feel challenged but be defined well enough so that you can achieve them. You must possess the appropriate knowledge, skills, and abilities needed to achieve the goal.
- ***Result Focused***: Actions should measure outcomes, not activities.
- ***Time specific***: Actions should be linked to a time frame that creates a practical sense of urgency or results in tension between the current reality and the expectation of the action. Without such tension, the action is unlikely to produce a relevant outcome.

Action plans shall be prepared and forwarded to the Lead Auditor no later than three weeks after the receipt of the issued audit report. The HSEQ manager, or designate, will approve action plans and follow up to ensure that corrective action has been implemented and is effective. When there is objective evidence that the corrective action is effective, the audit finding is closed out. If more work is needed to fully implement the action, the due date may be extended depending on the nature or complexity of the action in question.

AUDIT FINDINGS ANALYSIS AND REVIEW

Audit programs and action status reports are prepared monthly and submitted to management as part of the HSEQ KPI reporting program. At the end of each auditing cycle, all nonconformity reports established during the cycle are compiled, analyzed, and are presented at the management review meeting.

AUDITOR (EXTREME) BIAS—BEWARE OF REGISTRATION AUDITORS BEARING BOOKS

One of the things we wanted to achieve in this book is to profile real-world audit examples and scenarios based on our collective experience of working in the HSEQ field for in excess of thirty years each. To that end, this story demonstrates that sometimes challenges come from the most unlikely places, and then it's important to have built a system that is both compliant and suited to your organization, not somebody else's—even if that someone else happens to be a registration auditor.

In preparing for the transition from ISO 9001:2008 to ISO 9001:2015, the team of quality practitioners mapped out the transition plan. Based on a thorough gap analysis of the existing system against the new requirements, an understanding of corporate culture, and advice from a number of experienced third-party resources, it was determined that the transition would require diligent effort to incorporate what were viewed as some significant changes into the management system. It was important to get it right.

It was also important to take the time needed to update and revise the existing quality processes to make them both more meaningful and fully aligned with the requirements of the new standard. It was realized that with transition, there would be a period of adjustment and learning for both users of the standard and those who audit against its requirements (internal and external), as everyone made their way to competence with the standard's often vague and new requirements. This transition process to ISO 9001:2015 included the following activities which the team felt were prudent:

- Acquire a copy of the standard and digest it to try to get a practical sense of how the one-size-fits-all language could be adapted by the company.
- Determine what the key processes were which would need to be clearly managed.
- Determine, in a practical sense, what was needed to meet the new requirements regarding things like the context of the organization, risk-based thinking, and leadership.
- Consult with internal managers and provide an overview of the new version of the standard to determine how internal processes might be impacted or need to change based on the requirements of the standard.
- Conduct a session for the top-management team and profile for them the requirements of the new standard.
- Do a "desktop audit" to determine what internal processes, procedures, forms, and so on, already align with the requirements of the new standard and address any obvious gaps through a strategic action plan. The transition was completed, and the changes which were implemented fit the organization. During the audit, to their great surprise and astonishment, the registration auditor pulled out a book, written by an author he had an affinity for, and showed the auditees a table that he recommended as a good way to demonstrate the inputs and outputs of the company's processes.

Management had decided to do it a different way because (a) the system needed to fit the company's needs and realities, (b) nobody had a copy of that particular book anyway prior to the audit, and (c) the other books and professional references we consulted fit better with our culture and processes. After a fair bit of disagreement during the audit, and the registration auditor showing the book and the input/output chart to everyone he interviewed, it was decided to ask a question on the LinkedIn group ISO 9001 (which at the time had some 110,983 members) regarding the interpretation of section 4.4 of the ISO 9001:2015 Standard, which states: "4.4 Quality management system and its processes 4.4.1 The organization shall establish, implement, maintain and continually improve a quality management system, including the processes needed and their interactions, in accordance with the requirements of this International Standard. The organization shall determine the processes needed for the quality management system and their application throughout the organization and shall: a) determine the inputs required and the outputs expected from these processes."

The question was: Regarding the phrase "shall determine the inputs required and outputs expected from these processes," do the words input and output literally have to be in a process/procedure describing the process? Can it not be self-evident by reading the process/procedure what the inputs/outputs are without having to specifically spell them out using the actual words, input and output? (Even though 9.3.2 and 9.3.3 prescriptively define inputs and outputs of the management review process.)

Here are some of the numerous responses from a wide range of folks on this LinkedIn group (names have been removed, and only their commentary provided):

Every process consists of an input-activity-output; as such it should have some measure of success or achievement. The standard is simply requiring you to determine what you are expecting from that process, that is, how do you determine compliance?

- How you make it "demonstrable" is up to you. Certainly, you don't have to write essays that describe it—nobody at the sharp end will read them even if you do! For what it's worth, I use pictures like block diagrams, flowcharts, swim lanes, step action tables, Venn diagrams, and so on. I'm cautious with turtle diagrams as I find the target audience doesn't get much out of them.
- Turtle!, Terrapin! and Mutant ninjas! (This turtle diagram reference will be further mocked shortly).
- First, please check out clause 1 "Scope." As night follows day, unless every detail in 4.4.1 is "present and correct" and it's demonstrable, there is no tangible conforming customer-centric QMS. There is only a bunch of disjointed trivia. In the 2000/2008 version, it was clause 4.1, right at the top so that everything else flowed from it.
- You don't have to use the exact wording from the standard (but you may find you want to), nor directly incorporate the requirements into your procedure (but you would probably want to make explicit reference to where the requirements are handled).
- Defined to the degree necessary for your organization to achieve its intent (goals and objectives). If throughout your organization, each function understands "the process approach" and can answer an auditor's questions about what it takes for a process or function to achieve its intended function, and the goals and objectives of the organization are being met and you can also demonstrate that you are satisfying your customers, then the degree of documentation is up to the organization. Even if it is evident that the process or functions need those inputs and outputs defined, it is still up to you whether you use flow diagrams, turtle diagrams, or IDEF0-type diagrams. Your documentation could even be a detailed training program or include external training.
- The best thing to consider is what level of detail and what mechanism adds value. If it doesn't add value, then don't do it for the sake of an auditor. Get it? There are as many different interpretations of a standard as there are people who give their perspective and opinion. And with the changes

in 9001:2015, it will likely take a couple of years before there's general consensus, regardless of what the registration bodies or their auditors say or suggest. They are learning as they go as well. But I did find the Turtle!, Terrapin!, and Mutant ninjas! comment a welcome addition to the starchy conversation.

Sometimes humor in the serious world of HSEQ is a welcome diversion, if only temporarily. I also asked a question of the LinkedIn ISO 9001 group based on the following headline: "Auditor referencing a book during registration audit."

Here's what I asked the group: So, we've just finished our registration audit to 9001:2015 and the auditor was pulling out a book written on ISO 9001:2015 throughout the audit and referencing that we should buy/use this book in our transition to 2015. The audit concluded after three days—no nonconformances (which I assume means our processes demonstrated that we are meeting the requirements of ISO 9001:2015) but an opportunity for improvement to read the book he kept referencing, as he was of the opinion our QMS was "overdeveloped" and the book he was referencing should be used as the basis to "simplify" our QMS. Thoughts?

People did indeed have thoughts, and here are some of the comments received.

- There are possibilities for simplifying a management system to remove redundancies and eliminate waste. Usually, people close to processes provide value-added suggestions for continual improvement. A book is not always necessary to achieve these goals.
- The CB (certification body) duty is to review the auditor's report to ensure it meets their certification requirements before they release their certificate. This review includes conformity with ISO 17021 by default. As (name omitted) pointed out, there is a breach here that should have been picked up at the certification review step. So, I suggest you complain to the certification body and ask for evidence that indicates they have: (1) taken steps to correct the behavior of this particular auditor, (2) carried out an investigation to reveal the causal factors, (3) taken action accordingly to avoid recurrence and occurrence of similar behaviors elsewhere. Next time an auditor recommends a book, hand him mine and watch him spontaneously combust. Have an ambulance waiting. You should also copy this complaint to the CB's accreditation body, asking them what action they will take with respect to points 1, 2, and 3 above.
- We get audited by a variety of auditors for a number of reasons. I listen to all advice and suggestions; some are mentally filed in the round bin, while others have proved to be most helpful in making the company function

better. What was the book, by the way? PS: Congratulations on a successful transition—no NCs and an OFI to read a book equals good work. Maybe you should write a book; however, if it's a really good one, beware of auditors recommending it.

With tongue firmly planted in cheek, the response to this individual was as follows:

I have indeed written one with my partner (Integrated Management Systems), who is also a registration auditor. She would not dream of making any reference to it one way or another during a registration audit—whether it's good or not is a matter of opinion. And something else . . . while we were successful in the audit with no non-conformances identified, the majority of the Opportunities for Improvement written by the registration auditor were to write more procedures. While his opinion was that our QMS was "overdeveloped" his solution was to write more procedures. To say that this audit was not value added would be an understatement. But having said that, we will always continue to advocate for better, more professional and evidence-based auditing.

The moral of the story is that regardless of the standard, training, experience, qualifications, and personal approaches of the auditor, they are not clones. Some may be clowns, but all auditors are different, and your audit will reflect these differences. That said, any unprofessional or inappropriate behavior on the part of any auditor should be addressed by the auditee. As an auditee, you have that right. As an auditee, you should expect nothing less than unbiased, professional behavior. And you can be assured that the authors, if ever having the opportunity to audit your organization, would never bring their books into the audit process. Over a coffee, perhaps. During the audit—absolutely not. Believe it or not, we actually follow our own advice.

REFERENCES

This chapter has been adapted from Lawrence B. Cahill and Raymond W. Kane. *Environmental Health and Safety Audits*, 9th Edition. Government Institutes, 2010. It has been updated for this edition.

Wayne Pardy and Terri Andrews. *Integrated Management Systems: Leading Strategies and Solutions*, 2nd Edition. Bernan Press, 2019.

https://cdn.standards.iteh.ai/samples/70017/559078f9a2634aca84ff0a6aac1498f6/ISO-19011-2018.pdf

Appendix A1

Canadian Federation of Construction Safety Associations COR® Audit Program

We wanted to make available a real-world audit that reflected much of the content we've profiled in this book. To that end, we've included the requirements and processes of the Canadian Federation of Construction Safety Associations (CFCSA) COR® audit program. We feel that the audit methodology and process closely mirror, in a practical way, the HSEQ audit management processes and principles profiled in our book, so we thought it would be a great example to share with all readers. The authors would like to thank Sean Scott, Executive Director of the Construction Safety Association of Manitoba, and the CFCSA for their contribution to our HSEQ auditing book and the very detailed profile of the Certificate of Recognition (COR®) program audit for Canada's construction industry.

The CFCSA represents the united voice of all construction safety associations in every Canadian province and territory, who are funded by construction employers large and small to improve safety outcomes.

The CFCSA is responsible for the development and oversight of major safety programs operating across the country. These include the National COR® Accreditation Standard, and the National Construction Safety Officer (NCSO®), and National Health and Safety Administrator (NHSA™) designation programs.

The CFCSA also promotes awareness of construction health and safety practices and programs, facilitates information sharing, and collaboratively produces workplace health and safety training and information resources. As an organization with members in every jurisdiction, the CFCSA works to find common ground on important health and safety issues. By promoting the harmonization of safety standards and training across the country through collaboration and sharing of resources, the organization increases the reach and efficiency of programs and training materials, while reducing costs.

The following is the tool and process that the CFCSA has developed to work with provincial and territorial Construction Safety Associations with a shared interest in

- promoting awareness of construction health and safety;
- improving information sharing; and
- collaboratively producing workplace health and safety training standards/information resources.

TABLE OF CONTENTS

INTRODUCTION

The COR® accreditation program, owned and regulated by the CFCSA, has long been recognized as the national standard for an occupational health and safety management system in the Canadian construction industry.

COR® is an occupational health and safety accreditation program that verifies a fully implemented health and safety management system meeting national standards. The objectives of COR® are to provide industry employers with effective tools to develop, implement, assess, and promote continuous improvement of their health and safety management system to prevent or mitigate incidents and injuries, as well as their associated human and financial costs.

Originally established in 2000, COR® provides rigorous evaluations of an organization's health and safety management system. It encompasses hazard identification, risk assessment, and effective control measures, ensuring that Canadian firms are equipped to handle the unique challenges of the construction industry.

This program also provides companies with a competitive edge in reducing workplace incidents. COR® is one of the few health and safety accreditation programs offering empirical evidence to support its effectiveness in enhancing workplace safety and lowering injury rates. A key finding is that firms holding COR® accreditation experience an average of 18 percent lower injury rates compared to non-certified firms. This statistic is supported by comprehensive research papers, available on the CFCSA website (cfcsa.ca). These findings underscore the value of investing in COR® certification and its substantial contribution to the overall well-being of construction industry workers in Canada. In recognition of the value of COR®, seven of the eleven workers' compensation boards in Canada offer an annual incentive/rebate to companies that achieve COR®.

What Is Involved

To achieve COR® accreditation, an organization must establish, implement, monitor, and maintain a health and safety management system in accordance with the requirements of the CFCSA National COR® Accreditation Standard. Verification of the implementation of the health and safety management system is assessed through a series of formal audits.

The organization must allocate necessary financial, human, and organizational resources to plan, implement, monitor, review, correct, and continuously improve the health and safety management system. At a minimum, health and safety management systems involve the identification, communication, and control of hazards. The effective implementation of the health and safety management system also includes leadership commitment, hazard identification and risk control, worker participation, and correlating measures—the elements upon which a health and safety program is based.

The CFCSA COR® program is based on fourteen elements which must be included in an organization's health and safety management system.

1. Safety and Health Policy	7. Preventative Maintenance Program	13. Legislation
2. Hazard Assessment, Analysis, and Control	8. Training and Communication	14. Procurement and Contractor Management
3. Safe Work Practices	9. Inspections	15. **Provincial/Territorial Supplement**
4. Safe Job Procedures	10. Incident Investigation and Reporting	
5. Company Safety Rules	11. Emergency Preparedness	
6. Personal Protective Equipment	12. Statistics, Records, and Documentation	

**Each member of the CFCSA is the Authority Having Jurisdiction to grant COR® in its respective province/territory and has the discretion to make any additions to these national requirements. Additional jurisdictional requirements are typically included in a Provincial/Territorial Supplement (i.e., section 15).

AUDITING OVERVIEW

A company's health and safety management system is audited annually to confirm that National COR® Accreditation Standards are met. Audits are to be completed by a qualified and competent auditor and must follow the prescribed audit instrument of the CFCSA member. At minimum, the audit instrument must include the required health and safety program elements listed in the National COR® Accreditation Standard.

Verification of the implementation of these elements is assessed through a series of formal audits which include observations of the workplace, reviewing documentation, and interviewing employees.

For the audit to be successful, it must achieve a minimum score of 80 percent overall and 50 percent in each element. COR® is valid for a period not exceeding three years and must be validated annually.

The initial year of COR® accreditation requires the successful submission of

a) company internal/self-audit;
b) CFCSA external/independent audit.

Year two and three of COR® accreditation require the successful submission of

a) company internal/self-audit;
b) CFCSA verification review/CFCSA internal audit.

To assist CFCSA members, the CFCSA has created a harmonized audit instrument which is used as a template for the majority of Canadian jurisdictions.

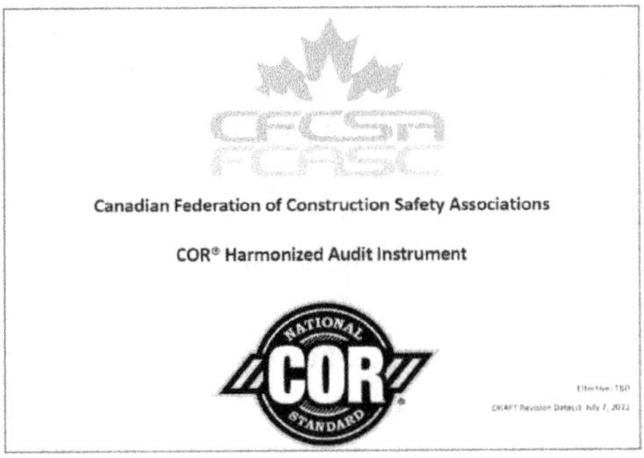

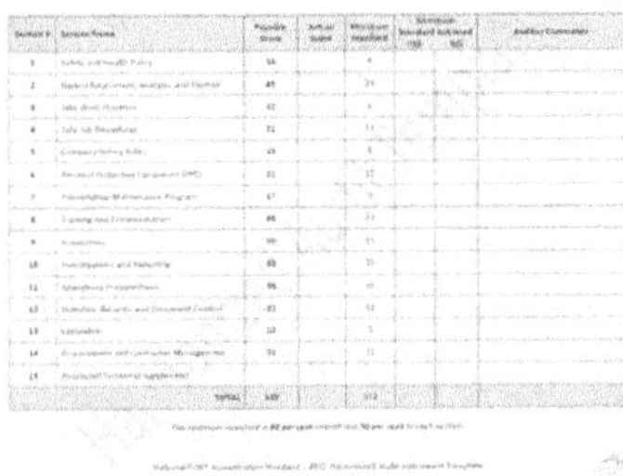

THE FIVE WS WITHIN THE COR® AUDIT PROCESS

What

An audit is an evaluation method used to identify successes and deficiencies according to an established standard. A safety audit is the examination of a company's health and safety management system to determine if it meets the National COR® Accreditation Standard. Via the collection of documentation, observations and interviews, information is gathered to verify that a standard is met and to effectively identify opportunities for improvement to the program or system.

The CFCSA-endorsed harmonized audit template aligns with the National COR® Accreditation Standard. Although COR® is recognized across Canada, a key benefit to helping companies navigate the legislative requirements specific to each province or territory is found in the Supplement section, section 15.

Why

An audit is used to verify the implementation of a safety and health management system to a given standard, as well as providing opportunity to improve the effectiveness and efficiency of a health and safety management system, including the written program and overall operations. Safety is an integral component of preventing or mitigating incidents and injuries, as well as their associated human and financial costs.

Safety audits provide an accurate picture of the implementation of a company's health and safety management system, indicating its effectiveness, and areas in which it may need improvement. A safety audit is an examination of a company's health and safety performance in an effort to

- determine a company's eligibility for COR®;
- identify opportunities for improvement regarding the health and safety management system and/or performance of a company's safety and health program.

When

The timing of the first audit is at the company's discretion; however, some submission requirements and recommendations help ensure the audit is being performed at an appropriate time of year for the company.

Things to consider prior to submitting a company's first self-audit:

1. Is at least 50 percent of the company workforce working at that time of year?
2. Is the audit being conducted during "peak season" or "slow season"?
3. Does the company perform seasonal work?
4. Will the audit coincide with the company's year-end reporting period?
5. When is the best time of year to perform an audit, so the company can ensure appropriate time is available?

Audit guidelines state that, at minimum, a company must have at least 50 percent of its workforce working and have sites available for visits in order to process the audit for certification. If the time of year in which the company submits the audit will not conform with one or both of these requirements, the audit would not be eligible for submission.

A company may wish to perform an audit during its slow season, but submitting during this time may present challenges to completing the audit each year moving forward. A general recommendation is that a company submit its audit at the beginning of or during its busier season. This ensures worksites are available for observation as well as workers for interviews.

If a company chooses to perform an audit close to the end of its slow season and submit it as work is starting to pick up, this will help ensure the audit can be performed and completed on time without worry that certification will lapse due to inability to meet submission standards.

When to submit an audit once a company has become COR® certified.

The month in which a company achieves COR® certification will be deemed its audit "anniversary month." To maintain certification, an audit is due from that company every year by the first of the month in which it was officially certified.

For example: If a company achieved COR® certification on April 15, 2022, it will be required to submit its next annual self-audit on or before April 1, 2023 and each subsequent year thereafter in order to maintain COR® certification.

A company's anniversary month generally does not change. Ensure that the time of year in which the first audit is submitted for a company is a consistent and appropriate time to ensure submission standards are met and that the audit can be completed on time.

CFCSA members understand that construction workflow is not always consistent. For this reason, a certified company is permitted to submit its audit up to four months in advance of its anniversary month to ensure sites are available and workers are working.

Where

Audits should be conducted at all areas of operation where the company is involved with work, including

- jobsites;
- offices;
- shops;
- storage areas;
- vehicles (primarily for delivery companies); and
- anywhere workers are performing work for the company.

A separate audit is not required on every company jobsite. The audit is being conducted on the company's health and safety management system and how it is functioning at multiple locations. A sampling of jobsites provides enough opportunities for observation for an auditor. It is recommended to visit an odd number of sites to determine a clear majority for each requirement evaluated. The more areas involved in the audit process, the more accurate the results will be. At minimum, if the company has three or fewer sites running at the time of the audit, all sites should be visited.

Who

The people involved in the audit process are critical to ensuring that the company's health and safety program is effective, efficient, and an integral part of the company's day-to-day business.

This may include but not be limited to the following people:

Internally:

- Owners/Employers
- Management
- Supervisors
- Workers
- Workplace safety committee members/worker safety representatives

Externally:

- CFCSA member (i.e., the provincial/territorial construction safety association)
- Subcontractors
- Other qualified persons (i.e., independent auditor)

The person conducting the audit must have the required training to properly perform an audit. This can be someone employed by the company being audited or a third-party auditor. In either case, they must be trained through a CFCSA member or an affiliate association. It is strongly recommended that a company complete the annual audit itself rather than hire external personnel. A company that audits itself will have a better understanding of the process and will be more successful in developing and implementing corrective actions identified through the audit process.

How to Perform an Audit

Auditors are given training, resources, and materials which they will apply during the audit process. The audit instrument and guidelines provide questions pertaining to the audit and details on what to look for—examples of what type of documentation, training, or observations would allow for points to be awarded, and interview questionnaires for different levels of the organization.

The three techniques used during the audit are:

- Documentation
- Observation
- Interview

These three techniques will assess and verify that what is being written (documentation), is being followed (observation) and understood (interview). They will be discussed in detail later in this workbook.

Activities Involved in the Audit Process

There are three major activities in the audit process. Each activity includes several steps:

1. Audit preparation
   - Inform participants
   - Locate necessary information
   - Gather tools
2. Performing the audit
   - Health and safety program preaudit review
   - Detailed audit
   - Documentation review
   - Site observation
   - Interviews

3. Reporting the results
   - Summarizing results
   - Analyzing results
   - Scoring the audit
   - Executive summary report
   - Corrective action plan
   - Close-out meeting

STEP ONE: AUDIT PREPARATION

Being organized and having the correct information/materials to conduct and record an audit efficiently will eliminate time wasted by searching for or acquiring knowledge and information after the fact.

Inform Participants

First, the auditor should inform all persons who will be participating in the audit—the company, organization, and/or site personnel—that an audit is about to take place. This may be done by email, telephone, or in-person. Make sure people understand the principles involved in the audit process so there are no surprises or misunderstandings.

Here are some examples of what effective auditors include during the initial contact with the company and the people involved:

1. The date or dates of the audit
2. The purpose of the audit
3. The people who will be involved
4. The types of activities that will occur
5. The way in which results will be communicated

Informing participants about what to expect ensures there are no surprises for both the auditor and the company. The goal of an audit is not to "catch" anyone doing something wrong or unsafe. Starting the audit with transparent dialogue encourages open communication.

The Date(s) of the Audit

The auditor should let people know which day(s) office, shop, and site visits, and observations and interviews will occur. This helps to ensure that employees will be working at the locations indicated. It also avoids disrupting time-sensitive work. Giving people the opportunity to organize and prepare for the audit will also help to alleviate undue stress and anxiety. The auditor should ask for the name(s) and contact information of the company's site supervisor(s) at each site and contact them directly to schedule site visits.

The auditor should call the supervisor or company representative in advance of the site visit to make scheduling arrangements. It is also a good idea to call the day before, or the day of the visit, in case there has been an unforeseen change.

When arranging site visits with supervisors, the auditor should ask any relevant questions. Are there any training or PPE requirements before entering the site? Where do visitors go once they are on site? Is there important information that may be necessary for the safety of the auditor and the safety of others?

The Purpose of the Audit

People tend to get nervous or worried when they hear the term "audit." In this context, the audit process is simply a tool used for the development, recognition, evaluation, and confirmation of a company's health and safety management system. The objectives of the COR® accreditation program and the audit process are to provide industry employers with an effective health and safety management system to reduce incidents and injuries, as well as their associated human and financial costs.

If people involved in the audit process are made aware that the audit is used for their benefit and not simply a "pass or fail" system, they can focus on how effectively their health and safety system is functioning and give them the opportunity to recognize areas which may require further attention.

Who Will Be Involved

The (internal) persons involved in the audit process should include:

- Owners/Employers
- Management
- Supervisors
- Workers
- Worker safety representatives
- Workplace safety committee members
- Subcontractors

When talking to the company representative and/or site supervisor, the auditor should get a good sense of how many people are on location and who should be included during the audit interviews. It is important to get a good representation of what people actually know and understand about their safety program, as well as areas of which they may be unclear.

The Types of Activities that Will Occur

Participants should be made aware that there are three main techniques used during the audit. These techniques will be covered in greater detail during step two of Performing the Audit.

1. Documentation
   Auditors should explain which types of documentation they will be looking for, to give the company time to organize and prepare them for the review. This can save time during the audit.
2. Observation
   The company should be told ahead of time what the auditor will look at during the observation process, to allow preparation for a walk-through. This gives the auditor the opportunity to see how the company's worksites and/or areas are maintained. The auditor will be looking at certain activities to verify they are in compliance with the relevant workplace health and safety regulation and company policy.
3. Interview
   Interviews can be intimidating. The auditor should put workers at ease and assure them that interviews are confidential and conducted to get an accurate reading of what people understand about their company health and safety program. Before the interview, explain that the intent is to gather information, share it with the company, and work toward a genuine understanding of their health and safety program, including their involvement in it.

   Letting those involved know in advance about these three techniques will help people prepare for the auditor and allow for an accurate representation of the worksite's daily activities so information can be communicated effectively.

How Results Will Be Communicated

In addition to informing participants of the activities involved prior to starting the audit process, the auditor should indicate that at the end of the audit, a summary of the results and corrective action recommendations will be available for review, at which time the results can be discussed and recommendations can be offered.

It is important for upper management to know what to expect before, during, and after the audit is completed. The auditor should let them know that a meeting will be requested once the audit is completed. Should they have any questions before then, they can contact the auditor.

The way in which results are summarized, scored, and recorded is covered in step two of Performing the Audit. A close-out meeting will be held with the company and the auditor to discuss results and review opportunities for improvement.

Locate Necessary Information

The auditor should gather as much background information as possible about the organization or areas that will be audited. An auditor who understands the people, processes, and projects involved in a company's work activities will have the ability to accurately identify how supportive the company's health and safety program is for the work they perform.

Key Information to Identify:

The company safety manual—the company safety manual will contain details specific to the company's procedures, policies, safety rules, PPE requirements, and work activities that will assist an auditor in recognizing what to look for during the audit. The company should provide a copy of this manual, which will make up the basis of the documentation review.

An organizational chart—reviewing a company's organizational chart helps the auditor to identify each individual's role and responsibilities within the company. A detailed organizational chart will help the auditor review the company's documentation, names, signatures, and initials to verify who is involved in which health and safety activities. The auditor should ask the company for a copy of its chart. If they don't have one, they should be asked to make one. An example can be found later in this workbook.

Previous records regarding the health and safety program—review audit/inspection reports that may be available or the previous audit corrective action plan (if applicable). Reviewing these reports helps the auditor to observe whether or not corrective actions have been completed for the items indicated as concerns. Inspection reports should also indicate areas which require attention. This allows the auditor to take note of these concerns during the audit process and identify how the safety management system is operating.

A description of the organization, area, or type of work performed—it is beneficial to give a company the opportunity to supply any additional details or information that would assist in understanding the organization. This allows the company to communicate and be involved in the audit process and builds a positive relationship between the company and the auditor. This information should be collected during the preaudit meeting, or when the auditor is contacting supervisors for site information.

The number of projects that are currently underway—it is good practice to ask a company for ALL of its current worksites and the general activities on each one. This information may help the auditor decide which sites would be best to visit to ensure an accurate assessment of the company's health and safety program relative to its activities.

NOTE: A description of the organization, area, or type of work; the number of projects currently underway; and other information specific to the company will be requested in the audit instrument.

During the audit process, documentation that has been generated within the past twelve months will be requested and will contribute to the evaluation of the company's current health and safety performance. This will be requested for every subsequent audit.

Gather Tools

The list below identifies tools, equipment, documents, and checklists to assist with performing the audit. There may also be some items required due to the nature of work, environment, or type of company that will be audited.

Gather the tools and people required:

- Appropriate personal protective equipment (PPE)
- Clipboard, note paper, pens, or pencils
- Any existing standards and policies applicable to the work
- Copies of the current workplace health and safety act, regulation and other appropriate industry standards
- The audit instrument
- Observational checklist(s)
- Interview questionnaires (bring enough copies of each)
- Management/supervisor
- Worker safety representative/safety committee member
- Employee
- Subcontractor

Given the type of hazards auditors may be exposed to during the audit, they may need special training before entering the site. This can be as simple as a site orientation provided by the person/company responsible for the site or even formal in-class training.

The COR® audit instrument, observational checklist, and interview questionnaires can be downloaded from CFCSA member websites and will be reviewed in detail further. These documents are designed to work together and alleviate stress and confusion when performing an audit.

Performing the Audit

The audit has three steps:

1. Pre-Audit Review
2. Detailed Audit
3. Reporting the Results

Step One: Preaudit Review

The preaudit review is an initial review of the company's health and safety manual/program documentation. This part of the audit does not look at the quality of the safety program. It simply identifies whether the various parts of the safety manual/program exist in a form that matches the requirements of the COR® audit instrument.

There are fourteen elements within the COR® harmonized audit template which verify if the company's health and safety program contains the required material. The preaudit review can be found in the audit instrument on the health and safety manual verification page. Whether the listed sections are available can be answered with a simple "yes" or "no."

Some items required for the verification portion of the audit may exist in different forms. They may not be contained in a corporate policy manual and more than one area may be contained in a single document. The auditors should seek out the information and organize it as if it were all part of one corporate manual or handbook.

If all elements/sections of information identified on the health and safety manual verification page can be located, the auditor can complete the detailed audit in step two. If certain sections of the basic safety program do not exist in any form, an auditor may pause the audit and encourage their development before proceeding.

> **NOTE:**
>
> **A COMPANY CANNOT PASS AN AUDIT IF ONE OR MORE OF THE REQUIRED ELEMENTS ARE MISSING.**

If the auditor decides to proceed with the audit even though some elements are missing from the health and safety program, some sections will be incomplete or may have to be scored as zero. This should be indicated in the results and recommendations so that corrective actions can be developed and put into place by the company.

Lastly, verification of the COR® compulsory competencies must be confirmed and documented at the bottom of the health and safety manual verification page. The information provided should include the participant's name and the date at which the courses were completed.

Required Training

Required competencies must be completed by an employee (or employees) of the company.

Each member of the CFCSA offers training modules to verify required competencies. The training modules provide a company with the information, resources, and ability to implement a health and safety management system (i.e., safety program) in alignment with the requirements of the National COR® Accreditation Program. The mandatory competencies required by the National COR® Accreditation Standard are as follows:

a) Health and Safety Program Development & Implementation
b) Leadership, Training & Communication
c) Safety Auditor Training
d) Hazard Identification & Risk Control

NOTE: The training competencies do not need to be a "standalone" course or training module. CFCSA members may choose to incorporate the required competencies into multiple courses. An employer must maintain at least one full-time employee with the required training.

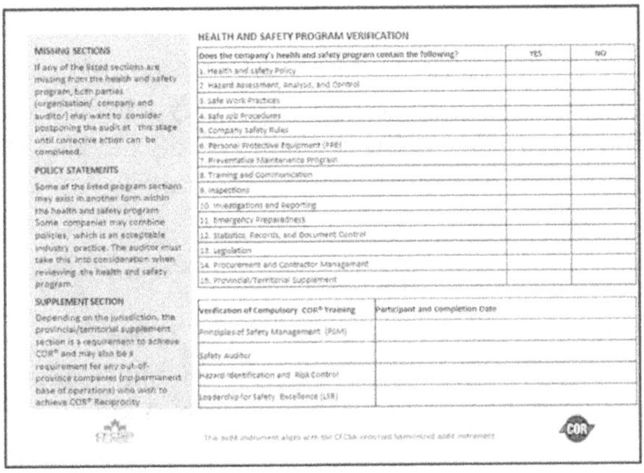

MISSING SECTIONS

If any of the listed sections are missing from the health and safety program, both parties (organization/ company and auditor) may want to consider postponing the audit at this stage until corrective action can be completed.

POLICY STATEMENTS

Some of the listed program sections may exist in another form within the health and safety program. Some companies may combine policies, which is an acceptable industry practice. The auditor must take this into consideration when reviewing the health and safety program.

SUPPLEMENT SECTION

Depending on the jurisdiction, the provincial/territorial supplement section is a requirement to achieve COR® and may also be a requirement for any out-of-province companies (no permanent base of operations) who wish to achieve COR® Reciprocity

HEALTH AND SAFETY PROGRAM VERIFICATION

Does the company's health and safety program contain the following?	YES	NO
1. Health and Safety Policy		
2. Hazard Assessment, Analysis, and Control		
3. Safe Work Practices		
4. Safe Job Procedures		
5. Company Safety Rules		
6. Personal Protective Equipment (PPE)		
7. Preventative Maintenance Program		
8. Training and Communication		
9. Inspections		
10. Investigations and Reporting		
11. Emergency Preparedness		
12. Statistics, Records, and Document Control		
13. Legislation		
14. Procurement and Contractor Management		
15. Provincial/Territorial Supplement		

Verification of Compulsory COR® Training	Participant and Completion Date
Principles of Safety Management (PSM)	
Safety Auditor	
Hazard Identification and Risk Control	
Leadership for Safety Excellence (LSE)	

STEP TWO: PERFORMING THE AUDIT

Performing the audit means using the audit instrument and associated checklists and forms. This step will include the following:

✓ Audit instrument section pages
✓ Layout and guidelines
✓ Verification techniques and how to apply them
- Documentation
- Observation
- Interview

The harmonized audit instrument is separated into fourteen major sections and an optional provincial/territorial supplement section. Each section reviews one major topic in a complete health and safety management system. The provincial/territorial supplement (section 15) assists companies in ensuring they meet their obligations as an employer working in the jurisdiction from which they are requesting COR®, including the legislative requirements as outlined in the provincial or territorial workplace health and safety act and regulation.

Audit Instrument Section Pages

Section number and name
The top of the table identifies the section number and the title of the section. This corresponds with the audit manual verification page.

Referencing Numbers

The numbers in the left-hand column are unique question identifiers for referencing documentation that will be used to verify whether requirements are being maintained during the audit. Referencing documents and using these numbers will be described in detail later in this guide.

Audit Question

The second column contains the audit questions. These questions outline the requirement to be verified in a short, easily communicated sentence. Questions will be specific to each section and related to the section they ask about.

Score Weighting

Each question will be assigned a point value identified in this column. This will be used when assessing and scoring results later and will be a key indicator in determining the importance of each question.

Safety and Health Program Verification		Score Weighting	Technique Employed			Points Awarded
1	Safety and Health Policy		D	O	I	
	Senior management shall establish, implement, monitor, and maintain a documented occupational safety and health policy appropriate to the scale and nature of the organization's operations and activities, and associated risks. *Does the employer have a written safety and health policy that:*					
1.1	Includes management's commitment to provide a safe and healthy work environment?	3				
1.2	Expresses a commitment to work in a spirit of consultation and cooperation with the workers?	3				
1.3	Addresses accountability and responsibility for safety and health for workplace parties?	4		AND		
1.4	Is signed by current senior management and appropriately dated?	2				
1.5	Is visibly posted in the workplace and/or made readily available to all workplace parties.	3		O	R	
1.6	Is communicated to workplace parties?	3				
	COR® total points possible/awarded	18				

National COR® Accreditation Standard – 2022 Harmonized Audit Instrument Template

VERIFICATION TECHNIQUES

Under "technique employed," there are three columns: D, O, and I—documentation, observation, and interview. These columns identify the three verification techniques used to assess the health and safety program of the company being audited. The shaded and unshaded boxes will identify which techniques apply to which questions. The question row should be connected with the technique column. Unshaded boxes will identify that a particular question requires a specific technique be used for verification.

- As information is verified using these techniques, the auditor should document the result in these boxes using ✓s and Xs only. Information on using the verification techniques and documenting the results will be covered later in this workbook.
- Boxes containing "AND" and "OR" will identify where multiple techniques are required or permitted to be used. Each technique that applies individually will be assessed during the audit. The application of the AND/OR questions will be relevant when scoring and will be discussed later in this workbook.
- When summarizing information during the audit, only a ✓ or an X can be placed in these boxes. Verifying these techniques is a "yes" or "no" response only, based on the assessment of information collected through the audit. Numbers/points are not placed in these columns.

Points Awarded

Once all techniques have been assessed and information has been gathered, the score for each question will be identified based on the analysis of the ✓s and Xs under the verification techniques and placed in this column. Each of these points are added to provide Total for Points Awarded in that section.

Audit Guidelines

The back of each section page offers guidelines to help an auditor award points for each question. These guidelines relate to the questions found on the section pages and can be identified using the reference number for each question. The guidelines will go into detail on the requirements for each question; provide examples of what to look for; and, where applicable, outline how points are to be awarded for each question.

These guidelines play a crucial role in performing the audit and should be reviewed often to ensure that the audit evaluations are being performed according to the standard.

1.0	**Guidelines - Safety and Health Policy**
1.1	The policy must state management's commitment to provide a safe and healthy work environment.
1.2	The policy must include a statement of the employer's commitment to work in a spirit of consultation and cooperation with their workers or clearly express the commitment to work jointly with their workforce in the development and implementation of their safety and health program.
1.3	The policy should include individual safety and health obligations and make reference to documented safety and health responsibilities of workplace parties (management, supervisors, workers, safety and health representatives, subcontractors, etc.). This information could be contained in a document separate from the company safety policy. - Award two (2) points for the written assignment of safety and health responsibilities. - Award two (2) points based on the majority of positive interview responses.
1.4	The policy must be signed by current senior management with a current date.
1.5	During worksite observations, verify the safety and health policy has been posted. If no suitable means of posting is available, points can be awarded if the majority of interviews confirm it is made readily available to workers (in the form of a handbook, safety and health manual, or other accessible electronic format).
1.6	The majority of interview responses must confirm that all personnel understand the safety and health policy.

USING THE AUDIT INSTRUMENT SECTION PAGES AND GUIDELINES

The following examples explain how it works:

Question 1.4 asks whether documentation "Is signed by current senior management and appropriately dated?"
The space under "O" and "I" are shaded, therefore documentation is the only method that can be used to determine compliance with this question. Through collection and review, determine if there is adequate documentation in compliance with this question and document these findings by putting a ✓ or an X in the white box under the "D" column.

Question 1.5 asks whether documentation "Is visibly posted in the workplace and/or made readily available to all workplace parties."
This question requires either observation OR interviews to verify if the health and safety policy is physically posted or available on the site. During a tour of the work areas, indicate compliance using an observational checklist for each site visited OR through interview questionnaires. The majority of responses for both would be identified here with a ✓ for positive, or an X for negative.

Evaluation and points are determined later. Regardless of AND/OR questions, each technique is evaluated separately. The combination of all the techniques and their analysis will be completed once all information has been collected and documented under the three technique columns.

Question 1.6 asks whether documentation "Is communicated to workplace parties?"
This question requires an interview response for verification only. In this case, if interviews confirm that the majority of company personnel knew the content of the policy, the auditor should place a ✓ in the box under the "I" column. To determine what a correct answer should look like, the auditor must become familiar with the policy and review the audit guideline.

Applying the Three Techniques: D—Documentation / O—Observation / I—Interview

The order in which these techniques are listed is the most efficient way for an auditor to perform an audit. The following approach will help the auditor perform the detailed audit quickly and easily.

Each technique will require the auditor to apply certain skills and evaluation criteria to properly evaluate the effectiveness of the health and safety management system. Below are instructions on how to use each technique; record-keeping and submission requirements; and how to troubleshoot grey areas.

Documentation Technique

Documentation is important because it is the only acceptable way for a company to demonstrate **due diligence**. This is the only allowable defense to an employer if charged with an offense under the workplace health and safety act. Due diligence means that the company did everything reasonably practicable to ensure the health and safety of workers and can confirm it through documentation.

The provincial or territorial workplace health and safety act and regulations are NOT the same as the criminal code, which assumes that a party is innocent until proven guilty. Workplace health and safety legislation assumes the opposite—one is presumed guilty until proven innocent. In law, this is called "reverse onus."

Documentation serves as a written plan and record of executing that plan. A receipt provides long-term proof that money was provided in exchange for goods and services. The same is true for a health and safety program: documentation serves as record of the plan, and whether or not the plan was followed.

Selecting Documentation

When selecting documentation for the audit, it is the auditor's responsibility to locate documentation that best represents the company's current health and safety activities. The audit questions will identify the information required. The audit guidelines related to each question will outline examples of documents and provide a further explanation of how documents are to be evaluated.

An audit is a snapshot in time. It is not intended to collect and evaluate all information that has been documented. The audit seeks enough information to make an informed evaluation and conclusion on the current state of the health and safety system and how it's performing.

IMPORTANT: Copies of originals should be made and provided in the audit. Original documents are part of company records and necessary for due diligence. Auditors **SHOULD NOT** provide originals within the audit submission. When an audit is submitted to a CFCSA member for COR® certification, it becomes part of the association records and will not be returned.

When selecting documentation for the audit, an auditor should keep the following in mind:

- Only a handful of copies will be necessary for each requirement.
- Providing too much documentation can cloud the assessment.
- Documents must be from the last twelve months.
- Audits are conducted on an annual cycle and therefore new documents from the last twelve months (e.g., June to June) must be provided every year to demonstrate continued adherence to the standards.

Although each section of the audit is based on an element or theme of information, it will be necessary to provide some of the same documents in multiple sections of the audit. For example, a new hire orientation will be most needed in section 8—Training and Communication, but it can also demonstrate requirements in sections 6 and 11. In these cases, an additional copy of the document should be supplied in each section where reference is required.

Documentation Types

Documentation can be used to verify:

1. Intent
2. Completion (action)

Intent: These are documents that act as a guideline on how to behave safely. Typically these documents include statements such as, "We will do/provide/maintain/ensure," which are most commonly found in policies. These are considered "documentation of intent." They are passive in nature, and once developed require little work to remain current or applicable. These documents are used for training and review purposes. Policies, directives, company rules, guidelines, and so on, are examples of documents of intent.

These documents are vital in a health and safety program, as they make up the structure of the program on which the health and safety management system is based.

Completion: These are documents for which a company/individual has performed an activity or action. These documents demonstrate that the document of intent is being fulfilled and are considered "documentation of completion." They typically involve the work of individuals to actively do something or regularly assess and document health and safety-related information. If a policy (document of intent) says hazard assessments will be completed prior to starting work, then the completed hazard assessment with names, signatures, identified hazards, and controls, would be the "document of completion."

In most cases, the guidelines will explain the type of documentation required as a verification technique for each question. For example: if an audit question asks if workers "have been trained in ____________," a policy statement saying workers "will" be trained is not acceptable. The company must provide a record of training via certificates, completed evaluations, and so on.

Assessing Documentation

Assessing documentation for compliance to audit questions requires an unbiased, impartial approach. Knowing the people who work for the company, or being familiar with their work, may affect one's judgment. An impartial third party should be able to look at the same document and come to the same conclusion. When assessing documentation, an auditor should evaluate it at face value and only conclude what can be clearly identified.

"Majority rules" means that the response that outweighs the other is the response that is documented. A majority means more than 50 percent. Where there is a "tie" it will be the responsibility of the auditor to either collect more information to identify an accurate and conclusive result or, where additional information is not available, assess the quality of the information provided and make an informed decision. The majority rule will carry over through the verification techniques when looking at observation and interview results.

For documentation questions, the auditor will provide a number of copies and make a majority rule conclusion on the sample provided. Using a sample of three, the auditor will average the evaluation for each question to determine an overall positive or negative response. It may be necessary to provide a few more examples to confidently conclude a majority response but an auditor should be mindful not to provide too many examples, which becomes less beneficial as more are provided.

The majority response is documented in the audit instrument with a ✓ or an X. Once documents have been located that effectively demonstrate requirements found in the audit, they must be appropriately referenced to clearly show where and how they demonstrate compliance. It is the responsibility of the auditor to demonstrate that they understand and are capable of assessing documentation accurately by referencing appropriately. This is where the question numbers come into play.

Each question has a unique identifying number. The first number identifies the section in which the question is located, and the second identifies the question number from that section, separated by a decimal. For example, reference number 2.8 would be from section 2 and is the eighth question in that section.

When a document demonstrates a requirement, it is the responsibility of the auditor to write that reference number directly beside the information on that document. Reference numbers are only required for documentation questions and only for information that is verified to be present. If a documentation question cannot be verified, there is no need to place a reference number on any documents.

Dos and Don'ts of Referencing Documentation

Do not line the top, bottom, or sides of a document with reference numbers.

- Reference numbers are used to quickly identify the applicable information for others to find. They also demonstrate the auditor's ability to accurately and fairly assess information. If reference numbers are placed far away from the information used to verify a positive response, the audit is not being performed to standard. This increases the chance that information will be missed or overlooked by a CFCSA auditor or the independent auditor when performing the audit. This also means an auditor's registered auditor status may not be achieved, or may be suspended pending repeat concerns.

Do not reference documentation for observation and interview questions.

- "Documentation required" questions are the only reference numbers that should be placed on documents. Each technique has its own method of verification. Referencing observation questions on completed documents is not an acceptable means of verifying those questions.
- Taking jobsite photos and referencing them in the audit is neither required nor beneficial. Observations are verified by the auditor who is physically on-site and sees those requirements being met. This is documented through an observational checklist. When the audit is submitted to a CFCSA member, the association will conduct its own audit and perform its own observations and interviews.

Documentation that is referenced and required for a specific section must be provided and referenced in that section.

- Referencing other sections is not acceptable. For example, if a document in section 8 can be used in section 2, copy that document again and provide it in both sections—appropriately referenced.

Documentation Technique—Review

- Only "documentation required" questions require supporting documentation to verify compliance.
- Use copies of originals only—do not provide originals in the audit, as they will not be returned.
- Provide only enough samples to verify a majority response.
- Do not oversupply documents.

- Where documentation requirements have been verified, reference numbers are placed on the document directly beside the information used to verify compliance.
- Lining the page with reference numbers is not an acceptable means of referencing.
- Majority rules when documenting results in the audit instrument.
- A good practice when performing an audit is to complete all documentation requirements in every section first, before moving on to the other techniques.
- Batching work is more efficient and saves time.
- Reviewing and assessing all documentation first will allow the auditor to gain a stronger understanding of the company program and safety behaviors before heading to site to observe and interview workers. It allows the auditor to identify information and requirements that could not be concluded or are missing and ask for this information on-site or when meeting with management.

OBSERVATION TECHNIQUE

Observation is the second verification technique used in the audit process and will require the auditor to OBSERVE active jobsites and work locations where workers are performing work. The jobsite is anywhere a worker is being compensated (paid) to be. This will include offices, shops, construction sites, vehicles, and so on.

Purpose

The purpose of the observation technique is to verify that what is written in policy and stated on paper is actually performed on-site. Safety is a conscious effort and by going to the site and observing activities and behaviors, the auditor can get a good account of the current state of compliance regarding the program.

Checklist

It may be cumbersome and inefficient to carry around the audit instrument on-site. For this reason, an observation checklist document has been developed including every observation question from every section. The reference numbers for each question in this document are consistent with the audit instrument.

An auditor will use one of these checklists **per site visited** and document all findings. Once completed, the results will be consolidated into the audit instrument, just as documentation was consolidated using the majority rules principle. Final results for each observation question will be documented under the "O" column in the instrument using a ✓ or an X during the summary portion of the audit process.

Visiting Sites

As with documentation, an auditor should look for a good representative sample. The auditor is not required to visit every active jobsite at the time of the audit. Typically, the auditor should visit at least three sites if available. If there are three (or fewer) sites available, they should visit all sites. If there are more sites, a representative sample is recommended. To make the summary of results easier, they should visit an odd number of sites to achieve a clear majority for each requirement evaluated.

When performing a site observation, it is recommended the auditor be escorted by the supervisor, safety representative, or any individual familiar with that location. This person is responsible for the auditor's safety and should be someone of whom questions can be asked, so they can help the auditor through the observation checklist to ensure nothing is overlooked.

REMEMBER: Auditors are not trying to "catch" anyone doing something unsafe. They are there to assess the health and safety management system and identify opportunities for improvement.

When performing observation, an auditor should look at the people, environment, material, equipment (PEME), and so on on-site. This will include checking whether certain documents are available on-site and workers have access to them. Auditors should review the guidelines for observation questions prior to heading to the site to educate themselves on what they are looking for.

Below is a summary of observations that are required according to the CFCSA harmonized audit instrument. The following checklist helps to organize and validate all observations that are required.

Interview Questionnaire – Employee

1.3	What are your safety and health responsibilities? How are you held accountable for them?
1.5	Where would you find a copy of the safety and health policy?
1.6	In your own words, what does the safety and health policy say?
2.1	Describe the process your company uses to conduct formal hazard assessments. What type of tasks are included in the formal hazard assessment process?
2.2	How are completed formal hazards assessments reviewed with you?
2.4	How are hazards reassessed as the job progresses or changes occur?
2.6	How are you involved in the hazard assessment process?
2.7	How have you been trained to identify and control hazards?
2.10	Who is responsible for implementation of controls?
3.2	Describe some of the key points of a safe work practice applicable to your work.
3.3	How do you have access to safe work practices when on site?
3.5	Can you give me an example of how a safe work practice has been reviewed or discussed?
4.2	Describe the step by step process of a safe job procedure for a critical task that is applicable to your work.
4.3	How do you have access to safe job procedures when on site?
4.5	Can you give me an example of how a safe job procedure has been reviewed or discussed?
5.2	Where can you find both company and project (work location) specific rules?
5.3	How are company safety rules provided or made available to you?
5.4	Can you give me an example of few company and/or site specific rules that you need to follow?
5.6	How are the company rules enforced?
6.1	How do you know what PPE is required to perform a specific task?
6.3	What type of training did you receive to understand the proper fitting, care and use of your PPE?
6.4	How do you have access to appropriate PPE when needed?
7.5	What is your company's system to remove defective tools or equipment from service?
8.2	After training, how are you evaluated for your retention of information regarding the company safety and health program?

2022 CFCSA Endorsed harmonized audit instrument in alignment with the national COR® accreditation standard

If the auditor can verify through observation that the policy is posted or made available, a ✓ or an X can be placed on this summary checklist. Later, all observations will be consolidated in the audit instrument by using the reference numbers for each question.

IMPORTANT: An auditor should keep good notes on all checklists and documents provided with the audit. Notes will eventually be used as comments on the successes and opportunities for improvement regarding the company's health and safety management system and will greatly assist in developing a corrective action plan, which is a requirement of the audit. Sometimes auditors will not be sure how to determine a positive or negative result. This is the reason notes are important. They should make note of the situation and make a conclusion at a later time when it can be looked into further.

A lot of work goes into an audit and it will be very difficult to remember the finer details of every ✓ or X concluded throughout the audit instrument. An auditor should take good notes, especially for observation and interview.

Also remember:

- Use the summary checklist provided for site observation.
- Get a guided tour of the worksite and work being performed.
- Majority rules when summarizing results into the audit instrument.

Interview Technique

The purpose of conducting interviews is to ensure that everyone involved in the program has an understanding of their role regarding health and safety at the company. What is written in documentation cannot always be observed during a site tour. This is why sitting down with workers and having a conversation about their role, the health and safety program, and what they should/would do in certain situations is vital when auditing an organization.

INTERVIEW QUESTIONNAIRES (CHECKLISTS)

Everyone who works for the company has the potential to be interviewed. Just like observation, there are checklists available to assist an auditor in performing interviews effectively. There are two types of interview questionnaires:

- Employee
- Management/supervisors

Choose the correct interview questionnaire based on the role the individual represents within the company.

Each questionnaire will follow the same template:

- The same reference numbers seen in the observation checklist and the audit instrument will be seen down the left-hand side.
- The second column includes the specific question to be asked for that requirement.
- Interview questions are asked differently from those in the audit instrument, because their intent is different.

Having a checklist of consistent questions ensures that everyone interviewed is asked the same question in the same way and helps maintain the standard of COR® certification across all companies.

Similar to the observation summary checklist, place a ✓ or an X following the question indicating a positive or negative response under one of these columns.

Interview notes or comments are also extremely important. The auditor may receive unexpected answers and information that may be challenging to evaluate until more information is gathered. Making a note and coming back to the question to determine positive or negative outcome is vital to a quality audit.

Below is a summary of interview question requirements within the CFCSA harmonized audit instrument. Utilizing a summary checklist will help to organize and validate interview responses.

Interview Questionnaire – Employee

1.3	What are your safety and health responsibilities? How are you held accountable for them?
1.5	Where would you find a copy of the safety and health policy?
1.6	In your own words, what does the safety and health policy say?
2.1	Describe the process your company uses to conduct formal hazard assessments. What type of tasks are included in the formal hazard assessment process?
2.2	How are completed formal hazards assessments reviewed with you?
2.4	How are hazards reassessed as the job progresses or changes occur?
2.6	How are you involved in the hazard assessment process?
2.7	How have you been trained to identify and control hazards?
2.10	Who is responsible for implementation of controls?
3.2	Describe some of the key points of a safe work practice applicable to your work.
3.3	How do you have access to safe work practices when on site?
3.5	Can you give me an example of how a safe work practice has been reviewed or discussed?
4.2	Describe the step by step process of a safe job procedure for a critical task that is applicable to your work.
4.3	How do you have access to safe job procedures when on site?
4.5	Can you give me an example of how a safe job procedure has been reviewed or discussed?
5.2	Where can you find both company and project (work location) specific rules?
5.3	How are company safety rules provided or made available to you?
5.4	Can you give me an example of few company and/or site specific rules that you need to follow?
5.6	How are the company rules enforced?
6.1	How do you know what PPE is required to perform a specific task?
6.3	What type of training did you receive to understand the proper fitting, care and use of your PPE?
6.4	How do you have access to appropriate PPE when needed?
7.5	What is your company's system to remove defective tools or equipment from service?
8.2	After training, how are you evaluated for your retention of information regarding the company safety and health program?

2022 CFCSA Endorsed harmonized audit instrument in alignment with the national COR® accreditation standard

8.5	How was your mandatory training verified or provided to you prior to starting work?
8.8	When was your orientation provided? Have you received a re-orientation?
8.12	How are you given the opportunity to give input and communicate safety and health concerns?
8.13	How often does your company hold scheduled safety meetings?
9.3	How are identified deficiencies assigned to individuals and corrected as required?
9.4	What specific method, form or checklist is used for pre-use inspections?
9.7	What is your role in the formal or informal inspection process?
9.8	How are the inspection reports posted and/or communicated to you?
10.1	What is the process for reporting an incident? What are your responsibilities?
10.4	Once an incident investigation has been completed, how are corrective actions implemented?
10.5	How are corrective actions communicated to you after an incident occurs?
10.6	What incidents do you report? Do you report near misses? Please give an example of a near miss?
11.4	How do you know who is a qualified to administer first aid on this site?
11.5	How do you alert everyone onsite in the event of an emergency? How do you contact appropriate personnel/agencies for emergency assistance?
11.9	Can you give me an example(s) of an emergency plan for this site? What are your specific roles and responsibilities?
11.12	How have site specific emergency plans been communicated to you?
13.1	Where are copies of relevant legislation on this site? *NOTE for AHJs – insert the name of required legislation*
13.2	Does your supervisor regularly discuss relevant regulations and legislation when assigning work? Can you give an example?
13.3	What are your legislated rights? Do you know how to exercise those rights?

2022 CFCSA Endorsed harmonized audit instrument in alignment with the national COR® accreditation standard

HOW MANY PEOPLE SHOULD BE INTERVIEWED?

The number of people to interview is subjective. Conduct enough interviews to acquire a clear and accurate majority response for all interview questions that are representative of the entire company.

A good guideline is to interview 10 percent of the workforce or at least five people on sites with fewer than fifty employees. On sites with more than 100 employees, a smaller percentage is acceptable. Normally twenty to twenty-five interviews will be sufficient. Interviews should take approximately 10 to 15 minutes each.

Who Should Be Interviewed?

All types of persons employed by the company should be interviewed. An auditor should strive for a representative sample of the company's current organizational structure, based on its organizational chart. For example, if 40 percent of the company is made up of workers/laborers, then 40 percent of the interviews should be conducted with those workers. It is a requirement of the audit that the owner or representatives of the ownership team (senior management) be interviewed as part of the certification audit.

Selecting Interviewees When On-site

Arriving at a worksite location, the auditor will first perform an observational tour and pay attention to the personnel and the type of work they are performing. Auditors may select certain individuals based on what they see. If a worker is working with a controlled product, WHMIS training will be especially important. Taking notes of these activities will allow the auditor to better connect information found in the audit, observed on-site, and communicated via interview.

An auditor should interview a good cross-section of company personnel to effectively document what the company knows about the health and safety program. A good approach is to ask the supervisor to identify the most senior and newest workers on-site that day. Interviewing these two extremes will allow the auditor to identify how the company is in training new workers and how they are communicating changes to existing workers who may have been with the company before the health and safety program was implemented. The remainder of the interviewees should be selected at random.

Dos and Don'ts When Conducting an Interview

The auditor should select the person to be interviewed.

- Do not allow the company to "prime" workers. Doing so may skew results.

All interviews must be held in private—no group interviews.

- The purpose of an interview is to see what individuals know and what they can communicate about the health and safety program. Group interviews prevent the auditor from getting individual results and may allow one worker to answer for all. Such results will not be accurate.

Take notes.

- A lot of information will be presented during interviews over the course of a few days or weeks. Documenting results is extremely important to the reporting process.
- Let the interviewee know that notes will be taken and why. This will help put them at ease as it can be intimidating to have a stranger documenting what they say. Communication skills will be covered further on in this workbook.

Interviews are confidential.

- Let the interviewee know that the interview process and individual results are confidential. No information about what they've said or how well they performed will be shared with the company, workplace health and safety officers, or anyone else. Interview results are consolidated, and the majority response (positive or negative) is communicated in the audit results.

Encourage questions at any time.

- Let interviewees know that they can ask questions at any time. If they don't understand a question, or are curious about the process, provide clarity where it is appropriate to do so.

Communication Skills

Good communication skills are essential to effectively gather information. The ability to understand and to be understood is key. Here are a few tips for the auditor to follow during the interview process:

- **Keep it simple**—use common terms and understandable language. People will feel more relaxed when they can answer and explain situations in their own words.
- **Listen carefully**—many people communicate important information in a matter-of-fact manner or offer unexpected responses. It is the responsibility of the auditor to seek clarity.
- **Recognize barriers**—never put people on the spot or make them feel intimidated. The goal of the audit is to evaluate the company's health and safety management system, not to interrogate individuals.

  If there are language barriers or issues with verbal communication, identify how the employer currently communicates with the individual. It may be necessary to adopt a similar method for the interview.
- **Discuss, don't dictate**—people will have a more positive experience and will be able to answer more appropriately if they feel they are a part of a conversation, rather than being drilled with questions.

  Interview subjects may be nervous or concerned about the process. It is the auditor's responsibility to put them at ease and facilitate an open and honest discussion about what they know and do regarding health and safety activities within the company.

- **Practice**—practicing interview techniques prior to the interview will help the auditor to be more relaxed and focus on positive communication.
  Part of practicing means knowing what a correct answer looks like. If auditors are unaware of a correct answer to a question, they will have a hard time documenting the results of the interview or asking important follow-up questions.
- **Acknowledge correct communication**—give credit where credit is due. Positive reinforcement and support for a job well done will encourage people to stay actively involved in their own health and safety, promote it to their coworkers and help to ensure a strong health and safety culture within the company.

Concluding an Interview

Just like observations, the auditor is responsible for taking the information available and analyzing it to determine compliance with the audit requirements. Two different answers can both be correct, depending on the situation.

Auditors should pose questions in a way that is understood by the interviewee, listen to the answers, and assess them to determine a positive or negative response. They may need to ask follow-up questions or reword the original question to ensure that interviewees are given an opportunity to share their knowledge. Getting comfortable with interviews starts with being familiar with the questions, how they're asked, and understanding the intent of the question.

Before ending an interview, the auditor should thank the participants for their time and effort, reaffirm the confidentiality of the interview, and give them one final opportunity for questions.

An auditor may not have a fully completed questionnaire identifying all positive or negative responses at the end of an interview, so good notes are important. Notes can be used to determine if the response received is correct (positive) or incorrect (negative). After an interview, it may be necessary to continue observation before leaving the worksite to verify responses.

Interview Technique—Review

Interviews provide the best information about the way in which health and safety is viewed and performed within an organization. An auditor should take good notes, be open to discussion, and ask for more information as needed.

An auditor should use the questionnaires to ensure consistency from interview to interview and make sure a cross-section of the company is interviewed. Auditors should remember that a correct answer can be different from person to person, and site to site. They should review documentation and conduct observations prior to performing interviews to become familiar with the company and its processes.

STEP THREE: REPORTING THE RESULTS

When auditing is complete via the three verification techniques, an auditor should consolidate and summarize the information collected into the audit instrument. This is where the referencing of documentation, checklists used, and notes fall into place.

Interviews will constitute the largest amount of information collected and summarized. Observations will follow a similar technique, and documentation will be a general review and verification that information has been transferred properly.

Interview Summary—Using the Interview Response Summary Tool

Interviews may generate a large number of interview questionnaires and will be evaluated according to majority rule. As interviews will result in the greatest diversity of information, this rule will be extremely important in summarizing results. It can be difficult to consolidate a large number of questionnaires into the audit instrument. To simplify this process and help ensure accurate information is concluded, use of the interview summary checklist is recommended.

The interview summary checklist helps to determine whether there are a majority of positive or negative responses to the interview questions. At a glance, the auditor will be able to verify whether or not the majority of people interviewed have a good understanding of their health and safety program for each question asked. During future audits, the auditor may want to look back at these documents to see if progress is being made in regard to the interview process.

Once all interview results have been logged, it will be easier to see where the majority of responses lie and transfer the final result for each question to the audit instrument. Remember, to look for a majority—MORE than half. If the majority of responses are negative, an X will be placed under the "I" column that corresponds with that particular question (using the reference numbers as guidance). The same rule applies for a majority positive response—a

✓ will be placed in the correct box. Where response to a question is exactly 50 percent positive and 50 percent negative, this is not a majority. The auditor must err on the side of caution and an X must be placed for that question.

Only a majority of positive responses can result in a ✓ in the audit instrument.

Where questions are split 50/50 and where possible, the auditor should perform additional interviews to break the tie and get a conclusive result. Where this is not possible, an X must be transferred to the audit instrument for that question.

Observation Summary

An observation summary will work the same way as an interview summary. At this stage, the auditor will have multiple observation checklists, one for each site visited. The majority rules here, also. The auditor can now consolidate all the ✓ and X observations in one checklist. They should tally up the majority responses and transfer those results into the audit instrument under the "O" column using the reference numbers as guidance.

As suggested, it is a good idea to visit an odd number of sites to ensure a majority response can be identified.

Documentation Summary

A documentation summary will use slightly different techniques. At this point, auditors have collected documentation, found the relevant information for questions identified in the audit, referenced those components of the document, and placed a ✓ in the corresponding box under the "D" column. They should now double check all references and fill in any gaps.

For every ✓ identified under the "D" column, a reference number is placed on a document in that section, appropriately communicating the requirement. Any blank boxes under the "D" column must now be filled in. If a document was found on-site or the company provided additional documentation, the new information can now be assessed, allowing completion of the remainder of the "D" column for all fourteen sections.

Check for Accuracy

If all audit procedures have been followed, all of the boxes under "D," "O," and "I" should be filled in with either a ✓ or an X.

For observation and interview, the auditor must verify that findings are accurate and, where information is missing, review checklists, or conduct further observations or interviews to conclude a result.

After completing the accuracy check, auditors may be able to answer "yes" in a few more places. The answers to the remaining questions will then be "no." They can then go back over the audit instrument section pages and place an X in the remaining blank boxes to indicate the verification of a negative response.

Analyzing Results

Now that all the data necessary for the audit has been collected, it is time to determine a score. As noted earlier, each question has a weighted score. This will identify the maximum points that can be awarded for each question of the audit.

For each question identified with a positive or negative response via ✓s and Xs the auditor can now evaluate the positive and negative results of each technique to determine a score. There are some rules to follow when scoring an audit to ensure an accurate result.

SCORING THE AUDIT—AWARDING POINTS

The final column in each section is for recording the points awarded for the questions. Now that all components of the audit have been verified, and there are ✓s or Xs in every box, the auditor can determine a score for each section. Points will be determined by the following rules:

For questions worth three points or less and using a single technique:

X = zero points ✓ = full points

For questions worth three points or less—using multiple techniques with "AND," both must be positive to award points:

✓	**AND**	*X = zero points*
X	**AND**	X = zero points
✓	**AND**	✓ = full points

For questions worth three points or less—using multiple techniques with "OR," if any one of the techniques is positive, points are awarded:

✓	**OR**	*X = full points*
X	**OR**	X = zero points
✓	**OR**	✓ = full points (not double)

For questions worth four points or more—using a single technique as well as "AND/OR" questions:

- Consult the guidelines to determine point distribution.
- Where the guidelines do not identify a split of points, follow the same rules as above.

The auditor should pay special attention to questions worth 4 points or more and use the guidelines to identify the way in which points can be awarded in these cases. Once points have been awarded for each question in a section, the sections may be added and a total recorded at the bottom of the page.

It is critical to only place ✓s or Xs in the D, O, and I columns. If the auditor attempts to score the audit before all information is collected, they may run into problems, forget to collect information, or calculate scores incorrectly. This can drastically affect the results of the audit. Only the final points awarded are placed in the far-right column.

Cor® Executive Summary Sheet

Once scores for all sections have been calculated, the auditor may transfer the results to the executive summary sheet. This sheet is the report card for the audit. It communicates "pass/fail" and scores in each section. The executive summary sheet does not communicate what was missing, nor does it make recommendations for improvement. This will be communicated through the audit corrective action plan.

Once all scores are entered, the auditor may determine if the minimum standard of 50 percent in each section has been met and identify this with a ✓ under "yes" or "no." If the auditor has any general comments about any section, they can be placed beside each section in the comments column. Generally, this column is used to identify the main issue/concern with that section. If a company primarily had an issue with documentation in section 2, that comment can be placed there. Further details and information regarding the performance of each section will be later identified through a written report or the audit corrective action plan.

Adding up the scores in all sections results in a final score. That total is transferred to the bottom of the page, and a percentage is calculated for the audit. As long as 50 percent or better was achieved in each section, and 80 percent or better was achieved overall, the auditor can identify that minimum standards have been achieved and set a goal for next year's audit. A realistic goal is approximately 5 percent improvement from one year to the next. This can change depending on the type of deficiencies that were noted through the audit process and the time and effort it will take to implement improvements.

8.5	How was your mandatory training verified or provided to you prior to starting work?
8.8	When was your orientation provided? Have you received a re-orientation?
8.12	How are you given the opportunity to give input and communicate safety and health concerns?
8.13	How often does your company hold scheduled safety meetings?
9.3	How are identified deficiencies assigned to individuals and corrected as required?
9.4	What specific method, form or checklist is used for pre-use inspections?
9.7	What is your role in the formal or informal inspection process?
9.8	How are the inspection reports posted and/or communicated to you?
10.1	What is the process for reporting an incident? What are your responsibilities?
10.4	Once an incident investigation has been completed, how are corrective actions implemented?
10.5	How are corrective actions communicated to you after an incident occurs?
10.6	What incidents do you report? Do you report near misses? Please give an example of a near miss?
11.4	How do you know who is a qualified to administer first aid on this site?
11.5	How do you alert everyone onsite in the event of an emergency? How do you contact appropriate personnel/agencies for emergency assistance?
11.9	Can you give me an example(s) of an emergency plan for this site? What are your specific roles and responsibilities?
11.12	How have site specific emergency plans been communicated to you?
13.1	Where are copies of relevant legislation on this site? *NOTE for AHJs – insert the name of required legislation*
13.2	Does your supervisor regularly discuss relevant regulations and legislation when assigning work? Can you give an example?
13.3	What are your legislated rights? Do you know how to exercise those rights?

2022 CFCSA Endorsed harmonized audit instrument in alignment with the national COR® accreditation standard

CFCSA
FCASC

COR® Audit—Corrective Action Plan

An audit corrective action plan is a critical component of an audit. Regardless of whether the company passes or fails an audit, there will always be opportunities for improvement. This is the place where the auditor can make those recommendations. At a minimum, a corrective action plan must

- identify deficient requirements of the audit, including audit reference numbers;
- make recommendations for improvement for each deficiency;
- assign responsibility for each action;
- set target dates for completion.

An action plan is a condensed version of the written report and is typically favored for that reason. An action plan can be submitted in any form or format but must contain the information stated above. Note that the corrective action plan must be signed off by the auditor, worker safety representative/safety committee member, and senior management just like the executive summary sheet. At the time of the close-out meeting, the action plan will be reviewed and signatures can be collected.

IMPORTANT: The corrective action plan developed by the auditor and presented to the company is to be considered suggestions for improvement based on the audit findings. The company is encouraged to either adopt or adapt the plan as they see fit. It is ultimately the company's responsibility to manage and improve the program in a way that best fits the organization.

Making Recommendations

When making a recommendation for improvement, it is important to provide enough detail and information to the company to effectively identify the area(s) of concern and adopt/implement the recommendations made. A good recommendation is procedural by nature and will identify the steps, in chronological order, on how to effectively and efficiently implement the changes.

For example:

A company was not awarded points for interview question 6.1—"Are activities requiring PPE documented and is specific criteria used to select appropriate PPE for those activities?"

The recommendation should lay out a plan for educating workers in all the methods and criteria used for selecting PPE. This can be done through updating orientations and developing topic-specific toolbox talks and can be reinforced through hazard identification and control methods.

The responsibility for updating orientations, writing new toolbox talks, and delivering toolbox talks should be clearly assigned to individuals, and timelines for implementation should be identified. This will be a good foundation for communication when there are questions regarding the plan, or when the company is following up on the corrective action plan to monitor progress.

The corrective action plan is not just for deficient components. It is a prime opportunity for the auditor to communicate any concerns they noted throughout the audit process or where questions resulted in a majority positive result, but only by a small margin. As a company grows and changes, these areas will become more and more important to the continued success of the program.

AUDIT CORRECTIVE ACTION PLAN

Date reviewed: ____________________

Audit Reference #	Recommendation	Assigned To	Target Completion Date	Date Completed

Reviewed: ____________________ Senior Management/Company Officer Signature ____________________ Auditor Signature ____________________ Worker Safety Rep./Safety Committee Co-Chair Signature

Close-out Meeting

Immediately after the audit is completed, the auditor should hold a close-out meeting. For larger organizations, an opening meeting is also held, and the close-out meeting usually has the same people in attendance.

At this time, the audit is reviewed in its entirety (section by section) from documentation review, sites visited, and number of interviews conducted.

Credit should be given where they have performed well and recommendations for improvement should be identified. This can be done by reviewing the corrective action plan developed as part of the audit. It is important to note that the company is expected to either accept and adopt the auditor's plan, or make its own based on the auditor's recommendations and what works for the organization.

It is common for companies to question the auditor's results and ask for examples and information so they have a better understanding of how they can improve. Notes from documentation, observation, and interview become indispensable here.

Once the meeting has concluded, the auditor should allow for questions and have the company's senior representative and worker representative identify a goal for the next audit, sign the audit summary sheet, and sign the corrective action plan. These signatures identify that the company has been presented with the results, that the auditor has communicated the reasons behind the findings, that they have been involved in the audit process, and that they have accepted the results as part of the record.

The agenda for this close-out meeting should be:

- Presentation of the written report or action plan.
- An overview of the audit and/or executive summary sheet.
- An identification of any immediate concerns that need to be addressed.
- Appropriate recommendations.
- A discussion of any other concerning issues.

Appendix A2

COR® Accreditation Standard

Audit Definitions and Interpretations

The following definitions are meant to assist auditors in interpreting the terminology within the CFCSA harmonized audit instrument template and to clarify the intent of the National COR® Accreditation Standard.

Auditors are reminded that the purpose of an audit is to analyze, interpret, and report on the system currently in place to manage the safety and health of a particular company.

Generally, this will focus on the implementation of an individual company's overall safety and health program. However, in circumstances where a company conducts its operations as a project manager, residential home builder, or prime contractor, the focus will shift to the implementation of the safety and health management system on the job site—which would include all contractors for whom it would be responsible.

PERSONNEL DEFINITIONS

Employee—a full-time or part-time person who is directly employed by the company (receiving a salary or hourly wage). This does not include persons working for a company on a fee-for-service basis (such as a subcontractor or consultant).

Employer—includes every person who, by themselves or through their representatives, employs or engages one or more workers.

Independent auditor—an impartial, independent auditor who performs an audit on a company that has requested or is renewing COR® certification. All external auditors are appointed and arranged by a member association of the CFCSA.

Internal auditor—a representative of a member association of the CFCSA who has been appointed to conduct an audit on a company that has requested COR® certification.

Management—a company representative who has the ability to make decisions, implement changes, direct the activities of others, and enforce the safety program. A manager can include a project manager, supervisor, lead hand, or others designated by the company.

Owner—the owner of land or premises to be used as a workplace.

Owner/operator—self-employed persons performing their own work operations.

Prime contractor—the person or company designated to be in charge of the entire work site. A prime contractor has the responsibility to develop, implement, and monitor a system to manage the safety and health performance of everyone at the work site.

Qualified person—a person whom the employer deems to be competent based on prior experience, knowledge, or training.

Senior management—the owner of a company or his/her authorized representative who has signing authority (for policies, procedures, purchases, etc.)

(Sub)-contractor—non-direct employees of a company performing duties on a contract basis. Subcontractors may be interviewed during the performance of an audit in residential construction or project management companies if there are few or no direct company employees on site. This definition includes self-employed persons.

Supervisor—an individual who has charge over a worksite and/or authority over other workers.

Supplier—an individual, company, or organization who provides/sells/leases/installs tools, equipment, materials, machines, devices, or biological or chemical substances to be used in a workplace.

Visitor—any person who is not directly employed at a worksite but who may enter the site (whether invited or uninvited) to deliver materials or conduct a formal or visual assessment.

Worker—an individual who does not have the authority to direct or manage the activities of others. Any person who is employed by an employer to perform a service, whether for gain or reward, or in hope of gain or reward.

Worker safety representative—an employee elected by fellow workers or designated by the employer to serve as a liaison between management and workers with respect to safety and health issues.

Workplace parties—all persons associated with a workplace. Includes, but is not limited to, the employer, prime contractor (constructor), owner, contractor(s), supervisor(s), worker(s), supplier(s), service provider(s), and visitor(s).

OTHER DEFINITIONS

Audit—a systematic process for obtaining evidence through documentation, observations, and interviews and objectively evaluating it to determine the extent to which predetermined criteria are fulfilled.

- **COMPANY INTERNAL/SELF-AUDIT**: Audit conducted by company representatives on their internal company safety and health management system, utilizing the prescribed audit instrument of the CFCSA member.
- **CFCSA VERIFICATION REVIEW**: Evaluation process used to verify the company's internal self-audit is complete and meets the required standards of the CFCSA member's prescribed method of verification and protocols.
- **CFCSA INTERNAL AUDIT**: An audit conducted by a CFCSA representative on the company safety and health management system, utilizing the prescribed audit instrument of the CFCSA member.
- **CFCSA EXTERNAL/INDEPENDENT AUDIT**: Audit conducted by an independent representative, external to the company being audited, who is authorized by a CFCSA member, utilizing the prescribed audit instrument of the CFCSA member.

Audit corrective action plan—a document within the audit instrument that aids the auditor in identifying weaknesses, setting goals, and assigning personnel to correct deficiencies for the company's next audit.

Authority Having Jurisdiction—an organization responsible for enforcing the minimum standards within its jurisdiction. (COR® is formally registered and trademarked. Although COR® is a national standard, COR® certification must be validated in each individual jurisdiction by the provincial/territorial Authority Having Jurisdiction. For the purposes of this National COR® Accreditation Standard, only a CFCSA member is permitted to grant and/or validate COR®.)

Close-out meeting—a meeting that involves the auditor and members from the company audited (usually upper management and a worker safety and health representative).

Current—other than policies (within three years), current documentation requires a date of no longer than one year prior to the current date.

Critical task—a task that has a high probability of severe injury, loss, or adverse effect if not performed properly. A critical task must have a written step-by-step safe work procedure in which employees must be trained.

Directive—written instructions or guidelines that indicate how to perform an action, reach a goal, or conduct company operations.

Documentation—supplying paperwork (completed hazard assessment forms, orientations, etc.) to prove a company's due diligence as required by law.

Due diligence—taking all reasonable precautions, under the particular circumstances, to prevent injuries and/or incidents in the workplace along with the ability to confirm this by means of documentation.

Executive summary sheet—a comprehensive evaluation form, including points awarded; verification of minimum standards met; and positive and negative comments for each audit section.

Hazard—any circumstance or condition that poses the risk of an accident or injury.

Hazard assessment—a thorough examination of an operation to identify the actual and potential hazards prior to work commencing and whenever the work or work environment changes.

Incident—any unplanned and unwanted event which results in, or could have resulted in, damage or injury.

Incident investigation—determination and analysis of the facts of the incident to establish the causes and the corrective measures required.

Internal audit—an audit performed by a representative of a CFCSA member as the second step toward the achievement or renewal of COR® certification.

Interview—a formal meeting in which people are asked predetermined questions by the auditor to test their knowledge of the company's safety and health program.

Job-specific training—includes both formal and informal training conducted by a qualified person that is required by employees in order to perform specific work tasks (i.e., confined space entry, aerial lift operation). This training can be delivered either in-house or by an outside agency.

Manufacturers' recommendations—written information supplied by the manufacturer providing details on recommended procedures for the use, care, or maintenance of tools, equipment, or vehicles.

Musculoskeletal injury (MSI)—an injury or disorder of the muscles, tendons, ligaments, joints, nerves, blood vessels, or related soft tissue.

Near-miss—an unplanned event that did not result in loss, damage, injury, or illness, but had the potential to do so.

Observation—the act or faculty of observing a worksite.

Personnel—the entire makeup of a company's workforce.

Policy—a written, signed statement that communicates management's intent, objectives, requirements, responsibilities, and standards.

Reverse onus—a clause within a statute that shifts the burden of proof onto the individual specified to disprove an element of information.

Safe job procedure—a step-by-step set of instructions outlining how to conduct a task or operate tools/equipment safely from beginning to end.

Safe work practice—generalized guidelines (dos and don'ts) on how to perform a task or an operation safely (i.e., tools, equipment, material handling).

Safety management—a systematic, organized process to identify, communicate, and control hazards to reduce the human and financial costs of workplace incidents.

Toolbox talk/tailgate meeting—a safety meeting required to be held and documented weekly for 15 minutes or biweekly for 30 minutes.

ACRONYMS

COR®—Certificate of Recognition
CFCSA—Canadian Federation of Construction Safety Associations
PPE—Personal Protective Equipment
WHMIS—Workplace Hazardous Materials Information System

Appendix B

ISO 45001

2018 Occupational Health and Safety Audit Tool

The authors would like to thank Ron Krebs of the Praxiom Research group for the most generous retirement gift which he so graciously offered the folks on LinkedIn. We're pleased to be able to provide some of these HSEQ audit resources here for those of you for whom the materials below might be applicable. Ron and Praxiom have been publishing these ISO ebooks for quite some time and the authors have also taken advantage of them from time to time. For any of you for whom ISO 45001 would be applicable, or who might have an integrated HSEQ management system to audit, the following guidance from Ron and the Praxiom Research Group would be beneficial.

Thanks for your contribution to the HSEQ community, Ron, and have a great retirement!

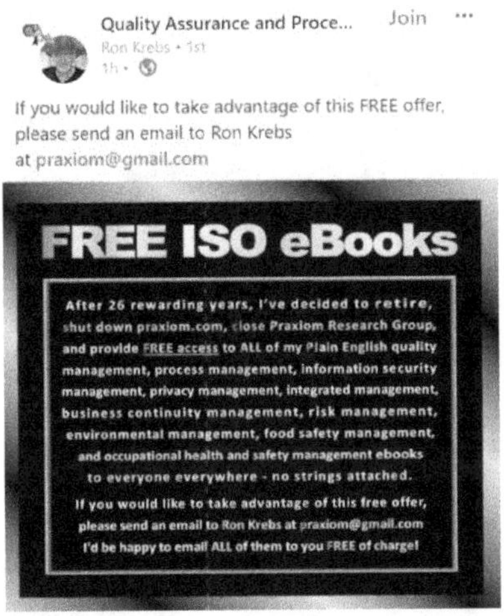
Quality Assurance and Proce...
Join
Ron Krebs • 1st
If you would like to take advantage of this FREE offer, please send an email to Ron Krebs at praxiom@gmail.com
FREE ISO eBooks
After 26 rewarding years, I've decided to retire, shut down praxiom.com, close Praxiom Research Group, and provide FREE access to ALL of my Plain English quality management, process management, information security management, privacy management, integrated management, business continuity management, risk management, environmental management, food safety management, and occupational health and safety management ebooks to everyone everywhere - no strings attached.
If you would like to take advantage of this free offer, please send an email to Ron Krebs at praxiom@gmail.com
I'd be happy to email ALL of them to you FREE of charge!

PART	TABLE OF CONTENTS	PAGE
1	Introduction to occupational health and safety audit tool	3
2	Profile of your occupational health and safety audit project	7
3	Mini occupational health and safety management audit tool	8
4	Assess how well you conform to ISO's contextual requirements	10
5	Assess how well you conform to ISO's leadership requirements	12
6	Assess how well you conform to ISO's planning requirements	19
7	Assess how well you conform to ISO's support requirements	37
8	Assess how well you conform to ISO's operational requirements	51
9	Assess how well you conform to ISO's evaluation requirements	58
10	Assess how well you conform to ISO's improvement requirements	67
11	Summary of your occupational health and safety audit results	71
12	Occupational health and safety terms and definitions	72

License agreement and contact information

ISO 45001:2018 OHS AUDIT TOOL

ISO 45001 2018 OHS AUDIT TOOL

1. INTRODUCTION TO OCCUPATIONAL HEALTH AND SAFETY AUDIT TOOL

INTERNATIONAL ORGANIZATION FOR STANDARDIZATION

ISO is the International Organization for Standardization. It was established in 1947 and is located in Geneva, Switzerland. Its purpose is to develop standards that facilitate and support international trade. ISO achieves this purpose through the support of its member bodies and through the work of its technical committees and subcommittees. The ISO 45001 2018 standard was developed by one of these committees: *ISO Project Committee 210*. ISO PC 283 is responsible for *"Occupational health and safety management systems"*.

ISO website: http://www.iso.org/

INTRODUCTION TO THE ISO 45001 2018 OH&S STANDARD

ISO 45001 2018 is an occupational health and safety (OH&S) management system standard. It defines a set of OH&S management system requirements. These requirements can be found in the following seven sections:

4. Context
5. Leadership
6. Planning
7. Support
8. Operations
9. Evaluation
10. Improvement

This first edition of ISO 45001 was published in March of 2018. This new ISO standard is based on the old OHSAS 18001 2007 OH&S standard which is now obsolete.

The purpose of this standard is to help organizations to prevent work-related injury and ill-health and to provide a safe and healthy workplace. According to ISO 45001, any organization can achieve these important objectives if it establishes an OH&S management system (OHSMS) and if it continually tries to improve the suitability, adequacy, and effectiveness of this system.

A *management system* is a set of interrelated or interacting elements that organizations use to implement their policies, to achieve their objectives, and to manage their processes. These elements include structures, programs, procedures, practices, plans, rules, roles, regulations, responsibilities, relationships, contracts, agreements, documents, records, methods, tools, technologies, and resources.

An *occupational health and safety management system (OHSMS)* is either a standalone management system or one part of a larger management system. It is a set of interrelated or interacting elements that organizations use to implement their OH&S policies, to achieve their OH&S objectives, and to manage their OH&S processes. The basic purpose or intended outcome of an OHSMS is to prevent injury and ill health and to provide a safe and healthy workplace.

ISO 45001 2018 OHS AUDIT TOOL

1. INTRODUCTION TO OCCUPATIONAL HEALTH AND SAFETY AUDIT TOOL

SCOPE OF ISO 45001 2018 STANDARD

ISO 45001 applies to all types of organizations. It doesn't matter what they do or what size they are. It can help any organization to prevent work-related injury and ill-health and to provide a safe and healthy workplace. According to ISO 45001 2018, your organization's OHSMS must meet every requirement if you wish to claim that it complies with this standard. However, how you choose to meet ISO's requirements, and to what extent, will depend on and be influenced by many factors. It will depend on your organization's context, its structure, its activities, its objectives, its compliance obligations, and its products and services and will be influenced by its OH&S risks and opportunities. Consequently, OH&S management systems can vary quite a bit.

The *scope of the standard* should not be confused with the *scope of your OH&S management system (OHSMS)*. ISO 45001 2018 section 4.3, below, explains how to define the scope of an OHSMS.

PURPOSE OF OUR AUDIT TOOL

ISO 45001 2018 section 9.2.1 expects you to *"conduct internal audits at planned intervals to provide information on whether the OH&S management system conforms to the requirements of this document"* (i.e., the ISO 45001 standard). Our audit tool will help you meet this requirement. It will show you how to determine whether or not your OH&S management system conforms to the requirements of ISO 45001 2018.

OUR AUDIT APPROACH

Our audit tool will pinpoint the gaps that exist between ISO's OH&S management standard and your organization's OH&S practices and processes. Once you've filled all the gaps, you can be sure that you conform to (or comply with) ISO 45001 2018 and that you've done everything you possibly can to enhance the effectiveness of your organization's OH&S management practices and processes.

AUDIT QUESTIONS

Since ISO 45001 has seven main sections, our audit tool uses seven questionnaires. These questionnaires will allow you to:

4. Assess how well you conform to contextual requirements.
5. Assess how well you conform to leadership requirements.
6. Assess how well you conform to planning requirements.
7. Assess how well you conform to support requirements.
8. Assess how well you conform to operational requirements.
9. Assess how well you conform to evaluation requirements.
10. Assess how well you conform to improvement requirements.

People often distinguish between compliance and conformance. For them, *compliance* is compulsory while *conformance* is voluntary. While ISO 45001 is a voluntary standard, it becomes compulsory when you decide to apply it. That's why we've chosen to use these two terms interchangeably.

ISO 45001 2018 OHS AUDIT TOOL

1. INTRODUCTION TO OCCUPATIONAL HEALTH AND SAFETY AUDIT TOOL

Our audit tool starts with section 4 because the ISO 45001 OH&S management requirements start in section 4. We've preserved this numbering system in order to make it easy to cross-reference the original ISO 45001 standard with our material. However, at the detailed level we have added a numbering system that you won't find in the original standard. We have sequentially numbered all questions within each of the 7 sections (4 to 10) that make up the core of the standard. We have done this in order to make it easier for you to work with our questionnaires.

In addition, we have used paragraph indents to distinguish between general questions and specific questions. This approach makes it easy to see how our questionnaires are structured. In most cases, a general question is immediately followed by several specific questions which usually help clarify what the general question means. If you're not sure what a general question is asking, just keep reading. In most cases, the more detailed questions will clarify what the general questions are trying to ask.

And if you're still confused, perhaps our plain English OH&S definitions will help (see section 12, below).

AUDIT METHOD

For each audit question, three answers are possible: YES, NO, or N/A (to save space we use Y, N, X). A YES answer means you're in compliance with the standard, a NO answer means you're not in compliance, while an N/A answer means that a question is not applicable in your case. NO answers identify gaps that exist between the standard and your OH&S practices and processes while N/A answers point to items that may be ignored or excluded.

All gaps must be filled and all N/A answers must be justified and explained before you can officially say that your OH&S management system (OHSMS) complies with (or conforms to) the new ISO 45001 standard.

Once you've completed all seven questionnaires, study your NO answers, your own comments, and our questions and then use this information to formulate actions or steps that need to be taken in order to bring your organization's practices and processes into compliance with the standard. Use this information to develop your own unique *ISO 45001 OHSMS Compliance Plan*.

Before you start your audit, please fill out the form entitled *Profile of your ISO 45001 OH&S audit project* (section 2, below). First record the name of the organization being audited, its address, and a brief description of the actual scope or focus of the audit. Also record the names of your audit team members and your start date. Once you've completed the audit, use the same form to record when the audit was finished, who reviewed the audit and when, and any review comments (if any).

You can also summarize your audit results quantitatively if you wish (see section 11). The idea here is to measure how compliant your OH&S management practices and processes actually are. And if you carry out regular audits, you can also use our approach to measure whether or not your OH&S management practices and processes are improving over time.

ISO 45001 2018 OHS AUDIT TOOL

1. INTRODUCTION TO OCCUPATIONAL HEALTH AND SAFETY AUDIT TOOL

This is how it works. For each section of the audit, count the number of YES answers and the number of NO answers and record the totals in the form provided in section 11, below. To calculate the average compliance score for each section, simply divide the total YES answers by the total YES+NO answers. To calculate the average score for the entire audit, do the same for the grand totals.

MINI AUDIT TOOL

We've also provided a mini audit questionnaire (section 3, below) that you can use to carry out a quick occupational health and safety management audit or to decide what general areas need more detailed attention. If you're not clear about what one of these general questions is talking about, simply go to our more detailed audit tool and study the relevant section.

ISO 45001 2018 OHS AUDIT TOOL

2. PROFILE OF YOUR OCCUPATIONAL HEALTH AND SAFETY AUDIT PROJECT

SCOPE OF YOUR OH&S AUDIT

NAME OF ORGANIZATION BEING AUDITED	ADDRESS OF ORGANIZATION BEING AUDITED
AREAS BEING AUDITED	ADDRESS OF YOUR AUDIT

SCOPE OF YOUR AUDIT

AUDITORS

AUDIT MANAGER	AUDIT STAFF

AUDIT SCHEDULE

AUDIT START DATE	AUDIT FINISH DATE

AUDIT REVIEWER

AUDIT REVIEWED BY	DATE AUDIT REVIEWED

REVIEW COMMENTS

ISO 45001 2018 OHS AUDIT TOOL

3. MINI OCCUPATIONAL HEALTH AND SAFETY MANAGEMENT AUDIT TOOL

4. ASSESS HOW WELL YOU CONFORM TO ISO'S CONTEXTUAL REQUIREMENTS			
4.1	Do you understand your organization and its unique external and internal context?	Y N X	
4.2	Do you clarify the needs and expectations of workers and other interested parties?	Y N X	
4.3	Did you define the scope of your occupational health and safety management system?	Y N X	
4.4	Did you establish, and do you maintain an occupational health and safety management system?	Y N X	
5. ASSESS HOW WELL YOU CONFORM TO ISO'S LEADERSHIP REQUIREMENTS			
5.1	Do you provide leadership by accepting responsibility for occupational health and safety?	Y N X	
5.2	Do you provide leadership by establishing, implementing, and maintaining an OH&S policy?	Y N X	
5.3	Do you provide leadership by assigning organizational roles, responsibilities, and authorities?	Y N X	
5.4	Do you provide leadership by consulting with workers and encouraging their participation?	Y N X	
6. ASSESS HOW WELL YOU CONFORM TO ISO'S PLANNING REQUIREMENTS			
6.1	Do you formulate actions to address your organization's risks and opportunities?	Y N X	
6.1.1	Did you plan the establishment and documentation of your OHSMS?	Y N X	
6.1.2	Do you identify your hazards and assess OH&S risks and opportunities?	Y N X	
6.1.2.1	Did you develop a process to identify your organization's hazards?	Y N X	
6.1.2.2	Did you develop a process to assess your organization's risks?	Y N X	
6.1.2.3	Did you develop a process to assess your organization's opportunities?	Y N X	
6.1.3	Did you develop a process to manage your legal and other requirements?	Y N X	
6.1.4	Do you plan actions and figure out how to implement and evaluate them?	Y N X	
6.2	Do you formulate OH&S objectives and develop plans to achieve them?	Y N X	
6.2.1	Do you establish OH&S objectives at relevant functions and levels?	Y N X	
6.2.2	Do you plan how to achieve your organization's OH&S objectives?	Y N X	
7. ASSESS HOW WELL YOU CONFORM TO ISO'S SUPPORT REQUIREMENTS			
7.1	Do you support your organization's OHSMS by providing the necessary resources?	Y N X	
7.2	Do you support your organization's OHSMS by ensuring that people are competent?	Y N X	
7.3	Do you support your organization's OHSMS by making people aware of their duties?	Y N X	

ORGANIZATION:		YOUR LOCATION:	
COMPLETED BY:		DATE COMPLETED:	
REVIEWED BY:		DATE REVIEWED:	

ISO 45001 2018 OHS AUDIT TOOL

3. MINI OCCUPATIONAL HEALTH AND SAFETY MANAGEMENT AUDIT TOOL

7.4	Do you support your organization's OHSMS by controlling your communications?	Y	N	X	
7.4.1	Do you support your organization's OHSMS by creating communication processes?	Y	N	X	
7.4.2	Do you support your organization's OHSMS by facilitating internal communications?	Y	N	X	
7.4.3	Do you support your organization's OHSMS by establishing external communications?	Y	N	X	
7.5	Do you support your organization's OHSMS by managing documented information?	Y	N	X	
7.5.1	Do you support your organization's OHSMS by including necessary documents and records?	Y	N	X	
7.5.2	Do you support your organization's OHSMS by managing the use of documents and records?	Y	N	X	
7.5.3	Do you support your organization's OHSMS by controlling relevant documents and records?	Y	N	X	
8. ASSESS HOW WELL YOU CONFORM TO ISO'S OPERATIONAL REQUIREMENTS					
8.1	Have you established and do you maintain processes needed to meet OHSMS requirements?	Y	N	X	
8.1.1	Have you established processes for managing occupational health and safety?	Y	N	X	
8.1.2	Have you established processes for managing hazards and controlling risks?	Y	N	X	
8.1.3	Have you established processes for managing changes and controlling impacts?	Y	N	X	
8.1.4	Have you established processes for managing contractors and service providers?	Y	N	X	
8.1.4.1	Have you developed procurement processes that meet your OHSMS requirements?	Y	N	X	
8.1.4.2	Do you expect contractors and their workers to meet your OHSMS requirements?	Y	N	X	
8.1.4.3	Do you maintain outsourcing arrangements that meet your OHSMS requirements?	Y	N	X	
8.2	Have you established all necessary emergency preparedness and response processes?	Y	N	X	
9. ASSESS HOW WELL YOU CONFORM TO ISO'S EVALUATION REQUIREMENTS					
9.1	Have you established processes to monitor, measure, analyze, and evaluate your OHSMS?	Y	N	X	
9.1.1	Have you established processes to monitor, measure, analyze, and evaluate performance?	Y	N	X	
9.1.2	Have you established processes to evaluate compliance with legal and other requirements?	Y	N	X	
9.2	Have you determined internal OH&S audit requirements, responsibilities, and methods?	Y	N	X	

ORGANIZATION:		YOUR LOCATION:	
COMPLETED BY:		DATE COMPLETED:	
REVIEWED BY:		DATE REVIEWED:	

ISO 45001 2018 OHS AUDIT TOOL

3. MINI OCCUPATIONAL HEALTH AND SAFETY MANAGEMENT AUDIT TOOL

9.2.1	Do you audit the conformance of your organization's OHSMS at planned intervals?	Y N X	
9.2.2	Did you establish and do you maintain an internal OHSMS audit programme?	Y N X	
9.3	Do you review the suitability, adequacy, and effectiveness of your OHSMS?	Y N X	
10. ASSESS HOW WELL YOU CONFORM TO ISO'S IMPROVEMENT REQUIREMENTS			
10.1	Do you identify improvement opportunities, and do you take action to achieve intended outcomes?	Y N X	
10.2	Have you established processes to investigate and respond to OH&S incidents and nonconformities?	Y N X	
10.3	Do you try to enhance the suitability, adequacy, and effectiveness of your organization's OHSMS?	Y N X	

Answer each of the above questions. Three answers are possible: Y (yes), N (no), and X (eXclude). Y means you're in compliance, N means you're not in compliance, while X means that this question can be excluded because it's not applicable in your situation. Y answers and X answers require no further action, while N answers point to things that need to be done to improve the overall performance of your process. Also, please use the column on the right to record your notes, and in the spaces below, enter the name and location of your organization, who completed this page, who reviewed it, and the dates.

ORGANIZATION:		YOUR LOCATION:	
COMPLETED BY:		DATE COMPLETED:	
REVIEWED BY:		DATE REVIEWED:	

ISO 45001 2018 OHS AUDIT TOOL

4. ASSESS HOW WELL YOU CONFORM TO ISO'S CONTEXTUAL REQUIREMENTS

	4.1 UNDERSTAND YOUR ORGANIZATION AND ITS UNIQUE EXTERNAL AND INTERNAL CONTEXT				
1	Did you identify and do you understand your organization's unique context?	Y	N	X	
2	Did you identify and did you understand your organization's context before you established its occupational health and safety management system (OHSMS)?	Y	N	X	
3	Did you consider the external issues that are relevant to your organization's purpose and did you think about the influence these issues could have on its OHSMS and the outcomes it intends to achieve?	Y	N	X	
4	Did you consider the internal issues that are relevant to your organization's purpose and did you think about the influence these issues could have on its OHSMS and the outcomes it intends to achieve?	Y	N	X	
	4.2 CLARIFY THE NEEDS AND EXPECTATIONS OF WORKERS AND OTHER INTERESTED PARTIES				
5	Do you identify groups and individuals that are relevant to your organization's OHSMS?	Y	N	X	
6	Do you identify the workers that are relevant to your organization's OHSMS?	Y	N	X	
7	Do you identify the interested parties that are relevant to your organization's OHSMS?	Y	N	X	
8	Do you determine the needs and expectations of workers and other interested parties?	Y	N	X	
9	Do you determine the needs and expectations of the workers that are relevant to the OHSMS?	Y	N	X	
10	Do you identify needs and expectations that are or could become worker requirements?	Y	N	X	
11	Do you determine the needs and expectations of the parties that are relevant to your OHSMS?	Y	N	X	
12	Do you identify needs and expectations that are or could become interested party requirements?	Y	N	X	
	4.3 DEFINE THE SCOPE OF YOUR OCCUPATIONAL HEALTH AND SAFETY MANAGEMENT SYSTEM				
13	Did you clarify boundaries, and did you think about what your OHSMS should apply to?	Y	N	X	
14	Did you use boundary and applicability information to define the scope of your OHSMS?	Y	N	X	
15	Did you consider all interested party requirements when you defined your scope?	Y	N	X	

ORGANIZATION:		YOUR LOCATION:	
COMPLETED BY:		DATE COMPLETED:	
REVIEWED BY:		DATE REVIEWED:	

ISO 45001 2018 OHS AUDIT TOOL

4. ASSESS HOW WELL YOU CONFORM TO ISO'S CONTEXTUAL REQUIREMENTS

16	Did you consider your external and internal context when you defined your scope?	Y	N	X	
17	Did you consider how external issues could influence intended OHSMS outcomes?	Y	N	X	
18	Did you consider how internal issues could influence intended OHSMS outcomes?	Y	N	X	
19	Did you define the scope of your occupational health and safety management system (OHSMS)?	Y	N	X	
20	Did you consider all the products that are under your organization's influence or control?	Y	N	X	
21	Did you include the products that could have an impact on your OH&S performance?	Y	N	X	
22	Did you consider all the services that are under your organization's influence or control?	Y	N	X	
23	Did you include the services that could have an impact on your OH&S performance?	Y	N	X	
24	Did you consider all the activities that are under your organization's influence or control?	Y	N	X	
25	Did you include the activities that could have an impact on your OH&S performance?	Y	N	X	
26	Did you include all the actual work activities that could have an impact on OH&S?	Y	N	X	
27	Did you include all the planned work activities that could have an impact on OH&S?	Y	N	X	
28	Did you document the scope of your occupational health and safety management system?	Y	N	X	
29	Do you control the documented information that defines the scope of your OHSMS?	Y	N	X	
30	Do you maintain your organization's OHSMS scope documents and records?	Y	N	X	
4.4 ESTABLISH AND MAINTAIN AN OCCUPATIONAL HEALTH AND SAFETY MANAGEMENT SYSTEM					
31	Did you establish an OHSMS in accordance with the ISO 45001 standard?	Y	N	X	
32	Did you establish the processes that your organization's OHSMS needs?	Y	N	X	
33	Did you specify how your organization's processes should interact?	Y	N	X	
34	Did you implement your OHSMS in accordance with the ISO 45001 standard?	Y	N	X	

ORGANIZATIO N:		YOUR LOCATION:	
COMPLETED BY:		DATE COMPLETED:	
REVIEWED BY:		DATE REVIEWED:	

ISO 45001 2018 OHS AUDIT TOOL

4. ASSESS HOW WELL YOU CONFORM TO ISO'S CONTEXTUAL REQUIREMENTS

35	Do you maintain your OHSMS in accordance with the ISO 45001 standard?	Y	N	X	
36	Do you improve your OHSMS in accordance with the ISO 45001 standard?	Y	N	X	

ORGANIZATION:		YOUR LOCATION:	
COMPLETED BY:		DATE COMPLETED:	
REVIEWED BY:		DATE REVIEWED:	

ISO 45001 2018 OHS AUDIT TOOL

5. ASSESS HOW WELL YOU CONFORM TO ISO'S LEADERSHIP REQUIREMENTS

5.1 PROVIDE LEADERSHIP BY ACCEPTING RESPONSIBILITY FOR OCCUPATIONAL HEALTH AND SAFETY					
1	Does your organization's top management accept responsibility for OH&S?	Y	N	X	
2	Do they accept responsibility for the prevention of work-related injury & ill-health?	Y	N	X	
3	Do they accept responsibility for the provision of safe and healthy workplaces?	Y	N	X	
4	Do they accept responsibility for maintaining safe and healthy activities?	Y	N	X	
5	Has your organization developed a corporate culture that supports OH&S?	Y	N	X	
6	Have you established a culture that encourages worker participation and consultation?	Y	N	X	
7	Have you established suitable worker participation and consultation processes?	Y	N	X	
8	Have you established and do you support worker health and safety committees?	Y	N	X	
9	Have you established a culture that expects personnel to achieve intended outcomes?	Y	N	X	
10	Does your culture expect personnel to achieve intended OHSMS outcomes?	Y	N	X	
11	Have you established a culture that protects workers from reprisals and retaliation?	Y	N	X	
12	Do you expect managers to protect workers from reprisals when they report incidents and hazards?	Y	N	X	
13	Do you expect managers to protect workers from reprisals when they report risks?	Y	N	X	
14	Does your top management demonstrate a sincere commitment to OH&S?	Y	N	X	
15	Do they ensure that OHSMS requirements are built into business processes?	Y	N	X	
16	Do they ensure that an occupational health and safety policy is formulated?	Y	N	X	
17	Do they make sure that this policy supports your strategic direction?	Y	N	X	
18	Do they ensure that occupational health and safety objectives are set?	Y	N	X	
19	Do they make sure that these objectives support your strategic direction?	Y	N	X	

ORGANIZATION:		YOUR LOCATION:	
COMPLETED BY:		DATE COMPLETED:	
REVIEWED BY:		DATE REVIEWED:	

ISO 45001 2018 OHS AUDIT TOOL

5. ASSESS HOW WELL YOU CONFORM TO ISO'S LEADERSHIP REQUIREMENTS

20	Do they ensure that your OHSMS achieves its intended outcomes?	Y	N	X	
21	Do they ensure that all necessary OHSMS resources are available?	Y	N	X	
22	Do they support the establishment of an OHSMS for your organization?	Y	N	X	
23	Do they provide the resources needed to implement your OHSMS?	Y	N	X	
24	Do they provide the resources needed to maintain your OHSMS?	Y	N	X	
25	Do they provide the resources needed to improve your OHSMS?	Y	N	X	
26	Does your top management communicate a firm commitment to OH&S?	Y	N	X	
27	Do they explain why occupational health and safety is important?	Y	N	X	
28	Do they explain why your organization's OHSMS must be effective?	Y	N	X	
29	Do they explain why OHSMS requirements must always be met?	Y	N	X	
30	Do they explain why your OHSMS must be continually improved?	Y	N	X	
31	Do they expect managers to be accountable for the OHSMS?	Y	N	X	
32	Do they expect your organization's top managers to accept responsibility for making sure that the OHSMS is effective?	Y	N	X	
33	Do they expect managers to demonstrate their leadership and commitment to the OHSMS within their own areas of responsibility?	Y	N	X	
34	Do they ask people to personally support the organization's OHSMS?	Y	N	X	
35	Do they ask people to help make the OHSMS as effective as possible?	Y	N	X	
5.2 PROVIDE LEADERSHIP BY ESTABLISHING, IMPLEMENTING, AND MAINTAINING AN OH&S POLICY					
36	Did your top management develop an occupational health and safety (OH&S) policy?	Y	N	X	
37	Is this OH&S policy appropriate to your organization and its particular context?	Y	N	X	

ORGANIZATION:		YOUR LOCATION:	
COMPLETED BY:		DATE COMPLETED:	
REVIEWED BY:		DATE REVIEWED:	

ISO 45001 2018 OHS AUDIT TOOL

5. ASSESS HOW WELL YOU CONFORM TO ISO'S LEADERSHIP REQUIREMENTS

38	Is this OH&S policy consistent with your organization's size and purpose?	Y	N	X	
39	Does your OH&S policy make a commitment to risk management?	Y	N	X	
40	Does your OH&S policy reflect the nature of your organization's OH&S risks?	Y	N	X	
41	Does your OH&S policy accommodate the scale and scope of your OH&S risks?	Y	N	X	
42	Does this OH&S policy provide a framework for managing OH&S objectives?	Y	N	X	
43	Does your OH&S policy provide a framework for establishing OH&S objectives?	Y	N	X	
44	Does your OH&S policy provide a framework for reviewing OH&S objectives?	Y	N	X	
45	Did your organization document its OH&S policy?	Y	N	X	
46	Did your organization define its OH&S policy?	Y	N	X	
47	Does your OH&S policy make a commitment to worker participation?	Y	N	X	
48	Does your OH&S policy make a commitment to consult with workers?	Y	N	X	
49	Does your policy make a commitment to consult with worker representatives?	Y	N	X	
50	Does your OH&S policy make a commitment to worker health and safety?	Y	N	X	
51	Does your policy make a commitment to provide safe and healthy working conditions?	Y	N	X	
52	Does your policy make a commitment to the prevention of work-related injuries?	Y	N	X	
53	Does your policy make a commitment to the prevention of work-related ill health?	Y	N	X	
54	Does your policy make a commitment to eliminate hazards and reduce OH&S risks?	Y	N	X	
55	Does your OH&S policy make a commitment to comply with requirements?	Y	N	X	
56	Does it make a commitment to comply with requirements about OH&S risks and hazards?	Y	N	X	

ORGANIZATION:		YOUR LOCATION:	
COMPLETED BY:		DATE COMPLETED:	
REVIEWED BY:		DATE REVIEWED:	

ISO 45001 2018 OHS AUDIT TOOL

5. ASSESS HOW WELL YOU CONFORM TO ISO'S LEADERSHIP REQUIREMENTS

57	Does it make a commitment to comply with all relevant legal OH&S requirements?	Y	N	X	
58	Does it make a commitment to comply with all relevant nonlegal OH&S requirements?	Y	N	X	
59	Does your OH&S policy make a commitment to continual improvement?	Y	N	X	
60	Does it make a commitment to continually improve your OH&S management?	Y	N	X	
61	Does it make a commitment to continually improve your OH&S performance?	Y	N	X	
62	Did your organization implement its OH&S policy?	Y	N	X	
63	Does your organization distribute its OH&S policy?	Y	N	X	
64	Is your OH&S policy available to all relevant interested parties?	Y	N	X	
65	Does your organization communicate its OH&S policy?	Y	N	X	
66	Do you communicate your policy within your own organization?	Y	N	X	
67	Does your organization maintain its OH&S policy?	Y	N	X	
68	Does your organization periodically review its OH&S policy?	Y	N	X	
69	Do you make sure that your policy continues to be relevant and appropriate?	Y	N	X	

5.3 PROVIDE LEADERSHIP BY ASSIGNING ORGANIZATIONAL ROLES, RESPONSIBILITIES, AND AUTHORITIES

70	Does your top management provide effective occupational health & safety leadership?	Y	N	X	
71	Does your top management assign all OHSMS roles, responsibilities, and authorities?	Y	N	X	
72	Did they assign responsibility and authority for ensuring that OHSMS complies with ISO 45001?	Y	N	X	
73	Did they assign responsibility and authority for reporting on the performance of your OHSMS?	Y	N	X	
74	Does your organization document its OHSMS roles, responsibilities, and authorities?	Y	N	X	

ORGANIZATION:		YOUR LOCATION:	
COMPLETED BY:		DATE COMPLETED:	
REVIEWED BY:		DATE REVIEWED:	

ISO 45001 2018 OHS AUDIT TOOL

5. ASSESS HOW WELL YOU CONFORM TO ISO'S LEADERSHIP REQUIREMENTS

75	Do you maintain documents that describe OHSMS roles, responsibilities, and authorities?	Y	N	X	
76	Does top management communicate OHSMS roles, responsibilities, and authorities?	Y	N	X	
77	Do they discuss OHSMS roles, responsibilities, and authorities at all organizational levels?	Y	N	X	
78	Do they expect workers to accept responsibility for the OH&S aspects they control?	Y	N	X	
5.4 PROVIDE LEADERSHIP BY CONSULTING WITH WORKERS AND ENCOURAGING THEIR PARTICIPATION					
79	Did you establish processes for consulting with people and encouraging their participation?	Y	N	X	
80	Did you establish a process for consulting with workers and worker representatives?	Y	N	X	
81	Did you develop a process that can be used to consult with nonmanagerial workers?	Y	N	X	
82	Can your consulting process be used at all organizational levels and in all functions?	Y	N	X	
83	Can your organization's consulting process be used to help plan its OHSMS?	Y	N	X	
84	Can your organization's consulting process be used to help develop its OHSMS?	Y	N	X	
85	Can your organization's consulting process be used to help implement its OHSMS?	Y	N	X	
86	Can your organization's consulting process be used to help evaluate its OHSMS?	Y	N	X	
87	Can your organization's consulting process be used to help improve its OHSMS?	Y	N	X	
88	Did you establish a process for encouraging people to participate in decision making?	Y	N	X	
89	Did you develop a process to encourage the participation of nonmanagerial workers?	Y	N	X	
90	Can your participative process be used at all organizational levels and in all functions?	Y	N	X	
91	Did you identify and remove obstacles or barriers to participation or minimize their impact?	Y	N	X	
92	Can your organization's participative process be used to help plan its OHSMS?	Y	N	X	
93	Can your organization's participative process be used to help develop its OHSMS?	Y	N	X	

ORGANIZATIO N:		YOUR LOCATION:	
COMPLETED BY:		DATE COMPLETED:	
REVIEWED BY:		DATE REVIEWED:	

ISO 45001 2018 OHS AUDIT TOOL

5. ASSESS HOW WELL YOU CONFORM TO ISO'S LEADERSHIP REQUIREMENTS

94	Can your organization's participative process be used to help implement its OHSMS?	Y	N	X	
95	Can your organization's participative process be used to help evaluate its OHSMS?	Y	N	X	
96	Can your organization's participative process be used to help improve its OHSMS?	Y	N	X	
97	Did you implement processes for consulting with people and encouraging their participation?	Y	N	X	
98	Do you consult with workers and worker representatives before you make OHSMS decisions?	Y	N	X	
99	Do you ask nonmanagerial workers to help establish your organization's OH&S policy?	Y	N	X	
100	Do you ask nonmanagerial workers to help clarify all relevant needs and expectations?	Y	N	X	
101	Do you ask them to help determine the needs and expectations of interested parties?	Y	N	X	
102	Do you ask nonmanagerial workers to help assign roles, responsibilities, and authorities?	Y	N	X	
103	Do you ask nonmanagerial workers to help figure out how to meet legal requirements?	Y	N	Y	
104	Do you ask nonmanagerial workers to help figure out how to meet other requirements?	Y	N	X	
105	Do you ask nonmanagerial workers to help establish your OH&S plans and objectives?	Y	N	X	
106	Do you ask nonmanagerial workers to help determine and develop suitable controls?	Y	N	X	
107	Do you ask nonmanagerial workers to help determine what needs to be monitored?	Y	N	X	
108	Do you ask nonmanagerial workers to help determine what needs to be measured?	Y	N	X	
109	Do you ask nonmanagerial workers to help determine what needs to be evaluated?	Y	N	X	
110	Do you ask nonmanagerial workers to help plan and establish audit programmes?	Y	N	X	
111	Do you ask non-managerial workers to help implement audit programmes?	Y	N	X	
112	Do you ask nonmanagerial workers to help maintain audit programmes?	Y	N	X	
113	Do you ask nonmanagerial workers to help generate continual improvement?	Y	N	X	

ORGANIZATIO N:		YOUR LOCATION:	
COMPLETED BY:		DATE COMPLETED:	
REVIEWED BY:		DATE REVIEWED:	

ISO 45001 2018 OHS AUDIT TOOL

5. ASSESS HOW WELL YOU CONFORM TO ISO'S LEADERSHIP REQUIREMENTS

114	Do you ask workers and worker representatives to participate in OHSMS decision making?	Y	N	X	
115	Do you ask nonmanagerial workers to help determine how participation can be done?	Y	N	X	
116	Do you ask nonmanagerial workers to help manage hazards, risks, and opportunities?	Y	N	X	
117	Do you ask nonmanagerial workers to help identify hazards, risks, and opportunities?	Y	N	X	
118	Do you ask nonmanagerial workers to help assess hazards, risks, and opportunities?	Y	N	X	
119	Do you ask nonmanagerial workers to help define actions to remove hazards and reduce risks?	Y	N	X	
120	Do you ask nonmanagerial workers to help clarify competence requirements and training needs?	Y	N	X	
121	Do you ask nonmanagerial workers to help with training and evaluate training activities?	Y	N	X	
122	Do you ask nonmanagerial workers to help figure out what needs to be communicated?	Y	N	X	
123	Do you ask nonmanagerial workers to help figure out how communication should be done?	Y	N	X	
124	Do you ask nonmanagerial workers to help determine and develop control measures?	Y	N	X	
125	Do you ask nonmanagerial workers to help decide how controls should be implemented?	Y	N	X	
126	Do you ask nonmanagerial workers to help decide how controls should be used?	Y	N	X	
127	Do you ask nonmanagerial workers to help investigate incidents and nonconformities?	Y	N	X	
128	Do you ask nonmanagerial workers to help determine corrective actions?	Y	N	X	
129	Do you maintain processes for consulting with people and encouraging their participation?	Y	N	X	
130	Do you provide information needed to support and facilitate consultation and participation?	Y	N	X	
131	Do you provide clear, understandable, and relevant information about your OHSMS?	Y	N	X	
132	Do you provide resources needed to support and facilitate consultation and participation?	Y	N	X	
133	Do you provide mechanisms and training needed to support consultation and participation?	Y	N	X	

ORGANIZATIO N:		YOUR LOCATION:	
COMPLETED BY:		DATE COMPLETED:	
REVIEWED BY:		DATE REVIEWED:	

NOV 2018 PLAIN ENGLISH OCCUPATIONAL HEALTH & SAFETY AUDIT TOOL EDITION 1.0

PART 5 PAGE 19

ISO 45001 2018 OHS AUDIT TOOL

5. ASSESS HOW WELL YOU CONFORM TO ISO'S LEADERSHIP REQUIREMENTS

Answer each of the above questions. Three answers are possible: Y (yes), N (no), and X (eXclude). Y means you're in compliance,
N means you're not in compliance, while X means that this question can be excluded because it's not applicable in your situation.
Y answers and X answers require no further action, while N answers point to things that need to be done to improve the performance of your OH&S management activities. Also, please use the column on the right to record your notes, and in the
spaces below, enter the name and location of your organization, who completed this page, who reviewed it, and the dates.

ORGANIZATION:		YOUR LOCATION:	
COMPLETED BY:		DATE COMPLETED:	
REVIEWED BY:		DATE REVIEWED:	

ISO 45001 2018 OHS AUDIT TOOL

6. ASSESS HOW WELL YOU CONFORM TO ISO'S PLANNING REQUIREMENTS

6.1 FORMULATE ACTIONS TO ADDRESS YOUR ORGANIZATION'S RISKS AND OPPORTUNITIES

6.1.1 PLAN THE ESTABLISHMENT AND DOCUMENTATION OF YOUR OHSMS

1	Did you plan the establishment of your organization's OHSMS?	Y	N	X	
2	Did you plan the development of your organization's OHSMS?	Y	N	X	
3	Did you consider what you need to do to achieve intended outcomes?	Y	N	X	
4	Have you figured out what you need to do to give assurance that the OHSMS will be able to achieve intended outcomes?	Y	N	X	
5	Have you figured out what you need to do to prevent or reduce any undesired effects that your OHSMS could cause?	Y	N	X	
6	Have you figured out what you need to do to ensure that your OHSMS can and will be continually improved?	Y	N	X	
7	Did you think about what could influence OHSMS performance?	Y	N	X	
8	Did you consider how your context could influence the OHSMS?	Y	N	X	
9	Did you consider how external issues could affect your OHSMS?	Y	N	X	
10	Did you consider how internal issues could affect your OHSMS?	Y	N	X	
11	Did you consider how your requirements could influence the OHSMS?	Y	N	X	
12	Did you consider how legal requirements could influence the performance of the OHSMS?	Y	N	X	
13	Did you consider how other requirements could influence the performance of the OHSMS?	Y	N	X	
14	Did you consider how your interested parties could influence the OHSMS?	Y	N	X	
15	Did you consider how worker requirements could affect your OHSMS?	Y	N	X	
16	Did you consider how interested party requirements could affect your OHSMS?	Y	N	X	

ORGANIZATION:		YOUR LOCATION:	
COMPLETED BY:		DATE COMPLETED:	
REVIEWED BY:		DATE REVIEWED:	

ISO 45001 2018 OHS AUDIT TOOL

6. ASSESS HOW WELL YOU CONFORM TO ISO'S PLANNING REQUIREMENTS

17	Did you consider how your risks and opportunities could influence the OHSMS?	Y	N	X	
18	Did you consider the risks that could influence the performance of your OHSMS?	Y	N	X	
19	Did you consider how OH&S risks could influence the performance of the OHSMS?	Y	N	X	
20	Did you consider how other risks could influence the performance of the OHSMS?	Y	N	X	
21	Did you consider the opportunities that could influence the performance of your OHSMS?	Y	N	X	
22	Did you consider how OH&S opportunities could influence the performance of OHSMS?	Y	N	X	
23	Did you consider how other opportunities could influence the performance of OHSMS?	Y	N	X	
24	Did you consider how your hazards could influence the OHSMS?	Y	N	X	
25	Did you consider how your scope could influence the OHSMS?	Y	N	X	
26	Do you plan the modification of your organization's OHSMS?	Y	N	X	
27	Do you identify the risks and opportunities that emerge when changes are being considered?	Y	N	X	
28	Do you identify the risks and opportunities associated with changes in your organization?	Y	N	X	
29	Do you identify the risks and opportunities associated with changes in your OHSMS?	Y	N	X	
30	Do you identify the risks and opportunities associated with changes in your processes?	Y	N	X	
31	Do you assess the risks and opportunities that emerge when changes are being considered?	Y	N	X	
32	Do you assess risks and opportunities when planned changes are being considered?	Y	N	X	
33	Do you assess risks and opportunities before planned changes are implemented?	Y	N	X	
34	Do you assess the risks and opportunities associated with planned organizational changes?	Y	N	X	
35	Do you assess the risks and opportunities associated with planned changes in OHSMS?	Y	N	X	
36	Do you assess the risks and opportunities associated with planned changes in processes?	Y	N	X	

ORGANIZATION:		YOUR LOCATION:	
COMPLETED BY:		DATE COMPLETED:	
REVIEWED BY:		DATE REVIEWED:	

ISO 45001 2018 OHS AUDIT TOOL

6. ASSESS HOW WELL YOU CONFORM TO ISO'S PLANNING REQUIREMENTS

37	Do you assess risks and opportunities when unplanned changes have occurred?	Y	N	X	
38	Do you assess risks and opportunities after unplanned changes are implemented?	Y	N	X	
39	Do you assess risks and opportunities associated with unplanned organizational changes?	Y	N	X	
40	Do you assess the risks and opportunities associated with unplanned changes in OHSMS?	Y	N	X	
41	Do you assess the risks and opportunities associated with unplanned changes in processes?	Y	N	X	
42	Have you established and do you maintain OHSMS documents and records?	Y	N	X	
43	Do you document the OH&S risks and opportunities that need to be addressed?	Y	N	X	
44	Do you document the processes and actions needed to plan and manage your OHSMS?	Y	N	X	
45	Do you document processes and actions needed to address incidents and hazards?	Y	N	X	
46	Do you document processes and actions needed to address risks and opportunities?	Y	N	X	
47	Do you document processes and actions needed to address emergency situations?	Y	N	X	
48	Do you document processes and actions needed to address legal requirements?	Y	N	X	
49	Do you document processes and actions needed to address other requirements?	Y	N	X	
6.1.2 IDENTIFY YOUR HAZARDS AND ASSESS OH&S RISKS AND OPPORTUNITIES					
6.1.2.1 DEVELOP A PROCESS TO IDENTIFY YOUR ORGANIZATION'S HAZARDS					
50	Did you establish a hazard identification process?	Y	N	X	
51	Did you establish a way to identify existing hazards?	Y	N	X	
52	Did you establish a way to identify hazards related to people?	Y	N	X	
53	Did you establish a way to identify hazards related to human factors?	Y	N	X	
54	Did you establish a way to identify hazards related to human capabilities?	Y	N	X	

ORGANIZATIO N:		YOUR LOCATION:	
COMPLETED BY:		DATE COMPLETED:	
REVIEWED BY:		DATE REVIEWED:	

ISO 45001 2018 OHS AUDIT TOOL

6. ASSESS HOW WELL YOU CONFORM TO ISO'S PLANNING REQUIREMENTS

55	Did you establish a way to identify hazards related to human shortcomings?	Y	N	X	
56	Did you establish a way to identify hazards related to human errors and mistakes?	Y	N	X	
57	Did you establish a way to identify hazards related to human attitudes?	Y	N	X	
58	Did you establish a way to identify hazards related to the attitude workers have?	Y	N	X	
59	Did you establish a way to identify hazards related to the attitude onsite workers have?	Y	N	X	
60	Did you establish a way to identify hazards related to the attitude offsite workers have?	Y	N	X	
61	Did you establish a way to identify hazards related to the attitude managers have?	Y	N	X	
62	Did you establish a way to identify hazards related to the attitude visitors have?	Y	N	X	
63	Did you establish a way to identify hazards related to the attitude suppliers have?	Y	N	X	
64	Did you establish a way to identify hazards related to the attitude contractors have?	Y	N	X	
65	Did you establish a way to identify hazards related to the attitude community members have?	Y	N	X	
66	Did you establish a way to identify hazards related to human behaviors?	Y	N	X	
67	Did you establish a way to identify hazards related to how workers behave?	Y	N	X	
68	Did you establish a way to identify hazards related to how onsite workers behave?	Y	N	X	
69	Did you establish a way to identify hazards related to how offsite workers behave?	Y	N	X	
70	Did you establish a way to identify hazards related to how managers behave?	Y	N	X	
71	Did you establish a way to identify hazards related to how visitors behave?	Y	N	X	
72	Did you establish a way to identify hazards related to how suppliers behave?	Y	N	X	
73	Did you establish a way to identify hazards related to how contractors behave?	Y	N	X	
74	Did you establish a way to identify hazards related to how community members behave?	Y	N	X	

ORGANIZATION:		YOUR LOCATION:	
COMPLETED BY:		DATE COMPLETED:	
REVIEWED BY:		DATE REVIEWED:	

ISO 45001 2018 OHS AUDIT TOOL

6. ASSESS HOW WELL YOU CONFORM TO ISO'S PLANNING REQUIREMENTS

75	Did you establish a way to identify hazards related to social factors?	Y	N	X	
76	Do you consider the influence of workload and working hours?	Y	N	X	
77	Do you consider the influence of bullying and harassment?	Y	N	X	
78	Did you establish a way to identify hazards related to cultural factors?	Y	N	X	
79	Did you establish a way to identify hazards related to the values workers have?	Y	N	X	
80	Did you establish a way to identify hazards related to the values managers have?	Y	N	X	
81	Did you establish a way to identify hazards related to work?	Y	N	X	
82	Did you establish a way to identify hazards related to the workplace?	Y	N	X	
83	Did you establish a way to identify hazards related to work activities?	Y	N	X	
84	Did you establish a way to identify hazards related to how work is performed?	Y	N	X	
85	Did you establish a way to identify hazards related to routine work activities?	Y	N	X	
86	Did you establish a way to identify hazards related to nonroutine work activities?	Y	N	X	
87	Did you establish a way to identify hazards related to how work is organized?	Y	N	X	
88	Did you establish a way to identify hazards related to how work areas are designed?	Y	N	X	
89	Did you establish a way to identify hazards related to how areas are maintained?	Y	N	X	
90	Did you establish a way to identify hazards related to how work environments are organized?	Y	N	X	
91	Did you establish a way to identify hazards related to how environments are maintained?	Y	N	X	
92	Did you establish a way to identify hazards related to incidents?	Y	N	X	
93	Did you establish a way to identify hazards related to internal incidents?	Y	N	X	
94	Did you establish a way to identify hazards related to external incidents?	Y	N	X	

ORGANIZATION:		YOUR LOCATION:	
COMPLETED BY:		DATE COMPLETED:	
REVIEWED BY:		DATE REVIEWED:	

ISO 45001 2018 OHS AUDIT TOOL

6. ASSESS HOW WELL YOU CONFORM TO ISO'S PLANNING REQUIREMENTS

95	Did you establish a way to identify hazards related to emergencies?	Y	N	X	
96	Did you establish a way to identify hazards related to previous emergencies?	Y	N	X	
97	Did you establish a way to identify hazards related to potential emergencies?	Y	N	X	
98	Did you establish a way to identify hazards related to processes?	Y	N	X	
99	Did you establish a way to identify hazards related to operating processes?	Y	N	X	
100	Did you establish a way to identify hazards related to how processes are performed?	Y	N	X	
101	Did you establish a way to identify hazards related to how processes are maintained?	Y	N	X	
102	Did you establish a way to identify hazards related to how processes are designed?	Y	N	X	
103	Did you have a way to identify hazards related to how operating processes are designed?	Y	N	X	
104	Did you have a way to identify hazards related to how operating procedures are designed?	Y	N	X	
105	Did you establish a way to identify hazards related to products?	Y	N	X	
106	Did you establish a way to identify hazards related to product design?	Y	N	X	
107	Did you establish a way to identify hazards related to product testing?	Y	N	X	
108	Did you establish a way to identify hazards related to product research?	Y	N	X	
109	Did you establish a way to identify hazards related to product development?	Y	N	X	
110	Did you establish a way to identify hazards related to product construction?	Y	N	X	
111	Did you establish a way to identify hazards related to product maintenance?	Y	N	X	
112	Did you establish a way to identify hazards related to product production?	Y	N	X	
113	Did you establish a way to identify hazards related to product assembly?	Y	N	X	
114	Did you establish a way to identify hazards related to product delivery?	Y	N	X	

ORGANIZATION:		YOUR LOCATION:	
COMPLETED BY:		DATE COMPLETED:	
REVIEWED BY:		DATE REVIEWED:	

ISO 45001 2018 OHS AUDIT TOOL

6. ASSESS HOW WELL YOU CONFORM TO ISO'S PLANNING REQUIREMENTS

115	Did you establish a way to identify hazards related to product disposal?	Y	N	X	
116	Did you establish a way to identify hazards related to services?	Y	N	X	
117	Did you establish a way to identify hazards related to service design?	Y	N	X	
118	Did you establish a way to identify hazards related to service testing?	Y	N	X	
119	Did you establish a way to identify hazards related to service delivery?	Y	N	X	
120	Did you establish a way to identify hazards related to service support?	Y	N	X	
121	Did you establish a way to identify hazards related to service updates?	Y	N	X	
122	Did you establish a way to identify hazards related to service disposal?	Y	N	X	
123	Did you establish a way to identify hazards related to raw materials?	Y	N	X	
124	Did you establish a way to identify hazards related to raw material suppliers?	Y	N	X	
125	Did you establish a way to identify hazards related to infrastructure?	Y	N	X	
126	Did you establish a way to identify hazards related to buildings and facilities?	Y	N	X	
127	Did you establish a way to identify hazards related to utilities and services?	Y	N	X	
128	Did you establish a way to identify hazards related to tools and equipment?	Y	N	X	
129	Did you establish a way to identify hazards related to how equipment is designed?	Y	N	X	
130	Did you establish a way to identify potential hazards?	Y	N	X	
131	Did you establish a way to identify hazards related to actual or potential changes?	Y	N	X	
132	Did you establish a way to identify hazards related to organizational changes?	Y	N	X	
133	Did you establish a way to identify hazards related to changes in activities?	Y	N	X	
134	Did you establish a way to identify hazards related to changes in processes?	Y	N	X	

ORGANIZATION:		YOUR LOCATION:	
COMPLETED BY:		DATE COMPLETED:	
REVIEWED BY:		DATE REVIEWED:	

ISO 45001 2018 OHS AUDIT TOOL

6. ASSESS HOW WELL YOU CONFORM TO ISO'S PLANNING REQUIREMENTS

135	Did you establish a way to identify hazards related to changes in operations?	Y	N	X	
136	Did you establish a way to identify hazards related to changes in personnel?	Y	N	X	
137	Did you establish a way to identify hazards related to changes in infrastructure?	Y	N	X	
138	Did you establish a way to identify hazards related to changes in raw materials?	Y	N	X	
139	Did you establish a way to identify hazards related to changes in equipment?	Y	N	X	
140	Did you establish a way to identify hazards related to changes in suppliers?	Y	N	X	
141	Did you establish a way to identify hazards related to changes in systems?	Y	N	X	
142	Did you establish a way to identify hazards related to changes in your OHSMS?	Y	N	X	
143	Did you implement a hazard identification process?	Y	N	X	
144	Do you use your process to identify actual hazards?	Y	N	X	
145	Do you identify hazards related to people?	Y	N	X	
146	Do you identify hazards related to human factors?	Y	N	X	
147	Do you identify hazards that arise because of human attitudes?	Y	N	X	
148	Do you identify hazards that arise because of the attitude workers have?	Y	N	X	
149	Do you identify hazards that arise because of the attitude onsite workers have?	Y	N	X	
150	Do you identify hazards that arise because of the attitude offsite workers have?	Y	N	X	
151	Do you identify hazards that arise because of the attitude visitors have?	Y	N	X	
152	Do you identify hazards that arise because of the attitude managers have?	Y	N	X	
153	Do you identify hazards that arise because of the attitude suppliers have?	Y	N	X	
154	Do you identify hazards that arise because of the attitude contractors have?	Y	N	X	

ORGANIZATION:		YOUR LOCATION:	
COMPLETED BY:		DATE COMPLETED:	
REVIEWED BY:		DATE REVIEWED:	

ISO 45001 2018 OHS AUDIT TOOL

6. ASSESS HOW WELL YOU CONFORM TO ISO'S PLANNING REQUIREMENTS

155	Do you identify hazards that arise because of the attitude community members have?	Y	N	X	
156	Do you identify hazards that arise because of human behaviors?	Y	N	X	
157	Do you identify hazards that arise because of how workers behave?	Y	N	X	
158	Do you identify hazards that arise because of how onsite workers behave?	Y	N	X	
159	Do you identify hazards that arise because of how offsite workers behave?	Y	N	X	
160	Do you identify hazards that arise because of how visitors behave?	Y	N	X	
161	Do you identify hazards that arise because of how managers behave?	Y	N	X	
162	Do you identify hazards that arise because of how suppliers behave?	Y	N	X	
163	Do you identify hazards that arise because of how contractors behave?	Y	N	X	
164	Do you identify hazards that arise because of how community members behave?	Y	N	X	
165	Do you identify hazards related to social factors?	Y	N	X	
166	Do you identify hazards that arise because of workload assignments?	Y	N	X	
167	Do you identify hazards that arise because of the way people are treated?	Y	N	X	
168	Do you identify hazards related to cultural factors?	Y	N	X	
169	Do you identify hazards related to the workplace?	Y	N	X	
170	Do you identify hazards related to work areas?	Y	N	X	
171	Do you identify hazards that arise in work areas under your control?	Y	N	X	
172	Do you identify hazards that arise because of how work areas are designed?	Y	N	X	
173	Do you identify hazards that arise because of how work areas are maintained?	Y	N	X	
174	Do you identify hazards that arise in work areas not under your control?	Y	N	X	
175	Do you identify hazards that arise in the vicinity of the workplace?	Y	N	X	

ORGANIZATION:		YOUR LOCATION:	
COMPLETED BY:		DATE COMPLETED:	
REVIEWED BY:		DATE REVIEWED:	

ISO 45001 2018 OHS AUDIT TOOL

6. ASSESS HOW WELL YOU CONFORM TO ISO'S PLANNING REQUIREMENTS

176	Do you identify hazards in nearby areas not under your control?	Y	N	X	
177	Do you identify hazards related to work activities?	Y	N	X	
178	Do you identify hazards that arise because of how work activities are performed?	Y	N	X	
179	Do you identify hazards that arise because of how routine activities are performed?	Y	N	X	
180	Do you identify hazards that arise because of how nonroutine activities are performed?	Y	N	X	
181	Do you identify hazards that arise because of how work activities are organized?	Y	N	X	
182	Do you identify hazards that arise because of how routine activities are organized?	Y	N	X	
183	Do you identify hazards that arise because of how nonroutine activities are organized?	Y	N	X	
184	Do you identify hazards related to the work environment?	Y	N	X	
185	Do you identify hazards that arise because of how work environment is organized?	Y	N	X	
186	Do you identify hazards that arise because of how work environment is maintained?	Y	N	X	
187	Do you identify hazards related to incidents?	Y	N	X	
188	Do you identify hazards related to internal incidents?	Y	N	X	
189	Do you identify hazards related to external incidents?	Y	N	X	
190	Do you identify hazards related to emergencies?	Y	N	X	
191	Do you identify hazards related to actual emergency situations?	Y	N	X	
192	Do you identify hazards related to potential emergency situations?	Y	N	X	
193	Do you identify hazards related to processes?	Y	N	X	
194	Do you identify hazards related to operating processes?	Y	N	X	
195	Do you identify hazards that arise because of how processes are performed?	Y	N	X	
196	Do you identify hazards that arise because of how processes are maintained?	Y	N	X	

ORGANIZATION:		YOUR LOCATION:	
COMPLETED BY:		DATE COMPLETED:	
REVIEWED BY:		DATE REVIEWED:	

ISO 45001 2018 OHS AUDIT TOOL

6. ASSESS HOW WELL YOU CONFORM TO ISO'S PLANNING REQUIREMENTS

197	Do you identify hazards that arise because of how processes are organized?	Y	N	X	
198	Do you identify hazards that arise because of how processes are designed?	Y	N	X	
199	Do you identify hazards related to products?	Y	N	X	
200	Do you identify hazards related to product design?	Y	N	X	
201	Do you identify hazards related to product testing?	Y	N	X	
202	Do you identify hazards related to product research?	Y	N	X	
203	Do you identify hazards related to product development?	Y	N	X	
204	Do you identify hazards related to product construction?	Y	N	X	
205	Do you identify hazards related to product maintenance?	Y	N	X	
206	Do you identify hazards related to product production?	Y	N	X	
207	Do you identify hazards related to product assembly?	Y	N	X	
208	Do you identify hazards related to product delivery?	Y	N	X	
209	Do you identify hazards related to product disposal?	Y	N	X	
210	Do you identify hazards related to services?	Y	N	X	
211	Do you identify hazards related to service design?	Y	N	X	
212	Do you identify hazards related to service testing?	Y	N	X	
213	Do you identify hazards related to service delivery?	Y	N	X	
214	Do you identify hazards related to service support?	Y	N	X	
215	Do you identify hazards related to service updates?	Y	N	X	
216	Do you identify hazards related to service disposal?	Y	N	X	
217	Do you identify hazards related to raw materials?	Y	N	X	

ORGANIZATION:		YOUR LOCATION:	
COMPLETED BY:		DATE COMPLETED:	
REVIEWED BY:		DATE REVIEWED:	

ISO 45001 2018 OHS AUDIT TOOL

6. ASSESS HOW WELL YOU CONFORM TO ISO'S PLANNING REQUIREMENTS

218	Do you identify hazards that arise because of how raw materials are stored?	Y	N	X	
219	Do you identify hazards that arise because of how raw materials are handled?	Y	N	X	
220	Do you identify hazards that arise because of how raw materials are transported?	Y	N	X	
221	Do you identify hazards related to infrastructure?	Y	N	X	
222	Do you identify hazards that arise because of how infrastructure is designed?	Y	N	X	
223	Do you identify hazards that arise because of how buildings are designed?	Y	N	X	
224	Do you identify hazards that arise because of how equipment is designed?	Y	N	X	
225	Do you identify hazards that arise because of how infrastructure is organized?	Y	N	X	
226	Do you identify hazards that arise because of how facilities are organized?	Y	N	X	
227	Do you identify hazards that arise because of how infrastructure is maintained?	Y	N	X	
228	Do you identify hazards that arise because of how buildings are maintained?	Y	N	X	
229	Do you identify hazards that arise because of how equipment is maintained?	Y	N	X	
230	Do you use your process to identify potential hazards?	Y	N	X	
231	Do you identify the potential hazards that organizational changes could cause?	Y	N	X	
232	Do you identify the potential hazards that changes in activities could cause?	Y	N	X	
233	Do you identify the potential hazards that changes in personnel could cause?	Y	N	X	
234	Do you identify the potential hazards that changes in processes could cause?	Y	N	X	
235	Do you identify the potential hazards that changes in infrastructure could cause?	Y	N	X	
236	Do you identify the potential hazards that changes in materials could cause?	Y	N	X	
237	Do you identify the potential hazards that changes in suppliers could cause?	Y	N	X	
238	Do you identify the potential hazards that changes in systems could cause?	Y	N	X	

ORGANIZATION:		YOUR LOCATION:	
COMPLETED BY:		DATE COMPLETED:	
REVIEWED BY:		DATE REVIEWED:	

ISO 45001 2018 OHS AUDIT TOOL

6. ASSESS HOW WELL YOU CONFORM TO ISO'S PLANNING REQUIREMENTS

239	Do you identify the potential hazards that changes in your OHSMS could cause?	Y	N	X	
240	Do you consider the impact that changes in OHSMS could have on operations?	Y	N	X	
241	Do you consider the impact that changes in OHSMS could have on processes?	Y	N	X	
242	Do you consider the impact that changes in OHSMS could have on activities?	Y	N	X	
243	Do you maintain a hazard identification process?	Y	N	X	
244	Do you document the results of your hazard identification process?	Y	N	X	
245	Do you keep your hazard identification documents up to date?	Y	N	X	
246	Do you document changes in knowledge and information about hazards?	Y	N	X	
6.1.2.2 DEVELOP A PROCESS TO ASSESS YOUR ORGANIZATION'S RISKS					
247	Did you establish processes to assess your organization's risks?	Y	N	X	
248	Did you establish a process to assess the OH&S risks related to hazards?	Y	N	X	
249	Do you consider the effectiveness of your organization's existing controls?	Y	N	X	
250	Did you establish a process to assess the other risks related to your OHSMS?	Y	N	X	
251	Did you implement processes to assess your organization's risks?	Y	N	X	
252	Did you implement a process to assess the OH&S risks related to your hazards?	Y	N	X	
253	Do you consider the effectiveness of existing controls when risks are assessed?	Y	N	X	
254	Did you implement a process to assess the other risks related to your OHSMS?	Y	N	X	
255	Do you identify and assess the risks related to the establishment of an OHSMS?	Y	N	X	
256	Do you identify and assess the risks related to the implementation of an OHSMS?	Y	N	X	
257	Do you identify and assess the risks related to the operation of your OHSMS?	Y	N	X	
258	Do you identify and assess the risks related to the maintenance of your OHSMS?	Y	N	X	

ORGANIZATION:		YOUR LOCATION:	
COMPLETED BY:		DATE COMPLETED:	
REVIEWED BY:		DATE REVIEWED:	

ISO 45001 2018 OHS AUDIT TOOL

6. ASSESS HOW WELL YOU CONFORM TO ISO'S PLANNING REQUIREMENTS

259	Do you document processes to assess your organization's risks?	Y	N	X	
260	Do you document your risk assessment criteria and your methodologies?	Y	N	X	
261	Do you document the scope, nature, and timing of risk assessments?	Y	N	X	
262	Do you maintain processes to assess your organization's risks?	Y	N	X	
263	Do you maintain a process to assess the OH&S risks related to your hazards?	Y	N	X	
264	Do you maintain and retain documents that describe your OH&S risk assessment process?	Y	N	X	
265	Do you maintain and retain documents and records that describe your methodology?	Y	N	X	
266	Do you maintain documents and records that describe your risk assessment criteria?	Y	N	X	
267	Do you maintain a process to assess the other risks related to your OHSMS?	Y	N	X	
6.1.2.3 DEVELOP A PROCESS TO ASSESS YOUR OPPORTUNITIES					
268	Did you establish a process to assess your organization's opportunities?	Y	N	X	
269	Did you establish a process to assess your organization's OH&S opportunities?	Y	N	X	
270	Did you establish a process to assess your organization's OHSMS opportunities?	Y	N	X	
271	Did you implement a process to assess your organization's opportunities?	Y	N	X	
272	Do you assess OH&S opportunities to improve your organization's OH&S performance?	Y	N	X	
273	Do you consider OH&S improvement opportunities whenever changes are being planned?	Y	N	X	
274	Do you identify opportunities whenever organizational changes are being considered?	Y	N	X	
275	Do you identify improvement opportunities whenever policy changes are being planned?	Y	N	X	
276	Do you identify improvement opportunities whenever process changes are being planned?	Y	N	X	
277	Do you identify improvement opportunities whenever activity changes are being planned?	Y	N	X	
278	Do you identify opportunities to adapt work to meet the needs and expectations of workers?	Y	N	X	

ORGANIZATIO N:		YOUR LOCATION:	
COMPLETED BY:		DATE COMPLETED:	
REVIEWED BY:		DATE REVIEWED:	

ISO 45001 2018 OHS AUDIT TOOL

6. ASSESS HOW WELL YOU CONFORM TO ISO'S PLANNING REQUIREMENTS

279	Do you identify opportunities to improve how your organization's work is organized?	Y	N	X	
280	Do you identify opportunities to improve your organization's work environment?	Y	N	X	
281	Do you identify opportunities to eliminate your organization's hazards and reduce its risks?	Y	N	X	
282	Do you assess other opportunities to improve your organization's OHSMS performance?	Y	N	X	
283	Do you maintain a process to assess your organization's opportunities?	Y	N	X	
284	Do you maintain a process to assess your organization's OH&S opportunities?	Y	N	X	
285	Do you maintain a process to assess your organization's OHSMS opportunities?	Y	N	X	
6.1.3 DEVELOP A PROCESS TO MANAGE YOUR LEGAL AND OTHER REQUIREMENTS					
286	Did you establish a process to manage all relevant legal and other requirements that apply to hazards, OH&S risks, and the OHSMS?	Y	N	X	
287	Did you establish a way to identify all relevant legal and other requirements?	Y	N	X	
288	Do you make sure that the most up-to-date information is identified?	Y	N	X	
289	Did you establish a way to document all relevant legal and other requirements?	Y	N	X	
290	Do you make sure that the most up-to-date information is documented?	Y	N	X	
291	Did you establish a way to access all relevant legal and other requirements?	Y	N	X	
292	Do you make sure that the most up-to-date information is accessed?	Y	N	X	
293	Did you establish a way to apply all relevant legal and other requirements?	Y	N	X	
294	Do you make sure that the most up-to-date information is applied?	Y	N	X	
295	Did you establish a way to determine how requirements are applied?	Y	N	X	
296	Did you establish a way to determine what needs to be communicated?	Y	N	X	
297	Did you implement a process to manage all relevant legal and other requirements that apply to hazards, OH&S risks, and the OHSMS?	Y	N	X	

ORGANIZATIO N:		YOUR LOCATION:	
COMPLETED BY:		DATE COMPLETED:	
REVIEWED BY:		DATE REVIEWED:	

ISO 45001 2018 OHS AUDIT TOOL

6. ASSESS HOW WELL YOU CONFORM TO ISO'S PLANNING REQUIREMENTS

298	Do you consider legal and other requirements when you establish your OHSMS?	Y N X
299	Do you consider legal and other requirements when you implement your OHSMS?	Y N X
300	Do you consider legal and other requirements when you maintain your OHSMS?	Y N X
301	Do you consider legal and other requirements when you improve your OHSMS?	Y N X
302	Do you maintain a process to manage all relevant legal and other requirements that apply to hazards, OH&S risks, and the OHSMS?	Y N X
303	Do you document and record all relevant legal and other requirements?	Y N X
304	Do you make sure that these documents and records are kept up to date?	Y N X
6.1.4 PLAN ACTIONS AND FIGURE OUT HOW TO IMPLEMENT AND EVALUATE THEM		
305	Do you plan your occupational health and safety actions?	Y N X
306	Do you plan how you're going to address OH&S risks?	Y N X
307	Do you consider avoiding or reducing your risks?	Y N X
308	Do you consider eliminating the source of the risk?	Y N X
309	Do you consider retaining the risk or sharing it with others?	Y N X
310	Do you consider modifying the probabilities or consequences?	Y N X
311	Do you plan how you're going to address OH&S hazards?	Y N X
312	Do you consider eliminating or removing hazards?	Y N X
313	Do you consider using less hazardous methods?	Y N X
314	Do you consider using less hazardous materials?	Y N X
315	Do you consider using less hazardous processes?	Y N X
316	Do you consider using less hazardous operations?	Y N X

ORGANIZATION:		YOUR LOCATION:	
COMPLETED BY:		DATE COMPLETED:	
REVIEWED BY:		DATE REVIEWED:	

ISO 45001 2018 OHS AUDIT TOOL

6. ASSESS HOW WELL YOU CONFORM TO ISO'S PLANNING REQUIREMENTS

317	Do you consider using less hazardous equipment?	Y	N	X	
318	Do you consider using controls to protect people?	Y	N	X	
319	Do you consider using engineering controls to protect people?	Y	N	X	
320	Do you consider re-engineering or re-organizing work activities?	Y	N	X	
321	Do you consider using adequate personal protective equipment?	Y	N	X	
322	Do you consider using barriers, enclosures, and machine guards?	Y	N	X	
323	Do you consider using administrative controls to protect people?	Y	N	X	
324	Do you consider using training to help protect people?	Y	N	X	
325	Do you consider using access controls to protect people?	Y	N	X	
326	Do you consider using alarms and signage to protect people?	Y	N	X	
327	Do you consider using inspection and supervision to protect people?	Y	N	X	
328	Do you consider using procedures and instructions to protect people?	Y	N	X	
329	Do you plan how you're going to address OH&S emergencies?	Y	N	X	
330	Do you plan how you're going to prepare for emergencies?	Y	N	X	
331	Do you plan how you're going to respond to emergencies?	Y	N	X	
332	Do you plan how you're going to address OH&S requirements?	Y	N	X	
333	Do you plan how you're going to address legal requirements?	Y	N	X	
334	Do you plan how you're going to address other requirements?	Y	N	X	
335	Do you plan how you're going to address OH&S opportunities?	Y	N	X	
336	Do you consider increasing your risk to pursue an opportunity?	Y	N	X	
337	Do you plan how you're going to implement your actions?	Y	N	X	

ORGANIZATION:		YOUR LOCATION:	
COMPLETED BY:		DATE COMPLETED:	
REVIEWED BY:		DATE REVIEWED:	

ISO 45001 2018 OHS AUDIT TOOL

6. ASSESS HOW WELL YOU CONFORM TO ISO'S PLANNING REQUIREMENTS

338	Do you plan how to integrate these actions into your OHSMS?	Y	N	X	
339	Do you plan how to make actions part of OHSMS processes?	Y	N	X	
340	Do you plan how to build these actions into other processes?	Y	N	X	
341	Do you plan how you're going to evaluate your actions?	Y	N	X	
342	Do you plan how to evaluate the effectiveness of actions?	Y	N	X	

6.2 FORMULATE YOUR OH&S OBJECTIVES AND DEVELOP PLANS TO ACHIEVE THEM

6.2.1 ESTABLISH OH&S OBJECTIVES AT RELEVANT FUNCTIONS AND LEVELS

343	Do you clarify criteria for setting your OH&S objectives?	Y	N	X	
344	Do you ensure that objectives are consistent with your OH&S policy?	Y	N	X	
345	Do you ensure that objectives are measurable (whenever practicable)?	Y	N	X	
346	Do you set OH&S objectives at all relevant levels and functions?	Y	N	X	
347	Do you set objectives that take worker input into account?	Y	N	X	
348	Do you set objectives that meet applicable requirements?	Y	N	X	
349	Do you set objectives that address risks and opportunities?	Y	N	X	
350	Do you set objectives that address risk assessment results?	Y	N	X	
351	Do you set objectives that continually improve the OHSMS?	Y	N	X	
352	Do you set objectives that could improve OH&S performance?	Y	N	X	
353	Do you communicate your organization's OH&S objectives?	Y	N	X	
354	Do you monitor your organization's OH&S objectives?	Y	N	X	
355	Do you update your organization's OH&S objectives?	Y	N	X	

ORGANIZATIO N:		YOUR LOCATION:	
COMPLETED BY:		DATE COMPLETED:	
REVIEWED BY:		DATE REVIEWED:	

ISO 45001 2018 OHS AUDIT TOOL

6. ASSESS HOW WELL YOU CONFORM TO ISO'S PLANNING REQUIREMENTS

6.2.2 PLAN HOW TO ACHIEVE YOUR ORGANIZATION'S OH&S OBJECTIVES					
356	Do you develop plans of action to achieve your OH&S objectives?	Y	N	X	
357	Do you figure out what actions will be taken to achieve objectives?	Y	N	X	
358	Do you figure out when actions must be carried out and completed?	Y	N	X	
359	Do you figure out who will be responsible for carrying out these actions?	Y	N	X	
360	Do you figure out what resources will be needed to perform these actions?	Y	N	X	
361	Do you consider how to integrate OH&S actions into your processes?	Y	N	X	
362	Do you figure out how to build OH&S actions into business processes?	Y	N	X	
363	Do you determine how to evaluate OH&S actions and OH&S results?	Y	N	X	
364	Do you monitor how well objectives are being achieved?	Y	N	X	
365	Did you establish indicators to monitor progress?	Y	N	X	
366	Do you maintain and retain OH&S planning documents and records?	Y	N	X	
367	Did you establish documents and records that define OH&S objectives?	Y	N	X	
368	Do you document the plans you've developed to achieve OH&S objectives?	Y	N	X	

Answer each of the above questions. Three answers are possible: Y (yes), N (no), and X (eXclude). Y means you're in compliance, N means you're not in compliance, while X means that this question can be excluded because it's not applicable in your situation. Y answers and X answers require no further action, while N answers point to things that need to be done to improve the performance of your OH&S management activities. Also, please use the column on the right to record your notes, and in the spaces below, enter the name and location of your organization, who completed this page, who reviewed it, and the dates.

ORGANIZATION:		YOUR LOCATION:	
COMPLETED BY:		DATE COMPLETED:	
REVIEWED BY:		DATE REVIEWED:	

ISO 45001 2018 OHS AUDIT TOOL

7. ASSESS HOW WELL YOU CONFORM TO ISO'S SUPPORT REQUIREMENTS

	7.1 SUPPORT YOUR ORGANIZATION'S OHSMS BY PROVIDING THE NECESSARY RESOURCES				
1	Do you determine the resources that your OHSMS needs?	Y	N	X	
2	Did you identify the resources that are needed to establish your OHSMS?	Y	N	X	
3	Did you identify the resources that are needed to implement your OHSMS?	Y	N	X	
4	Did you identify the resources that are needed to maintain your OHSMS?	Y	N	X	
5	Did you identify the resources that are needed to improve your OHSMS?	Y	N	X	
6	Do you provide the resources that your OHSMS needs?	Y	N	X	
7	Did you provide the resources that are needed to establish your OHSMS?	Y	N	X	
8	Did you provide the resources that are needed to implement your OHSMS?	Y	N	X	
9	Do you provide the resources that are needed to maintain your OHSMS?	Y	N	X	
10	Do you provide the resources that are needed to improve your OHSMS?	Y	N	X	
	7.2 SUPPORT YOUR ORGANIZATION'S OHSMS BY ENSURING THAT PEOPLE ARE COMPETENT				
11	Do you clarify your organization's OH&S competence requirements?	Y	N	X	
12	Do you identify those workers who can affect OH&S performance?	Y	N	X	
13	Do you determine the OH&S competence requirements of these workers?	Y	N	X	
14	Do you confirm that these workers know how to identify OH&S hazards?	Y	N	X	
15	Do you confirm the OH&S competence of your organization's workers?	Y	N	X	
16	Do you confirm that workers have the OH&S competence they need?	Y	N	X	
17	Do you confirm that they have the appropriate OH&S experience?	Y	N	X	
18	Do you confirm that they have the appropriate OH&S education?	Y	N	X	

ORGANIZATION:		YOUR LOCATION:	
COMPLETED BY:		DATE COMPLETED:	
REVIEWED BY:		DATE REVIEWED:	

ISO 45001 2018 OHS AUDIT TOOL

7. ASSESS HOW WELL YOU CONFORM TO ISO'S SUPPORT REQUIREMENTS

19	Do you confirm that they have the appropriate OH&S training?	Y	N	X	
20	Do you acquire competence whenever shortcomings are discovered?	Y	N	X	
21	Do you acquire competence whenever workers fail to meet your organization's OH&S competence requirements?	Y	N	X	
22	Do you consider helping your workers to improve?	Y	N	X	
23	Do you consider providing suitable training?	Y	N	X	
24	Do you consider offering mentoring services?	Y	N	X	
25	Do you consider hiring competent workers?	Y	N	X	
26	Do you consider hiring competent employees?	Y	N	X	
27	Do you consider hiring competent contractors?	Y	N	X	
28	Do you consider reassigning unsuitable workers?	Y	N	X	
29	Do you document the competence of workers who influence OH&S?	Y	N	X	
30	Do you retain your documentation and use it as evidence to show that workers have the competence they need?	Y	N	X	
31	Do you control all personnel records of OH&S competence?	Y	N	X	
32	Do you evaluate the effectiveness of actions taken to acquire competence?	Y	N	X	
7.3 SUPPORT YOUR ORGANIZATION'S OHSMS BY MAKING PEOPLE AWARE OF THEIR DUTIES					
33	Do you make workers aware of your organization's OHSMS?	Y	N	X	
34	Do you make workers aware of your organization's OH&S policy?	Y	N	X	
35	Do you make workers aware of your organization's OH&S objectives?	Y	N	X	
36	Do you make workers aware of your organization's OH&S hazards?	Y	N	X	
37	Do you make workers aware of your organization's OH&S risks?	Y	N	X	

ORGANIZATIO N:		YOUR LOCATION:	
COMPLETED BY:		DATE COMPLETED:	
REVIEWED BY:		DATE REVIEWED:	

ISO 45001 2018 OHS AUDIT TOOL

7. ASSESS HOW WELL YOU CONFORM TO ISO'S SUPPORT REQUIREMENTS

38	Do you make workers aware of your organization's OH&S incidents?	Y	N	X	
39	Do you make workers aware of the incidents that are relevant to them?	Y	N	X	
40	Do you make workers aware of your organization's OH&S practices?	Y	N	X	
41	Do you make workers aware of what they may do to protect themselves?	Y	N	X	
42	Do you make sure that workers know that they may remove themselves from work situations that present an imminent and serious danger to their life or health?	Y	N	X	
43	Do you make sure that workers know that arrangements have been made to protect them from retaliation if they choose to remove themselves from dangerous situations?	Y	N	X	
44	Do you make workers aware of your organization's OH&S investigations?	Y	N	X	
45	Do you make workers aware of the investigations that are relevant to them?	Y	N	X	
46	Do you make workers aware of actions being considered and being taken?	Y	N	X	
47	Do you make workers aware of your organization's OH&S performance?	Y	N	X	
48	Do you make workers aware of the contribution they can and do make?	Y	N	X	
49	Do you explain why they need to meet all OHSMS requirements?	Y	N	X	
50	Do you explain what could happen if they fail to meet OHSMS requirements?	Y	N	X	
51	Do you describe the implications of failing to meet OHSMS requirements?	Y	N	X	
52	Do you describe the consequences of failing to meet OHSMS requirements?	Y	N	X	
53	Do you explain why it's important to improve OH&S performance?	Y	N	X	
54	Do you explain how workers can enhance OHSMS effectiveness?	Y	N	X	

7.4 SUPPORT YOUR ORGANIZATION'S OHSMS BY CONTROLLING YOUR COMMUNICATIONS

7.4.1 SUPPORT YOUR ORGANIZATION'S OHSMS BY CREATING COMMUNICATION PROCESSES

55	Do you consider your organization's OHSMS communication needs?	Y	N	X	

ORGANIZATION:		YOUR LOCATION:	
COMPLETED BY:		DATE COMPLETED:	
REVIEWED BY:		DATE REVIEWED:	

ISO 45001 2018 OHS AUDIT TOOL

7. ASSESS HOW WELL YOU CONFORM TO ISO'S SUPPORT REQUIREMENTS

56	Do you ensure that OHSMS communications take diversity into account?	Y N X	
57	Do you ensure that OHSMS communications take gender into account?	Y N X	
58	Do you ensure that OHSMS communications take culture into account?	Y N X	
59	Do you ensure that OHSMS communications take literacy into account?	Y N X	
60	Do you ensure that OHSMS communications take language into account?	Y N X	
61	Do you ensure that OHSMS communications take disabilities into account?	Y N X	
62	Do you ensure that OHSMS communications are reliable and consistent?	Y N X	
63	Do you make sure that your OHSMS communications are consistent with the information generated by your organization's OHSMS?	Y N X	
64	Do you plan how you're going to manage OHSMS communications?	Y N X	
65	Do you plan how to manage communications about OHSMS requirements?	Y N X	
66	Do you plan how to manage communications about legal requirements?	Y N X	
67	Do you plan how to manage communications about other requirements?	Y N X	
68	Did you establish processes to manage your OHSMS communications?	Y N X	
69	Did you establish processes to manage your internal communications?	Y N X	
70	Do you figure out what your internal communications need to say?	Y N X	
71	Do you figure out how internal communications should be handled?	Y N X	
72	Do you figure out when internal communications should be carried out?	Y N X	
73	Do you figure out who should receive your internal communications?	Y N X	
74	Do you figure out what levels should receive communications?	Y N X	

ORGANIZATION:		YOUR LOCATION:	
COMPLETED BY:		DATE COMPLETED:	
REVIEWED BY:		DATE REVIEWED:	

ISO 45001 2018 OHS AUDIT TOOL

7. ASSESS HOW WELL YOU CONFORM TO ISO'S SUPPORT REQUIREMENTS

75	Do you figure out what functions should receive communications?	Y	N	X	
76	Did you establish processes to manage your external communications?	Y	N	X	
77	Do you figure out what your external communications need to say?	Y	N	X	
78	Do you consider the views of your external interested parties?	Y	N	X	
79	Do you figure out how external communications should be handled?	Y	N	X	
80	Do you figure out when external communications should be carried out?	Y	N	X	
81	Do you figure out who should receive your external communications?	Y	N	X	
82	Do you figure out how communications with visitors should be handled?	Y	N	X	
83	Do you figure out how communications with contractors should be handled?	Y	N	X	
84	Do you figure out how communications with interested parties should be handled?	Y	N	X	
85	Did you implement and do you apply your OHSMS communications processes?	Y	N	X	
86	Do you respond to relevant communications about your organization's OHSMS?	Y	N	X	
87	Do you maintain your organization's OHSMS communications processes?	Y	N	X	
88	Do you control information that documents your OHSMS communications?	Y	N	X	
89	Do you retain information that documents your OHSMS communications?	Y	N	X	
7.4.2 SUPPORT YOUR ORGANIZATION'S OHSMS BY FACILITATING INTERNAL COMMUNICATIONS					
90	Did you establish OHSMS communications within and throughout your organization?	Y	N	X	
91	Do you discuss your OHSMS with people at all organizational levels and functions?	Y	N	X	
92	Do you discuss changes to your OHSMS at all organizational levels and functions?	Y	N	X	
93	Do you enable workers to contribute to the continual improvement of the OHSMS?	Y	N	X	

ORGANIZATION:		YOUR LOCATION:	
COMPLETED BY:		DATE COMPLETED:	
REVIEWED BY:		DATE REVIEWED:	

ISO 45001 2018 OHS AUDIT TOOL

7. ASSESS HOW WELL YOU CONFORM TO ISO'S SUPPORT REQUIREMENTS

	7.4.3 SUPPORT YOUR ORGANIZATION'S OHSMS BY ESTABLISHING EXTERNAL COMMUNICATIONS				
94	Did you establish OHSMS communications between your organization and external parties?	Y	N	X	
95	Do you use your communications process to control your external communications?	Y	N	X	
96	Do you make sure that OHSMS communications take legal requirements into account?	Y	N	X	
97	Do you make sure that OHSMS communications take other requirements into account?	Y	N	X	
	7.5 SUPPORT YOUR ORGANIZATION'S OHSMS BY MANAGING DOCUMENTED INFORMATION				
	7.5.1 SUPPORT YOUR ORGANIZATION'S OHSMS BY INCLUDING NECESSARY DOCUMENTS AND RECORDS				
98	Do you figure out how extensive documented OHSMS information should be?	Y	N	X	
99	Do you consider your activities when you establish documents and records?	Y	N	X	
100	Do you consider your size when you establish documents and records?	Y	N	X	
101	Do you consider your workers when you establish documents and records?	Y	N	X	
102	Do you consider the competence of your organization's workers?	Y	N	X	
103	Do you consider your requirements when you establish documents and records?	Y	N	X	
104	Do you consider the need to fulfil your legal and other requirements?	Y	N	X	
105	Do you consider your processes when you establish documents and records?	Y	N	X	
106	Do you consider the complexity of your organization's processes?	Y	N	X	
107	Do you consider your products when you establish documents and records?	Y	N	X	
108	Do you consider your services when you establish documents and records?	Y	N	X	
109	Do you select all the documented information that your OHSMS needs?	Y	N	X	
110	Do you select all the internal documents and records that OHSMS needs?	Y	N	X	

ORGANIZATION:		YOUR LOCATION:	
COMPLETED BY:		DATE COMPLETED:	
REVIEWED BY:		DATE REVIEWED:	

ISO 45001 2018 OHS AUDIT TOOL

7. ASSESS HOW WELL YOU CONFORM TO ISO'S SUPPORT REQUIREMENTS

111	Do you include all the documented information required by ISO 45001?	Y	N	X	
112	Do you include information that documents your OH&S policy?	Y	N	X	
113	Do you include information that documents your requirements?	Y	N	X	
114	Do you include information that documents your legal requirements?	Y	N	X	
115	Do you include information that documents your other requirements?	Y	N	X	
116	Do you include information that documents your OH&S hazards?	Y	N	X	
117	Do you include information that documents actions needed to address hazards?	Y	N	X	
118	Do you include information that documents your risks and opportunities?	Y	N	X	
119	Do you include information that documents risk management processes?	Y	N	X	
120	Do you include information that documents risk management methods?	Y	N	X	
121	Do you include information that documents your risk identification methods?	Y	N	X	
122	Do you include information that documents your risk assessment methods?	Y	N	X	
123	Do you include information that documents your risk assessment criteria?	Y	N	X	
124	Do you include information that documents risk management actions?	Y	N	X	
125	Do you include information that documents actions needed to address risks?	Y	N	X	
126	Do you include information that documents actions needed to address opportunities?	Y	N	X	
127	Do you include information that documents your OHSMS scope?	Y	N	X	
128	Do you include information that documents your OHSMS roles?	Y	N	X	
129	Do you include information that documents OHSMS authorities?	Y	N	X	
130	Do you include information that documents OHSMS responsibilities?	Y	N	X	

ORGANIZATION:		YOUR LOCATION:	
COMPLETED BY:		DATE COMPLETED:	
REVIEWED BY:		DATE REVIEWED:	

ISO 45001 2018 OHS AUDIT TOOL

7. ASSESS HOW WELL YOU CONFORM TO ISO'S SUPPORT REQUIREMENTS

131	Do you include information that documents the competence of workers?	Y	N	X	
132	Do you include information that documents your OHSMS communications?	Y	N	X	
133	Do you include information that documents your OH&S objectives?	Y	N	X	
134	Do you include information that documents plans to achieve OH&S objectives?	Y	N	X	
135	Do you include information that documents your OH&S processes?	Y	N	X	
136	Do you include information that proves that processes are carried out as planned?	Y	N	X	
137	Do you include information that documents emergency responses?	Y	N	X	
138	Do you include information on the plans for responding to potential emergency situations?	Y	N	X	
139	Do you include information on the processes for responding to potential emergency situations?	Y	N	X	
140	Do you include information on the actions needed to address emergency situations?	Y	N	X	
141	Do you include information that documents your nonconformities?	Y	N	X	
142	Do you include documented information that describes OH&S incidents?	Y	N	X	
143	Do you include information that describes subsequent actions taken?	Y	N	X	
144	Do you include information that describes corrective actions taken?	Y	N	X	
145	Do you include information that describes the results achieved?	Y	N	X	
146	Do you include information that describes the effectiveness of actions taken?	Y	N	X	
147	Do you include information that describes the effectiveness of corrective actions?	Y	N	X	
148	Do you include information that documents your OHSMS results?	Y	N	X	
149	Do you include information that documents your monitoring results?	Y	N	X	
150	Do you include information that documents your measuring results?	Y	N	X	

ORGANIZATIO N:		YOUR LOCATION:	
COMPLETED BY:		DATE COMPLETED:	
REVIEWED BY:		DATE REVIEWED:	

ISO 45001 2018 OHS AUDIT TOOL

7. ASSESS HOW WELL YOU CONFORM TO ISO'S SUPPORT REQUIREMENTS

151	Do you include information that documents measuring equipment?	Y	N	X	
152	Do you include information that documents maintenance results?	Y	N	X	
153	Do you include information that documents verification results?	Y	N	X	
154	Do you include information that documents calibration results?	Y	N	X	
155	Do you include information that documents your analytical results?	Y	N	X	
156	Do you include information that documents your evaluation results?	Y	N	X	
157	Do you include information that documents performance evaluation results?	Y	N	X	
158	Do you include information that documents compliance evaluation results?	Y	N	X	
159	Do you include information that documents your internal audit results?	Y	N	X	
160	Do you include information that shows that you implemented an audit programme?	Y	N	X	
161	Do you include information that documents your management review results?	Y	N	X	
162	Do you include information that documents continual OH&S improvements?	Y	N	X	
163	Do you select all the external documents and records that your OHSMS needs?	Y	N	X	
164	Do you include all documented information of external origin that your organization needs in order to plan its OHSMS?	Y	N	X	
165	Do you include all documented information of external origin that your organization needs in order to operate its OHSMS?	Y	N	X	
7.5.2 SUPPORT YOUR ORGANIZATION'S OHSMS BY MANAGING THE USE OF DOCUMENTS AND RECORDS					
166	Do you manage the creation and modification of documented information?	Y	N	X	
167	Do you make sure that your organization's OHSMS documents and records are properly identified and clearly described?	Y	N	X	
168	Do you monitor the use of names and descriptive titles?	Y	N	X	

ORGANIZATION:		YOUR LOCATION:	
COMPLETED BY:		DATE COMPLETED:	
REVIEWED BY:		DATE REVIEWED:	

ISO 45001 2018 OHS AUDIT TOOL

7. ASSESS HOW WELL YOU CONFORM TO ISO'S SUPPORT REQUIREMENTS

169	Do you monitor the use of dates and reference numbers?	Y	N	X	
170	Do you make sure that your organization's OHSMS documents and records are properly formatted and clearly presented?	Y	N	X	
171	Do you monitor the use of paper and electronic media?	Y	N	X	
172	Do you monitor the use of language and graphics?	Y	N	X	
173	Do you monitor the use of software products?	Y	N	X	
174	Do you make sure that your organization's OHSMS documents and records are properly reviewed and officially approved?	Y	N	X	
175	Do you monitor the adequacy of documents and records?	Y	N	X	
176	Do you monitor the suitability of documents and records?	Y	N	X	
7.5.3 SUPPORT YOUR ORGANIZATION'S OHSMS BY CONTROLLING RELEVANT DOCUMENTS AND RECORDS					
177	Do you figure out how your documented information should be controlled?	Y	N	X	
178	Do you think about how OHSMS documents and records should be created?	Y	N	X	
179	Do you make sure that documents and records are suitable for use?	Y	N	X	
180	Do you think about how your OHSMS documents and records should be identified?	Y	N	X	
181	Do you consider how internal documents and records are identified and described?	Y	N	X	
182	Do you consider how external documents and records are identified and described?	Y	N	X	
183	Do you think about how your OHSMS documents and records should be distributed?	Y	N	X	
184	Do you think about how your OHSMS documents and records should be stored?	Y	N	X	
185	Do you think about how your OHSMS documents and records should be retrieved?	Y	N	X	
186	Do you think about how your OHSMS documents and records should be accessed?	Y	N	X	

ORGANIZATION:		YOUR LOCATION:	
COMPLETED BY:		DATE COMPLETED:	
REVIEWED BY:		DATE REVIEWED:	

ISO 45001 2018 OHS AUDIT TOOL

7. ASSESS HOW WELL YOU CONFORM TO ISO'S SUPPORT REQUIREMENTS

187	Do you prevent unauthorized access to OHSMS documents and records?	Y	N	X	
188	Do you make sure that they are available for use where they are needed?	Y	N	X	
189	Do you make sure that they are available for use when they are needed?	Y	N	X	
190	Do you think about how your OHSMS documents and records should be used?	Y	N	X	
191	Do you think about how documents and records are used to plan your OHSMS?	Y	N	X	
192	Do you consider how internal documents and records are used to plan your OHSMS?	Y	N	X	
193	Do you consider how external documents and records are used to plan your OHSMS?	Y	N	X	
194	Do you think about how documents and records are used to operate your OHSMS?	Y	N	X	
195	Do you consider how internal documents and records are used to operate OHSMS?	Y	N	X	
196	Do you consider how external documents and records are used to operate OHSMS?	Y	N	X	
197	Do you think about how your OHSMS documents and records should be protected?	Y	N	X	
198	Do you ensure that documents and records are adequately protected?	Y	N	X	
199	Do you protect the integrity of your documents and records?	Y	N	X	
200	Do you prevent unauthorized or improper use?	Y	N	X	
201	Do you protect the confidentiality of documents and records?	Y	N	X	
202	Do you protect the legibility of documents and records?	Y	N	X	
203	Do you think about how changes in OHSMS documents and records should be managed?	Y	N	X	
204	Do you consider using version control to manage your OHSMS changes?	Y	N	X	
205	Do you think about how your OHSMS documents and records should be preserved?	Y	N	X	

ORGANIZATIO N:		YOUR LOCATION:	
COMPLETED BY:		DATE COMPLETED:	
REVIEWED BY:		DATE REVIEWED:	

ISO 45001 2018 OHS AUDIT TOOL

7. ASSESS HOW WELL YOU CONFORM TO ISO'S SUPPORT REQUIREMENTS

206	Do you think about how your OHSMS documents and records are maintained?	Y	N	X	
207	Do you think about how your OHSMS documents and records are disposed of?	Y	N	X	
208	Do you control all the documented information that your OHSMS needs?	Y	N	X	
209	Do you control all the internal documents and records that OHSMS needs?	Y	N	X	
210	Do you control all the documented information required by ISO 45001?	Y	N	X	
211	Do you control information that documents your OH&S policy?	Y	N	X	
212	Do you control information that documents your OH&S requirements?	Y	N	X	
213	Do you control information that documents your legal requirements?	Y	N	X	
214	Do you control information that documents your other requirements?	Y	N	X	
215	Do you control information that documents your OH&S hazards?	Y	N	X	
216	Do you control information that documents actions to address hazards?	Y	N	X	
217	Do you control information that documents your OH&S risks and opportunities?	Y	N	X	
218	Do you control information that documents risk management processes?	Y	N	X	
219	Do you control information that documents risk management methods?	Y	N	X	
220	Do you control information that documents your risk identification methods?	Y	N	X	
221	Do you control information that documents your risk assessment methods?	Y	N	X	
222	Do you control information that documents your risk assessment criteria?	Y	N	X	
223	Do you control information that documents risk management actions?	Y	N	X	
224	Do you control information that documents actions needed to address risks?	Y	N	X	

ORGANIZATION:		YOUR LOCATION:	
COMPLETED BY:		DATE COMPLETED:	
REVIEWED BY:		DATE REVIEWED:	

ISO 45001 2018 OHS AUDIT TOOL

7. ASSESS HOW WELL YOU CONFORM TO ISO'S SUPPORT REQUIREMENTS

225	Do you control information that documents actions needed to address opportunities?	Y	N	X	
226	Do you control information that documents your OH&S objectives?	Y	N	X	
227	Do you control information that documents plans to achieve OH&S objectives?	Y	N	X	
228	Do you control information that documents your OHSMS scope?	Y	N	X	
229	Do you control information that documents your OHSMS roles?	Y	N	X	
230	Do you control information that documents OHSMS authorities?	Y	N	X	
231	Do you control information that documents OHSMS responsibilities?	Y	N	X	
232	Do you control information that documents your workers' competence?	Y	N	X	
233	Do you control information that documents your OHSMS communications?	Y	N	X	
234	Do you control information that documents your OH&S processes?	Y	N	X	
235	Do you control information that proves that processes are carried out as planned?	Y	N	X	
236	Do you control information that documents OH&S emergency responses?	Y	N	X	
237	Do you control information on the plans for responding to potential emergency situations?	Y	N	X	
238	Do you control information on the processes for responding to potential emergency situations?	Y	N	X	
239	Do you control information on the actions needed to address emergency situations?	Y	N	X	
240	Do you control information that documents your nonconformities?	Y	N	X	
241	Do you control documented information that describes OH&S incidents?	Y	N	X	
242	Do you control information that describes subsequent actions taken?	Y	N	X	
243	Do you control information that describes corrective actions taken?	Y	N	X	

ORGANIZATION:		YOUR LOCATION:	
COMPLETED BY:		DATE COMPLETED:	
REVIEWED BY:		DATE REVIEWED:	

ISO 45001 2018 OHS AUDIT TOOL

7. ASSESS HOW WELL YOU CONFORM TO ISO'S SUPPORT REQUIREMENTS

244	Do you control information that describes the results achieved?	Y	N	X	
245	Do you control information that describes the effectiveness of actions taken?	Y	N	X	
246	Do you control information that describes the effectiveness of corrective actions?	Y	N	X	
247	Do you control information that documents your OHSMS results?	Y	N	X	
248	Do you control information that documents your monitoring results?	Y	N	X	
249	Do you control information that documents your measuring results?	Y	N	X	
250	Do you control information that documents measuring equipment?	Y	N	X	
251	Do you control information that documents equipment verification results?	Y	N	X	
252	Do you control information that documents equipment calibration results?	Y	N	X	
253	Do you control information that documents equipment maintenance results?	Y	N	X	
254	Do you control information that documents your analytical results?	Y	N	X	
255	Do you control information that documents your evaluation results?	Y	N	X	
256	Do you control information that documents performance evaluation results?	Y	N	X	
257	Do you control information that documents compliance evaluation results?	Y	N	X	
258	Do you control information that documents your internal audit results?	Y	N	X	
259	Do you control information that shows that an audit programme was implemented?	Y	N	X	
260	Do you control information that documents your management review results?	Y	N	X	
261	Do you control information that documents continual OH&S improvements?	Y	N	X	
262	Do you control all the external documents and records that your OHSMS needs?	Y	N	X	
263	Do you control all documented information of external origin that your organization needs in order to plan its OHSMS?	Y	N	X	

ORGANIZATION:		YOUR LOCATION:	
COMPLETED BY:		DATE COMPLETED:	
REVIEWED BY:		DATE REVIEWED:	

ISO 45001 2018 OHS AUDIT TOOL

7. ASSESS HOW WELL YOU CONFORM TO ISO'S SUPPORT REQUIREMENTS

264	Do you control all documented information of external origin that your organization needs in order to operate its OHSMS?	Y	N	X	

Answer each of the above questions. Three answers are possible: Y (yes), N (no), and X (eXclude). Y means you're in compliance, N means you're not in compliance, while X means that this question can be excluded because it's not applicable in your situation. Y answers and X answers require no further action, while N answers point to things that need to be done to improve the performance of your OH&S management activities. Also, please use the column on the right to record your notes, and in the spaces below, enter the name and location of your organization, who completed this page, who reviewed it, and the dates.

ORGANIZATION:		YOUR LOCATION:	
COMPLETED BY:		DATE COMPLETED:	
REVIEWED BY:		DATE REVIEWED:	

ISO 45001 2018 OHS AUDIT TOOL

8. ASSESS HOW WELL YOU CONFORM TO ISO'S OPERATIONAL REQUIREMENTS

8.1 ESTABLISH AND MAINTAIN PROCESSES NEEDED TO MEET OHSMS REQUIREMENTS

8.1.1 ESTABLISH PROCESSES FOR MANAGING OCCUPATIONAL HEALTH AND SAFETY

1	Do you plan your organization's OHSMS processes?	Y	N	X	
2	Do you develop processes to meet OHSMS requirements?	Y	N	X	
3	Did you establish criteria that your processes must meet?	Y	N	X	
4	Do you use your criteria to establish process controls?	Y	N	X	
5	Did you establish work practices that consider workers?	Y	N	X	
6	Do you adapt work to accommodate worker needs?	Y	N	X	
7	Did you implement your organization's OHSMS processes?	Y	N	X	
8	Do you coordinate your OHSMS with other organizations?	Y	N	X	
9	Do you coordinate how your OHSMS interacts with other organizations?	Y	N	X	
10	Do you coordinate how relevant parts interact at multi-employer workplaces?	Y	N	X	
11	Do you control your organization's OHSMS processes?	Y	N	X	
12	Do you use your criteria to control your processes?	Y	N	X	
13	Do you maintain your organization's OHSMS processes?	Y	N	X	
14	Do you maintain and retain OH&S documents and records?	Y	N	X	
15	Do you use documents and records to show that processes follow plans?	Y	N	X	

8.1.2 ESTABLISH PROCESSES FOR MANAGING HAZARDS AND CONTROLLING RISKS

16	Do you use a Hierarchy of Controls approach to manage OH&S hazards and risks?	Y	N	X	
17	Did you establish hierarchical processes for managing hazards and risks?	Y	N	X	

ORGANIZATION:		YOUR LOCATION:	
COMPLETED BY:		DATE COMPLETED:	
REVIEWED BY:		DATE REVIEWED:	

ISO 45001 2018 OHS AUDIT TOOL

8. ASSESS HOW WELL YOU CONFORM TO ISO'S OPERATIONAL REQUIREMENTS

18	Do you ensure that your processes incorporate a Hierarchy of Controls?	Y	N	X
19	Do you apply hierarchical processes for managing hazards and risks?	Y	N	X
20	Do you eliminate your organization's OH&S hazards and risks (whenever this is practically possible)?	Y	N	X
21	Do you substitute dangerous hazards and risks for less dangerous ones (if you can't eliminate them)?	Y	N	X
22	Do you consider using less hazardous materials?	Y	N	X
23	Do you consider using less hazardous processes?	Y	N	X
24	Do you consider using less hazardous operations?	Y	N	X
25	Do you consider using less hazardous equipment?	Y	N	X
26	Do you use engineering controls (whenever you can't eliminate hazards and risks or make substitutions)?	Y	N	X
27	Do you consider reorganizing how people carry out work?	Y	N	X
28	Do you consider isolating people from hazards and risks?	Y	N	X
29	Do you use administrative controls (whenever you can't use engineering controls, eliminate hazards and risks, or make appropriate substitutions)?	Y	N	X
30	Do you consider using training to protect people from hazards?	Y	N	X
31	Do you use personal protective equipment (whenever you can't use administrative or engineering controls, eliminate hazards and risks, or make effective substitutions)?	Y	N	X
32	Do you maintain hierarchical processes for managing hazards and risks?	Y	N	X
8.1.3 ESTABLISH PROCESSES FOR MANAGING CHANGES AND CONTROLLING IMPACTS				
33	Do you develop processes to manage changes that impact OH&S performance?	Y	N	X
34	Do you determine how both permanent and temporary changes should be managed?	Y	N	X

ORGANIZATION:		YOUR LOCATION:	
COMPLETED BY:		DATE COMPLETED:	
REVIEWED BY:		DATE REVIEWED:	

ISO 45001 2018 OHS AUDIT TOOL

8. ASSESS HOW WELL YOU CONFORM TO ISO'S OPERATIONAL REQUIREMENTS

35	Do you determine how planned changes should be implemented and controlled?	Y	N	X	
36	Do you determine how changes in products should be implemented and controlled?	Y	N	X	
37	Do you determine how new product launches should be implemented and controlled?	Y	N	X	
38	Do you determine how changes in existing products should be implemented and controlled?	Y	N	X	
39	Do you determine how changes in services should be implemented and controlled?	Y	N	X	
40	Do you determine how new service offerings should be implemented and controlled?	Y	N	X	
41	Do you determine how changes in existing services should be implemented and controlled?	Y	N	X	
42	Do you determine how changes in processes should be implemented and controlled?	Y	N	X	
43	Do you determine how new processes should be implemented and controlled?	Y	N	X	
44	Do you determine how process modifications should be implemented and controlled?	Y	N	X	
45	Do you determine how changes in requirements should be implemented and controlled?	Y	N	X	
46	Do you determine how changes in legal OH&S requirements should be managed?	Y	N	X	
47	Do you determine how changes in other OH&S requirements should be managed?	Y	N	X	
48	Do you determine how changes in knowledge should be implemented and controlled?	Y	N	X	
49	Do you determine how changes in knowledge about OH&S risks should be managed?	Y	N	X	
50	Do you determine how changes in knowledge about OH&S hazards should be managed?	Y	N	X	
51	Do you determine how changes in technology should be implemented and controlled?	Y	N	X	
52	Do you determine how new technologies should be implemented and controlled?	Y	N	X	
53	Do you determine how technological changes should be implemented and controlled?	Y	N	X	
54	Do you determine how changes in the workplace should be implemented and controlled?	Y	N	X	
55	Do you determine how changes in workforce should be implemented and controlled?	Y	N	X	

ORGANIZATION:		YOUR LOCATION:	
COMPLETED BY:		DATE COMPLETED:	
REVIEWED BY:		DATE REVIEWED:	

ISO 45001 2018 OHS AUDIT TOOL

8. ASSESS HOW WELL YOU CONFORM TO ISO'S OPERATIONAL REQUIREMENTS

56	Do you determine how changes in locations should be implemented and controlled?	Y	N	X
57	Do you determine how changes in conditions should be implemented and controlled?	Y	N	X
58	Do you determine how changes in equipment should be implemented and controlled?	Y	N	X
59	Do you determine how changes in surroundings should be implemented and controlled?	Y	N	X
60	Do you determine how unplanned changes should be reviewed and controlled?	Y	N	X
61	Do you figure out how you're going to review the consequences of unintended changes?	Y	N	X
62	Do you figure out how you're going to take action to mitigate adverse effects?	Y	N	X
63	Did you implement processes to manage changes that impact OH&S performance?	Y	N	X
64	Do you use your change management processes to control all relevant changes?	Y	N	X
65	Do you manage and control changes that could impact OH&S performance?	Y	N	X
66	Do you manage and control planned changes that could impact OH&S performance?	Y	N	X
67	Do you manage and control unplanned changes that could impact OH&S performance?	Y	N	X

8.1.4 ESTABLISH PROCESSES FOR MANAGING CONTRACTORS AND SERVICE PROVIDERS

8.1.4.1 DEVELOP PROCUREMENT PROCESSES THAT MEET YOUR OHSMS REQUIREMENTS

68	Did you establish a process to control the procurement of products and services?	Y	N	X
69	Do you ensure that purchased products and services comply with the OHSMS?	Y	N	X
70	Did you implement a process to control the procurement of products and services?	Y	N	X
71	Do you use your process to ensure that purchased products comply with the OHSMS?	Y	N	X
72	Do you use your process to ensure that purchased services comply with the OHSMS?	Y	N	X
73	Do you maintain a process to control the procurement of products and services?	Y	N	X

ORGANIZATIO N:		YOUR LOCATION:	
COMPLETED BY:		DATE COMPLETED:	
REVIEWED BY:		DATE REVIEWED:	

ISO 45001 2018 OHS AUDIT TOOL

8. ASSESS HOW WELL YOU CONFORM TO ISO'S OPERATIONAL REQUIREMENTS

8.1.4.2 EXPECT CONTRACTORS AND THEIR WORKERS TO MEET YOUR OHSMS REQUIREMENTS					
74	Do you use your procurement process to specify your organization's OH&S requirements?	Y	N	X	
75	Do you expect contractors and their workers to comply with your OHSMS requirements?	Y	N	X	
76	Do you consider using your contractual documents to specify OH&S requirements?	Y	N	X	
77	Do you consider using your contractual documents to specify your OH&S criteria?	Y	N	X	
78	Do you select contractors who agree to meet your organization's OHSMS requirements?	Y	N	X	
79	Do you use your procurement process to identify hazards and assess and control OH&S risks?	Y	N	X	
80	Do you identify hazards and control risks arising from contractors' activities and operations?	Y	N	X	
81	Do you identify hazards and control risks that could impact your organization's workers?	Y	N	X	
82	Do you identify hazards and control risks that could impact other interested parties?	Y	N	X	
83	Do you identify hazards and control risks arising from your internal activities and operations?	Y	N	X	
84	Do you identify hazards and control risks that could impact your contractors' workers?	Y	N	X	
8.1.4.3 MAINTAIN OUTSOURCING ARRANGEMENTS THAT MEET YOUR OHSMS REQUIREMENTS					
85	Do you consider how outsourced functions and processes should be controlled?	Y	N	X	
86	Do you make sure that outsourcing arrangements meet all relevant requirements?	Y	N	X	
87	Do you make sure that these arrangements are consistent with legal requirements?	Y	N	X	
88	Do you make sure that these arrangements are consistent with other requirements?	Y	N	X	
89	Do you make sure that these arrangements are consistent with OHSMS requirements?	Y	N	X	
90	Do you make sure that outsourcing arrangements support intended OHSMS outcomes?	Y	N	X	

ORGANIZATIO N:		YOUR LOCATION:	
COMPLETED BY:		DATE COMPLETED:	
REVIEWED BY:		DATE REVIEWED:	

ISO 45001 2018 OHS AUDIT TOOL

8. ASSESS HOW WELL YOU CONFORM TO ISO'S OPERATIONAL REQUIREMENTS

91	Do you define how outsourced functions and processes should be controlled?	Y N X	
92	Do you define arrangements that support the achievement of intended OHSMS outcomes?	Y N X	
93	Do you use your organization's OHSMS to specify the type of control that should be applied?	Y N X	
94	Do you use your organization's OHSMS to specify how much control should be applied?	Y N X	
95	Do you control your organization's outsourced functions and processes?	Y N X	
8.2 ESTABLISH ALL NECESSARY EMERGENCY PREPAREDNESS AND RESPONSE PROCESSES			
96	Did you establish processes to prepare for and respond to potential emergency situations?	Y N X	
97	Do you plan how you're going to prepare for and respond to potential emergencies?	Y N X	
98	Do you plan how you're going to support emergency response processes?	Y N X	
99	Do you plan how you're going to provide emergency support services?	Y N X	
100	Do you plan how you're going to provide emergency training services?	Y N X	
101	Do you plan how you're going to provide emergency first aid services?	Y N X	
102	Do you plan how you're going to provide emergency testing services?	Y N X	
103	Do you plan how you're going to carry out emergency exercises?	Y N X	
104	Do you plan how you're going to manage emergency communications?	Y N X	
105	Do you plan how you're going to communicate with your workers?	Y N X	
106	Do you plan how you're going to communicate with your visitors?	Y N X	
107	Do you plan how you're going to communicate with your contractors?	Y N X	
108	Do you plan how you're going to communicate with your local community?	Y N X	
109	Do you plan how you're going to communicate with your government authorities?	Y N X	

ORGANIZATION:		YOUR LOCATION:	
COMPLETED BY:		DATE COMPLETED:	
REVIEWED BY:		DATE REVIEWED:	

ISO 45001 2018 OHS AUDIT TOOL

8. ASSESS HOW WELL YOU CONFORM TO ISO'S OPERATIONAL REQUIREMENTS

110	Do you plan how you're going to communicate with your emergency response services?	Y	N	X	
111	Do you develop processes to prepare for and respond to potential emergencies?	Y	N	X	
112	Do you involve interested parties in the development of planned responses?	Y	N	X	
113	Do you consider the needs and capabilities of relevant interested parties?	Y	N	X	
114	Did you establish planned responses to potential OH&S emergency situations?	Y	N	X	
115	Did you implement processes to prepare for and respond to potential emergencies?	Y	N	X	
116	Do you prepare for and respond to all types of OH&S emergency situations?	Y	N	X	
117	Do you maintain processes to prepare for and respond to potential emergencies?	Y	N	X	
118	Do you support your emergency preparedness and response processes?	Y	N	X	
119	Do you deliver emergency training and awareness services?	Y	N	X	
120	Do you provide emergency exercise and testing services?	Y	N	X	
121	Do you manage emergency communication services?	Y	N	X	
122	Do you ensure that all workers know what to do in an emergency?	Y	N	X	
123	Do you make sure they understand their duties and responsibilities?	Y	N	X	
124	Do you evaluate your emergency preparedness and response performance?	Y	N	X	
125	Do you periodically test emergency preparedness and response capabilities?	Y	N	X	
126	Do you periodically perform emergency preparedness and response exercises?	Y	N	X	
127	Do you revise your emergency preparedness and response plans and processes?	Y	N	X	
128	Do you revise plans and processes after emergency situations have occurred?	Y	N	X	
129	Do you revise plans and processes whenever evaluations support this decision?	Y	N	X	
130	Do you revise emergency plans and processes whenever tests support this decision?	Y	N	X	

ORGANIZATION:		YOUR LOCATION:	
COMPLETED BY:		DATE COMPLETED:	
REVIEWED BY:		DATE REVIEWED:	

ISO 45001 2018 OHS AUDIT TOOL

8. ASSESS HOW WELL YOU CONFORM TO ISO'S OPERATIONAL REQUIREMENTS

131	Do you revise emergency plans and processes whenever exercises support this decision?	Y	N	X	
132	Do you document your emergency preparedness and response plans and processes?	Y	N	X	
133	Do you maintain and retain documents and records that describe your processes?	Y	N	X	
134	Do you maintain and retain documents and records that describe your plans?	Y	N	X	

Answer each of the above questions. Three answers are possible: Y (yes), N (no), and X (eXclude). Y means you're in compliance,
N means you're not in compliance, while X means that this question can be excluded because it's not applicable in your situation.
Y answers and X answers require no further action, while N answers point to things that need to be done to improve the
performance of your OH&S management activities. Also, please use the column on the right to record your notes, and in the
spaces below, enter the name and location of your organization, who completed this page, who reviewed it, and the dates.

ORGANIZATION:		YOUR LOCATION:	
COMPLETED BY:		DATE COMPLETED:	
REVIEWED BY:		DATE REVIEWED:	

ISO 45001 2018 OHS AUDIT TOOL

9. ASSESS HOW WELL YOU CONFORM TO ISO'S EVALUATION REQUIREMENTS

9.1 ESTABLISH PROCESSES TO MONITOR, MEASURE, ANALYZE, AND EVALUATE YOUR OHSMS

9.1.1 ESTABLISH PROCESSES TO MONITOR, MEASURE, ANALYZE, AND EVALUATE PERFORMANCE

1	Do you develop processes to examine OH&S performance?	Y	N	X	
2	Do you plan how you're going to examine your OH&S performance?	Y	N	X	
3	Do you plan how you're going to monitor your OH&S performance?	Y	N	X	
4	Do you figure out what needs to be monitored and do you select methods?	Y	N	X	
5	Do you determine your OH&S monitoring needs and requirements?	Y	N	X	
6	Do you select monitoring methods that can produce valid results?	Y	N	X	
7	Did you establish when OH&S monitoring should be done?	Y	N	X	
8	Do you plan how you're going to measure your OH&S performance?	Y	N	X	
9	Do you figure out what needs to be measured and do you select methods?	Y	N	X	
10	Do you determine your OH&S measurement needs and requirements?	Y	N	X	
11	Do you select measurement methods that can produce valid results?	Y	N	X	
12	Did you establish when OH&S measuring should be done?	Y	N	X	
13	Do you plan how you're going to analyze your OH&S performance?	Y	N	X	
14	Do you select analytical methods that are capable of producing valid results?	Y	N	X	
15	Do you decide when monitoring and measurement results should be analyzed?	Y	N	X	
16	Do you plan how you're going to evaluate your OH&S performance?	Y	N	X	
17	Do you select evaluation methods that are capable of producing valid results?	Y	N	X	
18	Did you establish criteria that you can use to evaluate your OH&S performance?	Y	N	X	

ORGANIZATIO N:		YOUR LOCATION:	
COMPLETED BY:		DATE COMPLETED:	
REVIEWED BY:		DATE REVIEWED:	

ISO 45001 2018 OHS AUDIT TOOL

9. ASSESS HOW WELL YOU CONFORM TO ISO'S EVALUATION REQUIREMENTS

19	Do you decide when monitoring and measurement results should be evaluated?	Y	N	X
20	Do you plan how you're going to communicate your OH&S performance?	Y	N	X
21	Do you decide when monitoring results should be communicated?	Y	N	X
22	Do you decide when measurement results should be communicated?	Y	N	X
23	Did you implement processes to examine OH&S performance?	Y	N	X
24	Do you monitor your organization's OH&S performance?	Y	N	X
25	Do you monitor progress towards the achievement of OH&S objectives?	Y	N	X
26	Do you monitor the effectiveness of your operational and other controls?	Y	N	X
27	Do you monitor the extent to which OH&S requirements are being met?	Y	N	X
28	Do you monitor the extent to which legal requirements are being met?	Y	N	X
29	Do you monitor the extent to which other requirements are being met?	Y	N	X
30	Do you monitor all of the activities and operations related to OH&S?	Y	N	X
31	Do you monitor activities and operations related to identified risks?	Y	N	X
32	Do you monitor activities and operations related to identified hazards?	Y	N	X
33	Do you monitor activities and operations related to identified opportunities?	Y	N	X
34	Do you measure your organization's OH&S performance?	Y	N	X
35	Do you measure progress towards the achievement of OH&S objectives?	Y	N	X
36	Do you measure the effectiveness of your operational and other controls?	Y	N	X
37	Do you measure the extent to which OH&S requirements are being met?	Y	N	X
38	Do you measure the extent to which legal requirements are being met?	Y	N	X

ORGANIZATIO N:		YOUR LOCATION:	
COMPLETED BY:		DATE COMPLETED:	
REVIEWED BY:		DATE REVIEWED:	

ISO 45001 2018 OHS AUDIT TOOL

9. ASSESS HOW WELL YOU CONFORM TO ISO'S EVALUATION REQUIREMENTS

39	Do you measure the extent to which other requirements are being met?	Y	N	X	
40	Do you measure all of the activities and operations related to OH&S?	Y	N	X	
41	Do you measure activities and operations related to identified risks?	Y	N	X	
42	Do you measure activities and operations related to identified hazards?	Y	N	X	
43	Do you measure activities and operations related to identified opportunities?	Y	N	X	
44	Do you analyze your organization's OH&S performance?	Y	N	X	
45	Do you analyze the results of your monitoring activities?	Y	N	X	
46	Do you analyze the results of your measuring activities?	Y	N	X	
47	Do you evaluate your organization's OH&S performance?	Y	N	X	
48	Do you evaluate OH&S performance against OH&S performance criteria?	Y	N	X	
49	Do you evaluate the effectiveness of your organization's OHSMS?	Y	N	X	
50	Do you communicate your organization's OH&S performance?	Y	N	X	
51	Do you use your communication processes to control communications?	Y	N	X	
52	Do you discuss your OH&S performance within your own organization?	Y	N	X	
53	Do you discuss your OH&S performance with relevant external parties?	Y	N	X	
54	Do you maintain processes to examine OH&S performance?	Y	N	X	
55	Do you maintain monitoring and measuring processes?	Y	N	X	
56	Do you maintain your monitoring and measuring equipment?	Y	N	X	
57	Do you use only verified or calibrated monitoring equipment?	Y	N	X	
58	Do you maintain your monitoring equipment (as appropriate)?	Y	N	X	

ORGANIZATION:		YOUR LOCATION:	
COMPLETED BY:		DATE COMPLETED:	
REVIEWED BY:		DATE REVIEWED:	

ISO 45001 2018 OHS AUDIT TOOL

9. ASSESS HOW WELL YOU CONFORM TO ISO'S EVALUATION REQUIREMENTS

59	Do you use only verified or calibrated measurement equipment?	Y	N	X
60	Do you maintain your measurement equipment (as appropriate)?	Y	N	X
61	Do you retain records that document equipment calibration activities?	Y	N	X
62	Do you retain records that document equipment verification activities?	Y	N	X
63	Do you retain records that document equipment maintenance activities?	Y	N	X
64	Do you maintain information management processes?	Y	N	X
65	Do you maintain your OH&S records and documents?	Y	N	X
66	Do you record analytical results and retain these records?	Y	N	X
67	Do you record evaluation results and retain these records?	Y	N	X
68	Do you record monitoring results and retain these records?	Y	N	X
69	Do you record measurement results and retain these records?	Y	N	X

9.1.2 ESTABLISH PROCESSES TO EVALUATE COMPLIANCE WITH LEGAL AND OTHER REQUIREMENTS

70	Did you establish processes for evaluating your organization's OH&S compliance?	Y	N	X
71	Do you develop processes for evaluating your organization's OH&S compliance?	Y	N	X
72	Did you establish methods for evaluating your organization's OH&S compliance?	Y	N	X
73	Do you plan how you're going to evaluate compliance with legal requirements?	Y	N	X
74	Do you plan how you're going to evaluate compliance with other requirements?	Y	N	X
75	Do you determine how often compliance evaluations should be carried out?	Y	N	X
76	Did you implement processes for evaluating your OH&S compliance?	Y	N	X
77	Do you evaluate compliance with legal and other requirements?	Y	N	X

ORGANIZATION:		YOUR LOCATION:	
COMPLETED BY:		DATE COMPLETED:	
REVIEWED BY:		DATE REVIEWED:	

ISO 45001 2018 OHS AUDIT TOOL

9. ASSESS HOW WELL YOU CONFORM TO ISO'S EVALUATION REQUIREMENTS

78	Do you determine the status of your organization's compliance?	Y	N	X	
79	Did you establish knowledge and understanding of your compliance?	Y	N	X	
80	Do you maintain knowledge about compliance with legal requirements?	Y	N	X	
81	Do you maintain knowledge about compliance with other requirements?	Y	N	X	
82	Do you take action whenever requirements are not being met?	Y	N	X	
83	Do you maintain processes for evaluating your OH&S compliance?	Y	N	X	
84	Do you maintain and retain a record of compliance evaluation results?	Y	N	X	

9.2 DETERMINE INTERNAL OH&S AUDIT REQUIREMENTS, RESPONSIBILITIES, AND METHODS

9.2.1 AUDIT THE CONFORMANCE OF YOUR ORGANIZATION'S OHSMS AT PLANNED INTERVALS

85	Do you conduct internal OHSMS conformance audits at planned intervals?	Y	N	X	
86	Do you determine if your organization's OHSMS meets requirements?	Y	N	X	
87	Do you see if your OHSMS meets the requirements of this ISO standard?	Y	N	X	
88	Do you see if your OHSMS meets your organization's own requirements?	Y	N	X	
89	Do you see if your OHSMS is applying your organization's OH&S policy?	Y	N	X	
90	Do you see if your OHSMS is achieving your organization's OH&S objectives?	Y	N	X	
91	Do you examine the effectiveness of your organization's OHSMS?	Y	N	X	
92	Do you see if your organization's OHSMS was effectively implemented?	Y	N	X	
93	Do you see if your organization's OHSMS is being effectively maintained?	Y	N	X	

9.2.2 ESTABLISH, IMPLEMENT, AND MAINTAIN AN INTERNAL OHSMS AUDIT PROGRAMME

94	Do you plan your organization's internal audit programme?	Y	N	X	

ORGANIZATIO N:		YOUR LOCATION:	
COMPLETED BY:		DATE COMPLETED:	
REVIEWED BY:		DATE REVIEWED:	

ISO 45001 2018 OHS AUDIT TOOL

9. ASSESS HOW WELL YOU CONFORM TO ISO'S EVALUATION REQUIREMENTS

95	Did you develop a programme that can find out if your OHSMS meets requirements?	Y N X
96	Did you make sure it can determine if it meets your organization's requirements?	Y N X
97	Did you make sure it can determine if it meets the ISO 45001 2018 requirements?	Y N X
98	Did you develop a programme that can determine if your OHSMS is effective?	Y N X
99	Did you establish an internal audit programme for your organization?	Y N X
100	Did you establish your audit methods and expectations?	Y N X
101	Did you establish internal audit norms and values?	Y N X
102	Do you expect internal auditors to be objective?	Y N X
103	Do you expect internal auditors to be impartial?	Y N X
104	Did you establish internal audit planning expectations?	Y N X
105	Do you expect auditors to consider the results of previous internal audits?	Y N X
106	Do you expect auditors to consider the importance of processes being audited?	Y N X
107	Did you establish internal audit duties and responsibilities?	Y N X
108	Do you expect auditors to specify criteria for each audit?	Y N X
109	Do you expect auditors to define the scope of each audit?	Y N X
110	Do you expect auditors to consult with interested parties?	Y N X
111	Do you expect auditors to report the results of each audit?	Y N X
112	Do you expect auditors to report results to management?	Y N X
113	Do you expect auditors to report results to interested parties?	Y N X
114	Do you expect auditors to report results to other workers?	Y N X

ORGANIZATIO N:		YOUR LOCATION:	
COMPLETED BY:		DATE COMPLETED:	
REVIEWED BY:		DATE REVIEWED:	

ISO 45001 2018 OHS AUDIT TOOL

9. ASSESS HOW WELL YOU CONFORM TO ISO'S EVALUATION REQUIREMENTS

115	Do you expect them to report to worker representatives?	Y	N	X	
116	Did you implement your organization's internal audit programme?	Y	N	X	
117	Do you carry out internal audits at planned intervals?	Y	N	X	
118	Do you select impartial and objective internal auditors?	Y	N	X	
119	Do you specify audit criteria for each internal audit?	Y	N	X	
120	Do you define the scope for each internal audit?	Y	N	X	
121	Do you take action to address OH&S nonconformities?	Y	N	X	
122	Do you continually improve OH&S performance?	Y	N	X	
123	Do you report audit results to the appropriate people?	Y	N	X	
124	Do you report internal audit results to management?	Y	N	X	
125	Do you report internal audit results to other workers?	Y	N	X	
126	Do you report results to worker representatives?	Y	N	X	
127	Do you maintain your organization's internal audit programme?	Y	N	X	
128	Do you retain documents and records about your programme?	Y	N	X	
129	Do you retain a record of your implementation activities?	Y	N	X	
130	Do you retain a record of your internal auditing results?	Y	N	X	

9.3 REVIEW THE SUITABILITY, ADEQUACY, AND EFFECTIVENESS OF YOUR ORGANIZATION'S OHSMS

131	Do you review your organization's OHSMS at regular intervals?	Y	N	X	
132	Do you review OHSMS suitability, adequacy, and effectiveness?	Y	N	X	
133	Do you review the status of your previous management reviews?	Y	N	X	

ORGANIZATION:		YOUR LOCATION:	
COMPLETED BY:		DATE COMPLETED:	
REVIEWED BY:		DATE REVIEWED:	

ISO 45001 2018 OHS AUDIT TOOL

9. ASSESS HOW WELL YOU CONFORM TO ISO'S EVALUATION REQUIREMENTS

134	Do you review the status of the actions that were previously taken?	Y	N	X
135	Do you review how well your OH&S objectives are being achieved?	Y	N	X
136	Do you review how well your OH&S policy is being implemented?	Y	N	X
137	Do you review relevant communications with interested parties?	Y	N	X
138	Do you review OH&S performance, including trends?	Y	N	X
139	Do you review trends in OH&S risks and opportunities?	Y	N	X
140	Do you review trends in audit results and audit activities?	Y	N	X
141	Do you review trends in OH&S incidents and nonconformities?	Y	N	X
142	Do you review trends in worker participation and consultation?	Y	N	X
143	Do you review trends in monitoring and measurement results?	Y	N	X
144	Do you review trends in corrective actions and improvements?	Y	N	X
145	Do you review trends in relevant compliance evaluation results?	Y	N	X
146	Do you review how well legal requirements are being met?	Y	N	X
147	Do you review how well other requirements are being met?	Y	N	X
148	Do you review changes in requirements, issues, risks, and opportunities?	Y	N	X
149	Do you review changes in external and internal issues relevant to your OHSMS?	Y	N	X
150	Do you review changes in the needs and expectations of interested parties?	Y	N	X
151	Do you review changes in your organization's OH&S requirements?	Y	N	X
152	Do you review all relevant changes in legal requirements?	Y	N	X
153	Do you review all relevant changes in other requirements?	Y	N	X

ORGANIZATION:		YOUR LOCATION:	
COMPLETED BY:		DATE COMPLETED:	
REVIEWED BY:		DATE REVIEWED:	

ISO 45001 2018 OHS AUDIT TOOL

9. ASSESS HOW WELL YOU CONFORM TO ISO'S EVALUATION REQUIREMENTS

154	Do you review changes in the risks that affect OH&S performance?	Y	N	X	
155	Do you review changes in your organization's OH&S opportunities?	Y	N	X	
156	Do you review potential continual improvement opportunities?	Y	N	X	
157	Do you review the strategic direction that your OHSMS is taking?	Y	N	X	
158	Do you review the adequacy of your OHSMS resources?	Y	N	X	
159	Do you review how well OHSMS is being maintained?	Y	N	X	
160	Do you generate appropriate management review outputs?	Y	N	X	
161	Do you draw conclusions about your organization's OHSMS?	Y	N	X	
162	Do you consider OHSMS suitability, adequacy, and effectiveness?	Y	N	X	
163	Do you consider how well OHSMS is achieving intended outcomes?	Y	N	X	
164	Do you identify ways of improving OHSMS integration with other processes?	Y	N	X	
165	Do you make decisions about your organization's OHSMS?	Y	N	X	
166	Do you consider continual improvement opportunities?	Y	N	X	
167	Do you consider whether you need to change your OHSMS?	Y	N	X	
168	Do you consider whether you need to change OHSMS resources?	Y	N	X	
169	Do you define actions to improve OH&S performance?	Y	N	X	
170	Do you consider how well OH&S policy is being implemented?	Y	N	X	
171	Do you take action whenever your policy isn't being applied?	Y	N	X	
172	Do you consider how well OH&S objectives are being achieved?	Y	N	X	
173	Do you take action whenever objectives aren't being achieved?	Y	N	X	

ORGANIZATION:		YOUR LOCATION:	
COMPLETED BY:		DATE COMPLETED:	
REVIEWED BY:		DATE REVIEWED:	

ISO 45001 2018 OHS AUDIT TOOL

9. ASSESS HOW WELL YOU CONFORM TO ISO'S EVALUATION REQUIREMENTS

174	Do you consider implications for your overall strategic direction?	Y	N	X	
175	Do you communicate relevant outputs of management reviews?	Y	N	X	
176	Do you share management review outputs with workers?	Y	N	X	
177	Do you share outputs with workers' representatives?	Y	N	X	
178	Do you document the results of your management reviews?	Y	N	X	
179	Do you retain your management review records?	Y	N	X	

Answer each of the above questions. Three answers are possible: Y (yes), N (no), and X (eXclude). Y means you're in compliance, N means you're not in compliance, while X means that this question can be excluded because it's not applicable in your situation. Y answers and X answers require no further action, while N answers point to things that need to be done to improve the performance of your OH&S management activities. Also, please use the column on the right to record your notes, and in the spaces below, enter the name and location of your organization, who completed this page, who reviewed it, and the dates.

ORGANIZATION:		YOUR LOCATION:	
COMPLETED BY:		DATE COMPLETED:	
REVIEWED BY:		DATE REVIEWED:	

ISO 45001 2018 OHS AUDIT TOOL

10. ASSESS HOW WELL YOU CONFORM TO ISO'S IMPROVEMENT REQUIREMENTS

10.1 IDENTIFY IMPROVEMENT OPPORTUNITIES AND TAKE ACTION TO ACHIEVE INTENDED OUTCOMES

1	Do you determine opportunities to improve OHSMS and achieve its intended outcomes?	Y	N	X	
2	Do you use performance evaluation results to identify opportunities to improve your organization's OHSMS and achieve its intended outcomes?	Y	N	X	
3	Do you use compliance evaluation results to identify opportunities to improve your organization's OHSMS and achieve its intended outcomes?	Y	N	X	
4	Do you use internal audit results to identify opportunities to improve your organization's OHSMS and achieve its intended outcomes?	Y	N	X	
5	Do you use management review results to identify opportunities to improve your organization's OHSMS and achieve its intended outcomes?	Y	N	X	
6	Do you take all necessary actions to improve OHSMS and achieve its intended outcomes?	Y	N	X	
7	Do you use performance evaluation results to improve your organization's OHSMS?	Y	N	X	
8	Do you use performance evaluation results to help achieve intended outcomes?	Y	N	X	
9	Do you use compliance evaluation results to improve your organization's OHSMS?	Y	N	X	
10	Do you use compliance evaluation results to help achieve intended outcomes?	Y	N	X	
11	Do you use internal audit results to improve your organization's OHSMS?	Y	N	X	
12	Do you use internal audit results to help achieve intended outcomes?	Y	N	X	
13	Do you use management review results to improve your organization's OHSMS?	Y	N	X	
14	Do you use management review results to help achieve intended outcomes?	Y	N	X	

10.2 ESTABLISH PROCESSES TO INVESTIGATE AND RESPOND TO OH&S INCIDENTS AND NONCONFORMITIES

15	Did you establish processes to manage OH&S incidents and nonconformities?	Y	N	X	
16	Did you implement processes to manage incidents and nonconformities?	Y	N	X	

ORGANIZATION:		YOUR LOCATION:	
COMPLETED BY:		DATE COMPLETED:	
REVIEWED BY:		DATE REVIEWED:	

ISO 45001 2018 OHS AUDIT TOOL

10. ASSESS HOW WELL YOU CONFORM TO ISO'S IMPROVEMENT REQUIREMENTS

17	Do you react to incidents and nonconformities in a timely manner?	Y	N	X
18	Do you take action to control your incidents and nonconformities?	Y	N	X
19	Do you take action to address incidents and correct nonconformities?	Y	N	X
20	Do you take action to deal with all relevant impacts and consequences?	Y	N	X
21	Do you investigate incidents and review nonconformities?	Y	N	X
22	Do you evaluate your incidents and nonconformities?	Y	N	X
23	Do you involve workers and other interested parties?	Y	N	X
24	Do you evaluate your organization's incidents?	Y	N	X
25	Do you determine the cause of the incident?	Y	N	X
26	Do you determine if similar incidents have occurred?	Y	N	X
27	Do you determine if similar incidents could recur?	Y	N	X
28	Do you determine if they could occur elsewhere?	Y	N	X
29	Do you evaluate your organization's nonconformities?	Y	N	X
30	Do you determine the cause of the nonconformity?	Y	N	X
31	Do you determine if similar nonconformities exist?	Y	N	X
32	Do you determine if similar nonconformities could recur?	Y	N	X
33	Do you determine if they could happen elsewhere?	Y	N	X
34	Do you evaluate the need to take corrective action?	Y	N	X
35	Do you examine the need to eliminate root causes?	Y	N	X
36	Do you review your incidents and nonconformities?	Y	N	X

ORGANIZATION:		YOUR LOCATION:	
COMPLETED BY:		DATE COMPLETED:	
REVIEWED BY:		DATE REVIEWED:	

ISO 45001 2018 OHS AUDIT TOOL

10. ASSESS HOW WELL YOU CONFORM TO ISO'S IMPROVEMENT REQUIREMENTS

37	Do you review related existing risk assessments?	Y	N	X	
38	Do you review existing assessments of OH&S risks?	Y	N	X	
39	Do you review existing assessments of other risks?	Y	N	X	
40	Do you develop suitable corrective actions to address root causes?	Y	N	X	
41	Do you decide if corrective action or other action should be taken?	Y	N	X	
42	Do you develop actions to address incidents and nonconformities?	Y	N	X	
43	Do you develop actions that address actual and potential effects?	Y	N	X	
44	Do you use a hierarchy of controls approach to select actions?	Y	N	X	
45	Do you consider eliminating causes whenever this is possible?	Y	N	X	
46	Do you consider using controls when you can't eliminate causes?	Y	N	X	
47	Do you consider using engineering controls when causes can't be removed?	Y	N	X	
48	Do you consider using administrative controls when engineering controls can't be used?	Y	N	X	
49	Do you consider using personal protective equipment whenever other actions can't be taken?	Y	N	X	
50	Do you take action to address incidents and nonconformities?	Y	N	X	
51	Do you use change management processes to control implementation?	Y	N	X	
52	Do you make changes to your OHSMS whenever this is necessary or desirable?	Y	N	X	
53	Do you assess OH&S risks that relate to new or changed hazards before acting?	Y	N	X	
54	Do you review the effectiveness of the actions that have been taken?	Y	N	X	
55	Do you review the effectiveness of your corrective actions?	Y	N	X	
56	Do you report OH&S incidents, nonconformities, actions, and results?	Y	N	X	

ORGANIZATION:		YOUR LOCATION:	
COMPLETED BY:		DATE COMPLETED:	
REVIEWED BY:		DATE REVIEWED:	

ISO 45001 2018 OHS AUDIT TOOL

10. ASSESS HOW WELL YOU CONFORM TO ISO'S IMPROVEMENT REQUIREMENTS

57	Do you maintain processes to manage incidents and nonconformities?	Y	N	X
58	Do you document your incidents, nonconformities, actions, and results?	Y	N	X
59	Do you document your organization's incidents and nonconformities?	Y	N	X
60	Do you retain your record of incidents and nonconformities?	Y	N	X
61	Do you document actions to address incidents and nonconformities?	Y	N	X
62	Do you retain a record of actions and corrective actions taken?	Y	N	X
63	Do you describe the results that were actually achieved?	Y	N	X
64	Do you assess how effective your actions actually were?	Y	N	X
65	Do you communicate your incidents, nonconformities, actions, and results?	Y	N	X
66	Do you share documented information with relevant interested parties?	Y	N	X
67	Do you share this information with your organization's workers?	Y	N	X
68	Do you share this information with worker representatives?	Y	N	X

10.3 ENHANCE THE SUITABILITY, ADEQUACY, AND EFFECTIVENESS OF YOUR ORGANIZATION'S OHSMS

69	Do you continually improve the suitability, adequacy, and effectiveness of your OHSMS?	Y	N	X
70	Do you improve your OHSMS by promoting a culture that actively supports OH&S?	Y	N	X
71	Do you promote a culture that supports the continual improvement of the OHSMS?	Y	N	X
72	Do you promote a culture that supports worker participation and communication?	Y	N	X
73	Do you support participation and communication with worker representatives?	Y	N	X
74	Do you promote a culture that supports the documentation of improvements?	Y	N	X
75	Do you expect relevant documents and records to be maintained and retained?	Y	N	X

ORGANIZATION:		YOUR LOCATION:	
COMPLETED BY:		DATE COMPLETED:	
REVIEWED BY:		DATE REVIEWED:	

ISO 45001 2018 OHS AUDIT TOOL

10. ASSESS HOW WELL YOU CONFORM TO ISO'S IMPROVEMENT REQUIREMENTS

Answer each of the above questions. Three answers are possible: Y (yes), N (no), and X (eXclude). Y means you're in compliance,
N means you're not in compliance, while X means that this question can be excluded because it's not applicable in your situation.
Y answers and X answers require no further action, while N answers point to things that need to be done to improve the
performance of your OH&S management activities. Also, please use the column on the right to record your notes, and in the
spaces below, enter the name and location of your organization, who completed this page, who reviewed it, and the dates.

ORGANIZATION:		YOUR LOCATION:	
COMPLETED BY:		DATE COMPLETED:	
REVIEWED BY:		DATE REVIEWED:	

ISO 45001 2018 OHS AUDIT TOOL

11. SUMMARY OF YOUR OCCUPATIONAL HEALTH AND SAFETY AUDIT RESULTS

PART	AUDIT QUESTIONNAIRE	YES	NO	YES + NO	SCORE (%)	RANK
4	Contextual Compliance Score					
5	Leadership Compliance Score					
6	Planning Compliance Score					
7	Support Compliance Score					
8	Operational Compliance Score					
9	Evaluation Compliance Score					
10	Improvement Compliance Score					
	GRAND TOTALS					
	AVERAGE ISO 45001 COMPLIANCE SCORE					

For each section of your audit, count the number of YES answers and record the total in the YES column and count the number of NO answers and record the total in the NO column. Then add the two numbers together and record the totals in the YES+NO column. To calculate the SCORE for each section, divide the total YES answers by the total YES+NO answers and multiply the result by 100 to get a percentage. To calculate the AVERAGE ISO 45001 2018 COMPLIANCE SCORE, use the GRAND TOTALS to do the same. RANK the 7 sections by assigning the number "1" to the highest score, the number "2" to the next highest score, and so on.

NOTES AND COMMENTS

ORGANIZATIO N:	YOUR LOCATION:
COMPLETED BY:	DATE COMPLETED:
REVIEWED BY:	DATE REVIEWED:

ISO 45001 2018 OHS AUDIT TOOL

11. SUMMARY OF YOUR OCCUPATIONAL HEALTH AND SAFETY AUDIT RESULTS

ORGANIZATION:		YOUR LOCATION:	
COMPLETED BY:		DATE COMPLETED:	
REVIEWED BY:		DATE REVIEWED:	

ISO 45001 2018 OHS AUDIT TOOL

12. OCCUPATIONAL HEALTH AND SAFETY TERMS AND DEFINITIONS

The following section on terminology is based on ISO 45001, section 3, *Terms and definitions*. We have translated these definitions into plain English in order to make them easier to understand. Our definitions are based not only on ISO's official definitions but also on how ISO 45001 actually uses these terms.

We've also defined several important terms that ISO 45001 uses but doesn't formally define, terms that are, nevertheless, essential to a proper understanding of the new ISO 45001 standard. For example, ISO 45001 uses the terms *risk assessment, risk criteria,* and *context of the organization*, but doesn't formally define what they mean. We've addressed this shortcoming by considering how the standard uses these terms and by using other definitions to construct a new definition.

We've also tried to make it easier to find definitions by listing them in alphabetical order.

Terms that aren't formally defined here tend to have their ordinary non-technical meanings. Whenever you're not sure about the meaning of a word, and it's not defined here, you may wish to consult a dictionary.

Acceptable risk

A risk is *acceptable* to a specific organization if it has been reduced to a level that it can tolerate given its obligations, policies, and basic purpose.

Audit

An *audit* is systematic evidence gathering process. Audits must be independent, and evidence must be evaluated objectively to determine how well audit criteria are being met. There are three types of audits: first-party, second-party, and third-party. First-party audits are internal audits while second- and third-party audits are external audits.

Organizations use first party audits to audit themselves. First party audits are used to provide input for management review and for other internal purposes. They're also used to declare that an organization meets specified requirements (this is called a self-declaration).

Second party audits are external audits. They're usually done by customers or by others on their behalf. However, they can also be done by regulators or any other external party that has an interest in an organization. Third party audits are external audits as well. However, they're performed by independent organizations such as registrars (certification bodies) or regulators.

Objective means factual. *Independence* can often be achieved by ensuring that auditors do not audit their own work.

ISO also distinguishes between *combined audits* and *joint audits*. When two or more management systems of different disciplines are audited together at the same time, it's called a *combined audit*; and when two or more auditing organizations cooperate to audit a single auditee organization it's called a *joint audit*.

For more information about auditing, see our ISO 19011 Auditing Library at http://www.praxiom.com/19011.htm

Competence

Competence means being able to apply knowledge and skill to achieve intended results. *Being competent* means having the knowledge and skill that you need and knowing how to apply it. It means that you're qualified to do the job.

Conformity

Conformity is the "fulfillment of a requirement". To conform means to meet or comply with requirements and a *requirement* is a need, expectation, or obligation. There are many types of requirements including occupational health and safety requirements, management requirements, product requirements, service requirements, contractual requirements, statutory requirements, and regulatory requirements.

ISO 45001 2018 OHS AUDIT TOOL

12. OCCUPATIONAL HEALTH AND SAFETY TERMS AND DEFINITIONS

Consultation When organizations engage in *consultation* it means that they seek and receive the views and opinions of others before making a decision. In the context of OH&S, organizations often consult managers, workers, health and safety committees, and workers' representatives before making decisions that could affect the health and safety of these groups.	*Consultation* is not the same as *participation*. While *consultation* means receiving the views and opinions of others before decisions are made, *participation* means getting people involved in the actual decision-making process itself.
Context of the organization An organization's *context* is its business environment. It includes all of the internal and external factors and conditions that affect its products and services, have an influence on its OHSMS, and are relevant to its purpose and strategic direction. An organization's *external context* includes all of the needs and expectations of interested parties, as well as its social, cultural, legal, technological, regulatory, and competitive environment. An organization's *internal context* includes its values, culture, knowledge, and performance. ISO 45001 expects you to consider your organization's internal and external context when you define the scope of its OHSMS and when you plan its design and development.	*OHSMS* is short for *occupational health and safety management system*.
Continual improvement In this context, *continual improvement* is a set of recurring activities that are carried out in order to enhance OH&S performance. Continual improvements can be achieved by carrying out audits, self-assessments, and management reviews. Continual improvements can also be realized by collecting data, analyzing information, setting objectives, and taking corrective actions.	*Continual improvements* do not have to occur continuously without interruption.
Contractor A *contractor* is an organization that provides services to another organization in accordance with an agreed set of terms, conditions, and specifications.	
Corrective action *Corrective actions* are steps that are taken to eliminate the causes of nonconformities and incidents in order to prevent recurrence. The corrective action process tries to make sure that existing nonconformities and incidents don't happen again.	ISO 45001 no longer uses the term *preventive action*. It has been replaced by risk planning.
Documented information The term *documented information* refers to information that must be controlled and maintained and its supporting medium. Documented information can be in any format and on any medium and can come from any source. Documented information includes information about the management system and related processes. It also includes all the information that organizations need to operate and all the information that they use to document the results that they achieve (aka records).	The term *documented information* is just a new name for what used to be called *documents* and *records*. ISO 45001 does not expect you to write an OH&S manual.

ISO 45001 2018 OHS AUDIT TOOL

12. OCCUPATIONAL HEALTH AND SAFETY TERMS AND DEFINITIONS

Effectiveness *Effectiveness* refers to the degree to which a planned *effect* is achieved. Planned activities are effective if these activities are actually carried out and planned results are effective if these results are actually achieved.	
Hazard A *hazard* is any situation, substance, activity, event, or environment that could potentially cause injury or ill health. More precisely: • *Hazardous situations* can cause injury or ill health. Examples of potentially hazardous situations include slippery or uneven walking surfaces, cramped working conditions, badly ventilated areas, high altitudes, noisy locations, poorly lit areas, and confined spaces. • *Hazardous substances* can cause injury or ill health. Examples of potentially hazardous substances include corrosive and toxic chemicals, flammable and explosive materials, dangerous gases and liquids, radioactive substances, particulates, poisons, bacteria, and viruses. • *Hazardous activities* can cause injury or ill health. Examples of potentially hazardous activities include dangerous tasks, unnatural movements and postures, heavy lifting, repetitive work, interpersonal conflicts, bullying, and intimidation. • *Hazardous events* can cause injury or ill health. Examples of potentially hazardous events include explosions, implosions, collisions, vibrations, fires, leaks, releases, chemical reactions, electric shocks, falling objects, loud noises, structural breakdowns, software failures, equipment malfunctions, and unscheduled shutdowns.	Hazards can also be classified as follows: • Chemical hazards • Biological hazards • Thermal hazards • Electrical hazards • Structural hazards • Acoustical hazards • Mechanical hazards • Radiological hazards • Psychological hazards
Hazard identification *Hazard identification* is a process that involves recognizing that an OH&S hazard exists and then describing its characteristics.	
Injury or ill health An *injury or ill health* is an adverse effect on someone's physical, mental, or cognitive condition. Adverse effects include disease, illness, and death.	
Incident An *incident* is a work-related occurrence or event during which: • injury, ill health, or fatality actually occurs, or • injury, ill health, or fatality could have occurred. An *accident* is a type of incident. It is a work-related event during which injury, ill health, or fatality actually occurs. It is a type of incident. A *close call, near miss, or near hit* is also a type of incident. It is a	*Incidents* and *nonconformities* are not the same thing. *Incidents* can occur on their own or in association with one or more *nonconformities*.

work-related event during which injury, ill health, or fatality could have occurred, but didn't actually occur.	
Interested party An *interested party* (or stakeholder) is anyone who can affect, be affected by, or believe that they are affected by a decision or activity. An *interested party* is a person, group, or organization that has an interest or a stake in a decision or activity.	
Legal requirements and other requirements In the context of this standard, a *requirement* is an OHSMS need, expectation, or obligation. It can be stated or implied by an organization, its customers, or other interested parties. *Legal requirements* are compulsory. Organizations must comply with them. *Other requirements*, may be compulsory or voluntary: organizations may be forced to comply with them, or they may choose to comply with them.	Legal and other requirements may include those found in collective agreements and those that apply to workers' representatives.
Management system A *management system* is a set of interrelated or interacting elements that organizations use to implement their policies, to achieve their objectives, and to manage their processes. These elements include structures, programs, procedures, practices, plans, rules, roles, responsibilities, relationships, contracts, agreements, documents, records, methods, tools, techniques, technologies, and resources. There are many types of management systems. Some of these include OH&S management systems, environmental management systems, financial management systems, information security management systems, business continuity management systems, emergency management systems, disaster management systems, food safety management systems, risk management systems, and, of course, occupational health and safety management systems. The scope or focus of a management system could be restricted to a function or section of an organization or it could include the entire organization. It could even include a function that cuts across several organizations.	
Measurement *Measurement* is a process that is used to determine a value. In most cases this value will be a quantity.	
Monitoring To *monitor* means to determine the status of an activity, process, or system at different stages or at different times. In order to determine status, you need to supervise and to continually check and critically observe the activity, process, or system that is being monitored.	
Nonconformity *Nonconformity* is a nonfulfillment or failure to meet a requirement. In the	

ISO 45001 2018 OHS AUDIT TOOL

12. OCCUPATIONAL HEALTH AND SAFETY TERMS AND DEFINITIONS

context of this standard, *nonconformity* refers to a failure to meet ISO 45001 requirements or a failure to meet your organization's own requirements.

Objective

An *objective* is the result you intend to achieve. *Objectives* can be strategic, tactical, or operational and can apply to an organization as a whole or to a system, process, project, product, or service. Objectives may also be referred to as targets, aims, goals, or intended outcomes. OH&S objectives are generally based on or derived from an organization's OH&S policy and must be consistent with it.

Occupational health and safety management system (OHSMS)

An *OHSMS* is either a standalone management system or one part of a larger management system. It is a set of interrelated or interacting elements that organizations use to implement their OH&S policies, to achieve their OH&S objectives, and to manage their OH&S processes. These elements include structures, programs, procedures, practices, plans, rules, roles, regulations, responsibilities, relationships, contracts, agreements, documents, records, methods, tools, techniques, technologies, and resources.

You can develop an OHSMS for your organization simply by meeting all ISO 45001 requirements. An *OHSMS* is only one type of management system. Other management systems include the following: environmental management system, OH&S management system, food safety management system, emergency management system, information security management system, and continuity management system.

Occupational health and safety objectives

OH&S objectives are specific OH&S results that organizations set for themselves and wish to achieve. Your organization's OH&S objectives should be both measurable and consistent with its OH&S policy.

Occupational health and safety opportunity

An *OH&S opportunity* is a circumstance or a set of circumstances that could lead to the improvement of OH&S performance.

Occupational health and safety performance

OH&S performance is all about results and effectiveness. Whenever organizations prevent injury and ill health and provide safe and healthy workplaces, they are achieving good results and being effective.

Occupational health and safety policy

An *occupational health and safety (OH&S) policy* statement should express top management's commitment to the prevention of work-related injury and ill-health and to the provision of a safe and healthy workplace. It should also make a commitment to the implementation, maintenance, and improvement of the occupational health & safety management system (OHSMS). And it should allow workers to set OH&S objectives and it should encourage action.

Your OH&S policy should be developed and documented by your top management, and should be communicated to all persons who work for or on behalf of your organization.

Occupational health and safety risk

ISO 45001 2018 defines *OH&S risk* as the *"combination of the likelihood of occurrence of a work-related hazardous event(s) or exposure(s) and the severity of injury or ill health that can be caused by the event(s) or exposure(s)."* ISO 45001 accepts the more traditional definition of risk and rejects the newer ISO 31000 definition (discussed below) when it defines OH&S risk. The more

A *high-risk event* would have a high likelihood of occurring and have a severe impact if it actually occurred.

traditional definition of risk combines three elements: it starts with a potential event and then combines its probability with its potential severity.	
Organization An *organization* can be a single person or a group that achieves its objectives by using its own functions, responsibilities, authorities, and relationships. It can be a company, corporation, enterprise, firm, partnership, charity, or institution and can be either incorporated or unincorporated and be either privately or publicly owned. It can also be an operating unit that is part of a larger entity.	
Outsource When an organization makes an arrangement with an outside organization to perform part of a function or process, it is referred to as *outsourcing. To outsource* means to ask an external organization to perform part of a function or process normally done in-house. While an outsourced organization is beyond the scope of your OHSMS, the outsourced process or function itself falls within the scope of your OHSMS.	
Participation When people are involved in decision making, it's called participation. Workers, workers' representatives, and health and safety committees are often asked to participate in organizational decision making.	Participation is not the same as consultation. While *consultation* means receiving the views and opinions of others before decisions are made, *participation* means getting people involved in the actual decision-making process itself.
Performance According to ISO, the term *performance* refers to a measurable result. It refers to the measurable results that activities, processes, products, services, systems and organizations are able to achieve.	Measurements can be quantitative or qualitative.
Policy A policy is a general commitment, direction, or intention and is formally stated by top management.	
Procedure A *procedure* is a way of carrying out a process or an activity.	Procedures may or may not be documented.
Process A *process* is a set of activities that are interrelated or that interact with one another. They transform inputs into outputs. *Processes* are interconnected because the output from one process often becomes the input for another process.	Processes may or may not be documented.
Requirement A *requirement* is a need, expectation, or obligation. It can be stated or implied by an organization, its customers, or other interested parties. A *specified requirement* is one that has been stated (in a document for	Voluntary requirements become obligatory requirements once an organization decides to comply with them.

example), whereas an *implied requirement* is a need, expectation, or obligation that is common practice or customary.

Risk

According to ISO 45001, *"risk is the effect of uncertainty"*. This cryptic definition is based on a similar definition of risk found in the ISO 31000 risk management standard. According to ISO 31000, *risk* is the *"effect of uncertainty on objectives"* and an effect is a positive or negative deviation from what is expected. Both definitions are essentially the same. The following will explain what this odd definition means.

ISO 31000 recognizes that all of us operate in an uncertain world. Whenever we try to achieve an objective, there's always the chance that things will not go according to plan. Every step has an element of risk that needs to be managed and every outcome is uncertain. Whenever we try to achieve an objective, we don't always get the results we expect. Sometimes we get positive results and sometimes we get negative results and occasionally we get both.

The traditional definition of risk combines three elements: it starts with a potential event and then combines its probability with its potential severity. A high-risk event would have a high likelihood of occurring and a severe impact if it actually occurred.

While ISO 31000 defines risk in a new and unusual way, the old and the new definitions are largely compatible. Both definitions talk about the same phenomena but from two different perspectives. ISO thinks of risk in goal-oriented terms while the traditional definition thinks of risk in event-oriented terms.

These two definitions can and do co-exist. They're two different ways of talking about the same phenomena. ISO provides a conceptual definition of risk while the traditional formulation operationalizes this general definition: it explains how to quantify risk. It argues that the amount or level of risk can be calculated by combining probability and severity.

ISO 45001 actually rejects this ISO 31000 definition of risk when it defines *OH&S risk*. Instead of accepting the ISO 31000 definition, ISO 45001 defines *OH&S risk* as the *"combination of the likelihood of occurrence of a work-related hazardous event(s) or exposure(s) and the severity of injury or ill health that can be caused by the event(s) or exposure(s)."*

Risk assessment

Risk assessment is a process that is made up of three separate processes: risk identification, risk analysis, and risk evaluation. *Risk identification* is a process that is used to find, recognize, and describe risks. *Risk analysis* is a process that is used to understand the nature, sources, and causes of the risks that you have identified and to estimate the level of risk. It is also used to study impacts and consequences and to examine the controls that exist. *Risk evaluation* is a process that is used to compare risk analysis results with risk criteria (see below) in order to determine whether or not a specified level of risk is acceptable or tolerable.

Risk criteria

Risk criteria are terms of reference and are used to evaluate the significance or importance of your organization's risks. They are used to determine whether a specified level of risk is acceptable or tolerable. Risk criteria should reflect your organization's values, policies, and objectives, should be based on its external

ISO 45001 2018 OHS AUDIT TOOL

12. OCCUPATIONAL HEALTH AND SAFETY TERMS AND DEFINITIONS

and internal context, should consider the views of stakeholders, and should be derived from standards, laws, policies, and other requirements.	
Top management The term *top management* normally refers to the people at the top of an organization. It refers to the people who provide resources and delegate authority and who coordinate, direct, and control organizations. However, if the scope of a management system covers only part of an organization, then the term *top management* refers, instead, to the people who direct and control that part of the organization.	The term *management* refers to all the *activities* that are used to coordinate, direct, and control organizations. In this context, the term *management* does not refer to people. It refers to what managers do.
Worker The term *worker* is defined as anyone who performs work or work-related activities that are under an organization's control. Workers include both managers and nonmanagers and include both employees and non-employees (i.e., contractors, agency workers, and external product and service providers). They could be permanent or part-time, regular or temporary, and paid or unpaid; all of these people are defined as *workers*.	
Workplace A *workplace* is a place where an organization's work is performed. A place is an organization's workplace only if it is under its control, at least to some extent. How much responsibility an organization has over OH&S depends on how much control it has over its workplace.	

ISO 45001 2018 OHS AUDIT TOOL

12. OCCUPATIONAL HEALTH AND SAFETY TERMS AND DEFINITIONS

Title	ISO 45001 2018 OHS AUDIT TOOL
Authors	Praxiom Product Development Team
Publisher	Praxiom Research Group Limited
Acknowledgment	Praxiom Research Group Limited gratefully acknowledges its reliance upon the ISO 45001 2018 standard published by the *International Organization for Standardization*.
Copyright	Copyright © 2018 by Praxiom Research Group Limited. All rights reserved. No part of this work may be reproduced or transmitted in any form, by any means (electronic, photocopying, recording, or otherwise) without the permission of Praxiom Research Group Limited (see Site License below for exceptions). Also, you may not modify, edit, or alter this work without the permission of Praxiom Research Group Limited. You may, however, add additional notes and comments whenever our publication allows you to do so.
License	Our publications are licensed for use at one physical site only. Once you've chosen your site or location, you may make as many copies of our publication as you need in order to carry out your work at that site. But you may not use your copy of our publication at other sites. If you need to work at other sites, you must purchase a Global Corporate License (twice the price of a regular license). However, if you're a consultant, you're not restricted to a single site. If you're a consultant, you may use our publication as often as you need to in the service of your clients. You do not need to purchase a new copy for each consulting project. However, your clients must buy their own copy. If you're a trainer, teacher, or professor, you may make as many copies as you need in order to teach your students. However, if your students wish to use our publication for professional or occupational purposes, they must buy their own copy. We retain ownership of our publication. This license agreement does not transfer title or ownership to you. You may not resell or republish our publication without the express permission of Praxiom Research Group Limited.
Liability	We have used our best efforts in preparing this publication. Praxiom Research Group Limited makes no representation or warranties with respect to the accuracy or completeness of the contents of this publication and specifically disclaims any implied warranties or merchantability or fitness for any particular purpose and shall in no event be liable for any loss of profit or any other commercial damage, including but not limited to special, incidental, consequential, or other damages.
Contact	Praxiom Research Group Limited http://www.praxiom.com/ support@praxiom.com 780-461-4514 First Edmonton Place, 14th Floor, 10665 Jasper Avenue, Edmonton, Alberta, Canada

Appendix C

SAMPLE Audit Notification and Plan

Quality Plus	**Audit Notification and Plan**	*Audit Number:*	
		Page 1 of	

To:		Date of Audit:	
From:		Notification Date:	
Location of Audit:		Revision:	#
Audit #:			

AUDIT TEAM:

Lead Auditor:
Additional Auditors:

1.0 PURPOSE

2.0 SCOPE

3.0 AUDIT SCHEDULE

<Date>

09h00–09h15	
09h15–12h00	
12h00–13h00	
13h00–15h30	
15h30–16h00	
16h00–16h30	

NOTE:

(a) Specific topics and interviews will be scheduled based on the availability of key personnel with the aim of minimizing disruption to the work processes. If you are or become aware of any conflicts or resource issues, please notify the Lead Auditor.
(b) Interview schedule will be finalized/updated during the Opening Meeting.
(c) Closing Meeting, if deemed necessary will be scheduled in consultation with the auditee management.

4.0 INTERVIEW LIST—POTENTIAL INTERVIEWEES

The auditee management team members with responsibility for the areas identified in the scope of this audit are asked to develop an interview list to ensure that the appropriate personnel are interviewed during the audit. Please forward the list to the Lead Auditor as soon as practical. It is understood by the audit team that the list will be subject to change based on schedules and personnel availability. Where two or more people perform the same or complementary functions, joint interviews can work to create synergies and save time. Please identify any such combinations during the Opening Meeting.

5.0 AUDIT BASIS

The auditors will be using the following standards or guidelines to assist them in carrying out the audit:

Examples:

a) Contract for Services
b) Internal Management System Procedures
c) ISO 9001 Quality Management Systems—Requirements

6.0 EXIT INTERVIEW, CLOSING MEETING, AND ACTION TRACKING

An exit interview has been scheduled for the end of the last day of the audit. The actual timing of the exit interview will be mutually agreed. Your management team is invited to meet with the audit team at that time. This is intended to be an opportunity for your management to informally review the findings with the audit team, prior to the auditors preparing their report.

Once the final audit report is ready it will be issued to a representative of your management team. If requested, a Closing Meeting will be scheduled at that time.

Corrective actions may be identified as a result of the audit. Progress on implementing the actions must be reported to the Lead Auditor who will track the actions and follow-up once they have been closed to ensure effective implementation.

7.0 REPORTING/DISTRIBUTION

The audit report will be issued to the distribution list below:

1. <>
2. <>
3. <>

8.0 DOCUMENTATION REQUIREMENTS—PRE-AUDIT

Auditee is requested to email the following documents to **<The Lead Auditor>**

9.0 COMMENTS OR QUESTIONS

If you have any comments, questions, or suggestions with respect to the information contained herein or the planning, execution, reporting, and/or distribution of the audit, please feel free to contact **<The Lead Auditor>**

Appendix D

Sample HSEQ Audit Report Template

Quality Plus	**HSEQ Audit Report**	Audit Number:	
		Page 1 of (will depend on the content of your audit report)	

To:	<Designated contact – Supplier>	Date of Audit:	dd-mmm-yyyy
From:		Report Date:	dd-mmm-yyyy
Location of Audit:	Supplier Address	Revision:	Draft
Audit #:	AUD-YY-XXXX		

Quality Plus

CONTENTS

1. Purpose
2. Scope
3. Audit Team/Personnel Interviewed
4. Summary
5. Administration and Tracking of Corrective Action
6. Findings

1/ Purpose		
2/ Scope		
3 A) Audit Team		
<as appropriate> Technical Specialist	<as appropriate>, HSE Auditor	<as appropriate>, Lead Auditor
3 B) Personnel Interviewed		
ID Personnel interviewed		
4/ Summary of Audit		

Summary Comments <By Area of Interest or Overall comment>

Health and Safety Management: <as appropriate>

Environmental Management: <as appropriate>

Security Management (Physical and IT): <as appropriate>

Technical Management: <as appropriate>

Quality Management: <as appropriate>

Numerical Summary of Audit Results

X Nonconformances **(NCR's)** and **Y** Opportunities for Improvement **(OFI's)** were identified by the audit team.

Lead Auditor	All Auditors / Specialists have contributed to, reviewed and accepted this report		Date
<as appropriate>	<as appropriate>	<as appropriate>	dd-mmm-yyyy

5/ Administration and Tracking of Corrective Action

Corrective Action Plan:

Presentation of Action Plan:

Tracking of Corrective Action for Nonconformances (NCR's): ____

Opportunities for Improvement (OI's __)

6/ Results (see below):

Result #	Results with Suggested Action – if appropriate	Due Date	Planned Corrective Action / Steward
	Brief title of issue: Description		

Appendix E

Quality Plus Integrated HSEQ Management System Audit Course

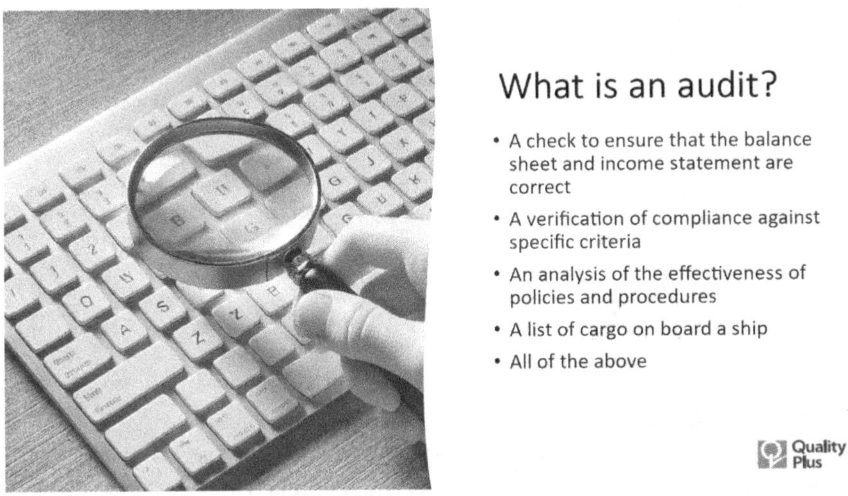

WHAT IS AN AUDIT?

Does a check to ensure that the balance sheet and income statement are correct qualify as an audit? Yes. Audits are performed to verify the accuracy and completeness of financial records.

What about an evaluation of compliance against specific criteria? Of course. Compliance is a core part of any type of audit.

Analysis of the effectiveness of policies and procedures? Right again. Once compliance has been established, the next step in a systems audit is often to evaluate effectiveness.

But a list of cargo on board a ship? Absolutely. Checking the ship's cargo can indeed be considered an early form of audit.

Audits have been around for a very long time. In early maritime history, verifying the type, quantity and condition of cargo, and matching it to the manifests, was a critical task. The audit ensured that the right goods were shipped and received at the other end of the voyage, that the ship and its crew were safe and that taxes were correctly calculated and paid. They reduced the risk of loss, theft, and errors that could lead to serious financial or legal implications for the owners of the vessel and the cargo.

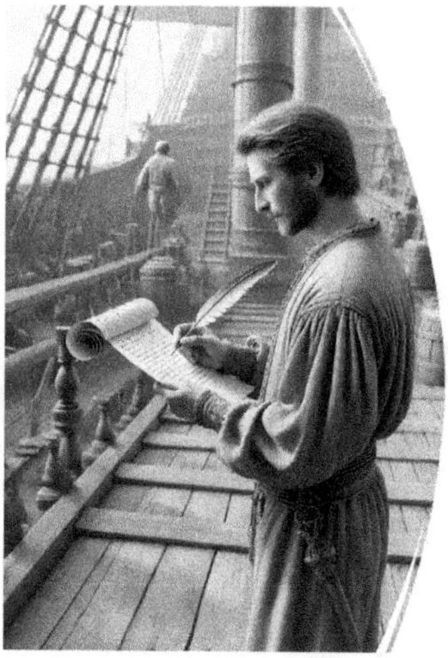

It can accurately be said that checking "a list of cargo on board a ship" constitutes a simple form of audit. Although these early cargo checks were not exactly audits in the contemporary sense, they were based on the concept of verifying against established criteria, a concept that is still central to modern auditing principles.

Quality Plus

Early examples of ship's audits trace back to ancient times. Around 2500 BCE, Egypt had organized maritime activity and carried out audits for commercial and taxation purposes. Later, the Phoenicians used a system of cargo checks to support their extensive maritime trade activities. Ancient Romans utilized systematic audits to enforce maritime laws and trade regulations. And in China, officials and merchants kept detailed records of trade goods along the Silk Road and maritime routes.

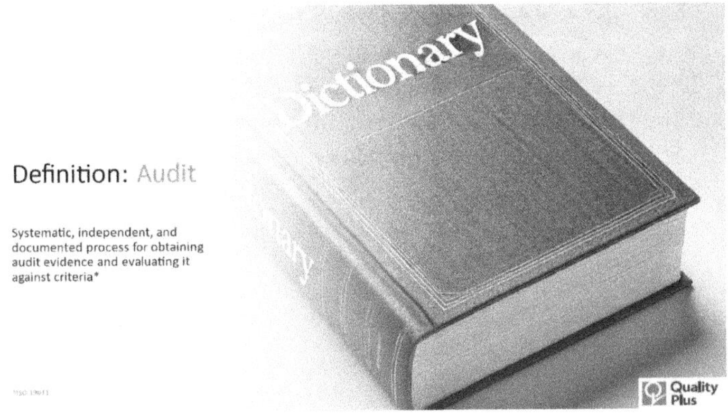

The International Organization for Standardization (ISO) defines an audit as a "systematic, independent, and documented process for obtaining audit evidence and evaluating it objectively to determine the extent to which the audit criteria are fulfilled."

Audits have evolved in complexity, application, and depth over the centuries, but the principles of auditing remain systematic, independent, documented, and objectively evaluated.

Audit criteria are requirements or benchmarks against which the audit is conducted and the audited information or activity is compared. This may include laws, regulations, standards, policies, procedures, contractual obligations, or other requirements.

The audit criteria are the reference points when determining compliance.

MANAGEMENT SYSTEM AUDITS

ISO 19011, the international standard for auditing management systems, establishes the framework for conducting management system audits. It applies to various types of management systems, including those for quality, environmental, and health and safety.

The management system audit framework has four main aspects:

- Principles of Auditing
- Managing the Audit Program
- Conducting the Audit
- Competence and Evaluation of Auditors

Regardless of the area and criteria to which the audit program is applied, these four aspects apply.

A management system audit is carried out for various purposes. While the determination of compliance is the primary objective, an audit serves several purposes. It is

- a management tool;
- a snapshot of how processes are being managed and procedures carried out, or how they have been in the past;
- a means to gather and use current and historic information in order to make projections of how effective the processes and procedures will be in the future;
- a tool for identifying risks and opportunities;
- a way to make informed decisions about the health of processes and the effectiveness of controls; and
- an opportunity for internal communication.

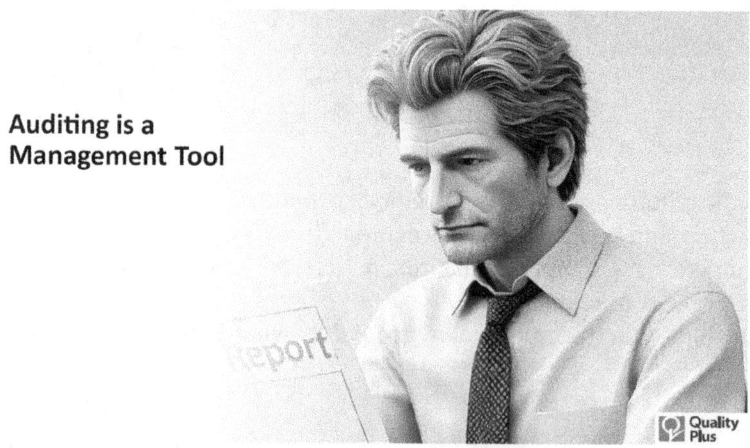

Auditing serves a lot of purposes. In the management system world, it is first and foremost, a management tool. It is not meant to be a means by which to assign blame but rather a way to evaluate the state of the management system and by extension, the business itself.

It is, therefore, part of the auditor's job to report to management, in terms management understands, the following:

- Are applicable requirements being met?
- Are there controls in place? Do they work? Is there room for improvement?
- Are there changes being implemented and will they impact the management system?
- What risks are present and are they being controlled?
- Are there issues which should be considered?
- Was there a constraint that restricted the depth or effectiveness of the audit?
- Is there anything that should be followed up and investigated?

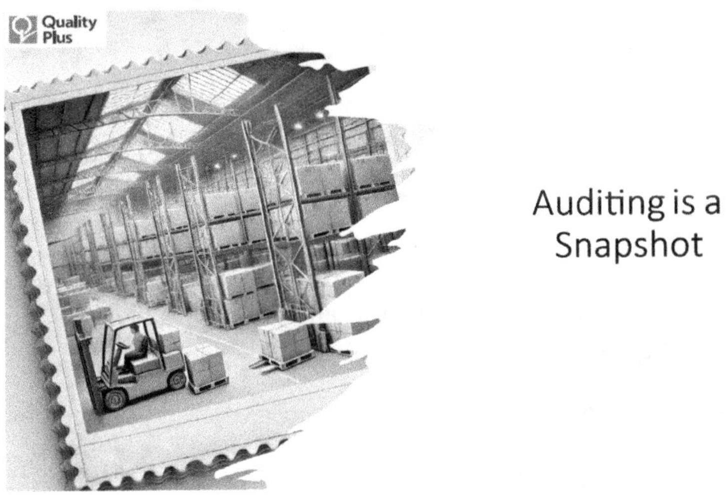

An audit examines processes, practices, records, and environments at a given point, within a specific sample size and area. It captures a moment in time, much like a photograph.

It is important to remember that like a photograph, it may not capture the entire picture. It is static and does not reflect the changes that occur after the audit is completed. Because something is absent during an audit doesn't mean it doesn't exist. Likewise, because something happens during an audit doesn't mean that it happens all the time. It is important, therefore, that auditors collect enough objective evidence, over a wide-enough sample size, to make the snapshot as representational as possible of the conditions that existed at the time it was taken.

Managers must consider this when interpreting the audit results. While the audit provides factual information, insights, and independent observations, analysis and investigation are often required to establish the true significance of the audit findings.

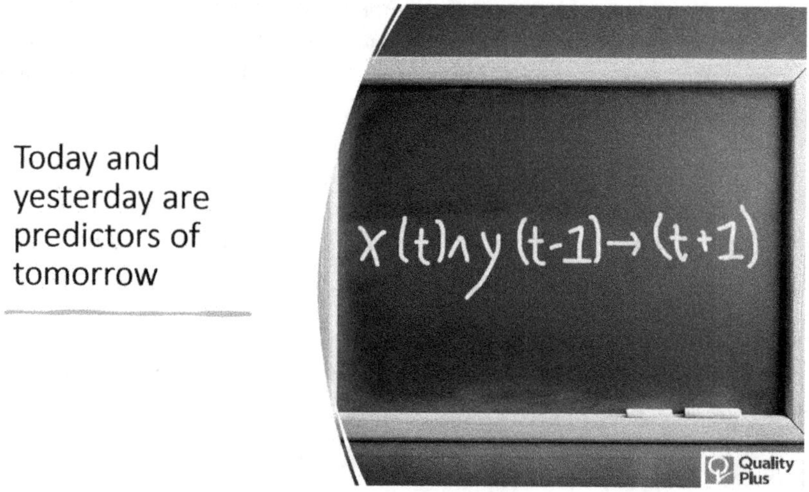

An audit involves the collection of data from two sources:

- Current—real-time data or information from recent operations. Auditors examine ongoing processes, practices, performance metrics, and compliance.
- Historical—past performance. Auditors review records of past operations, performance, compliance issues, and other historical data.

Once gathered, that data is analyzed to assess the current state of the management system and to make predictions about how things are likely to evolve in the future.

This involves:

- **Compliance and Performance Evaluation:** Comparing current and past records and practices against the audit criteria to determine compliance and effectiveness of the management system. Audit findings based on current and past performance include noncompliances/nonconformances, incidents, and observations.
- **Trend Analysis:** Examining current and historical data to identify patterns and trends upon which to make predictions about future performance and

potential issues. Audit findings which address potential future issues or opportunities are corrective actions, preventive actions, risks, and opportunities for continual improvement.

The predictive aspect of auditing is an important part of risk management and continuous improvement. By evaluating historical trends and current practices, potential risks to future performance can be identified. Audit recommendations can, therefore, include action to address current issues or action to address those that are likely to happen.

As a management tool, the audit process helps managers

- determine the extent of issues and the costs associated with correcting or accepting them;
- make informed decisions, based on factual information;
- establish priorities and assign resources where they are most beneficial to the organization;
- implement corrective action to eliminate or mitigate risks;
- ensure continuing compliance and acceptability of outputs; and
- improve processes and future performance.

So, as a snapshot, the audit captures an objective picture of the organization's current state, and collects data which can be used to predict and influence the future. Just like the immediate nature of an inspection allows the organization to correct real-time issues, the additional predictive aspect of an audit contributes to continual improvement and strategic planning.

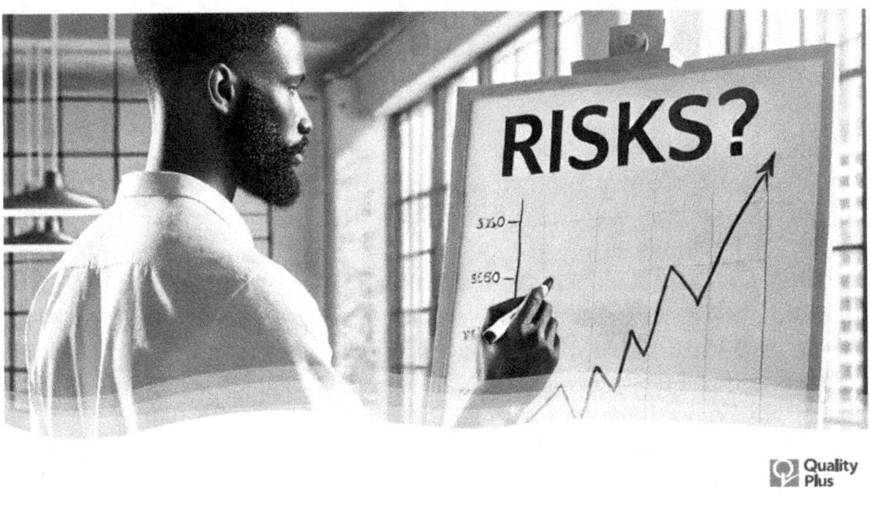

Auditing is a tool to identify risks and opportunities.

Management system audits involve comprehensive, systematic examination of systems, processes, procedures, and practices. This approach helps identify existing or potential noncompliances, inefficiencies and discrepancies between intended and actual performance which represent areas of risk.

On the other hand, not all audit findings are negative. Audits also identify opportunities for improvement or pockets of excellence. Audits can highlight positive practices that can be shared or applied in other areas of the organization. In this respect, audits trigger positive recognition and foster a culture of continuous improvement.

Because auditors are independent of the process being audited, they bring an objective point of view and a fresh eye which can enable them to spot risks or opportunities which might be overlooked.

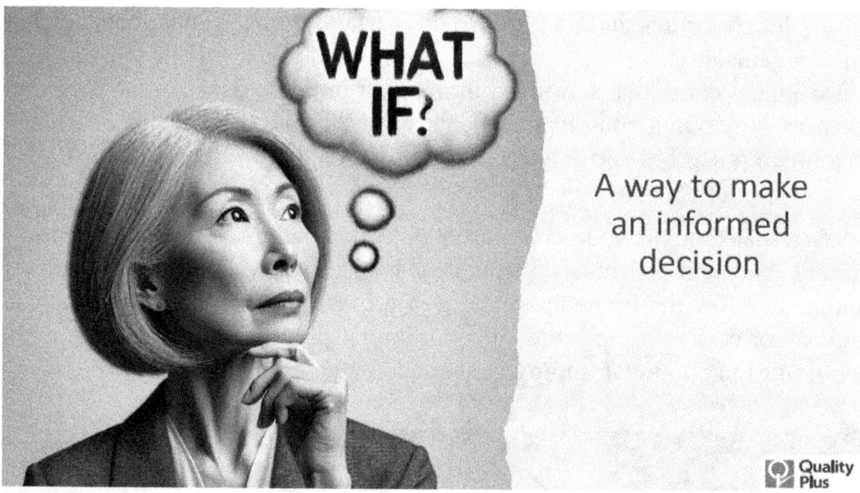

Audits employ an evidence-based approach to the collection of information. While audits can also provide valuable insight into the perceptions and opinions of auditees, they are, by definition, focused on collecting verifiable facts.

Auditors collect evidence about the compliance and effectiveness of the organization's processes and deliverables; performance against objectives and key performance indicators; nonconformances; risks and vulnerabilities; strengths and positive practices; stakeholder needs and satisfaction; and other factors which contribute to the organization's health and growth.

Analysis and trending of the collected data enhances the ability to make sound strategic decisions and plans, including those relating to

- business and goals and targets;
- company vision and strategic directions;
- resource allocation;
- alignment and efficiency of operations;
- prioritization of corrective action and continual improvements; and
- programs and initiatives.

Audits provide insights to remove or minimize subjectivity in decision-making.

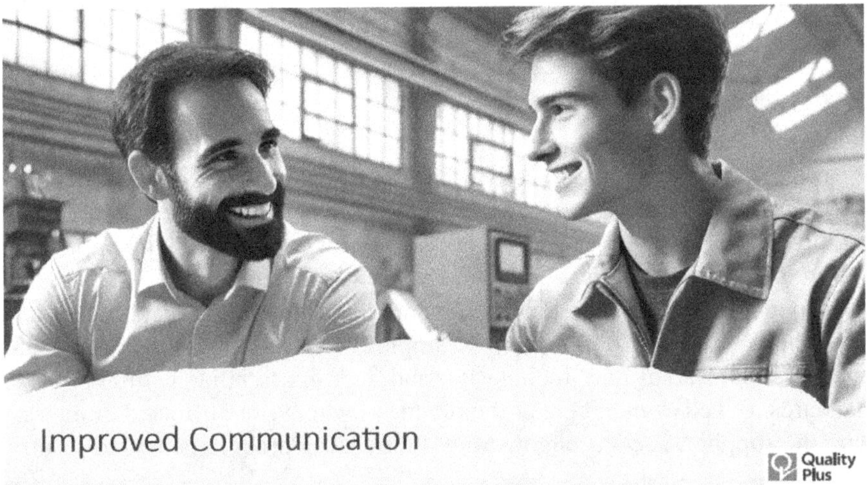

Audits are an opportunity for people to talk and share experiences and practices. In collecting data, auditors gain understanding of the whys and hows of the processes being examined. They also bring their own expertise and knowledge to the table.

An internal audit provides the opportunity for coworkers to share insights into how procedures and outcomes affect other processes and individuals. This promotes greater understanding between functions and often helps isolate issues, encourage cooperative problem-solving and migrate best practices.

Audits by external auditors can be learning experiences. While external auditors cannot breach another auditee's confidentiality, they can offer general information relating to industry practices and suggestions for improvement. In this way, audits become a way to benchmark against other similar organizations.

TYPES OF AUDITS

There are many types of audits, each with their own focus and approach. Management system audits can be separated into three distinct groupings:

1. First-Party Audits

Internal audits fall into this group. First-party audits are conducted by an organization on its own management system to verify compliance and evaluate the effectiveness of its processes and controls. They are conducted by internal auditors, who are independent of the process being audited.

First-party audits are the backbone of the audit process. Internal auditors have the time and knowledge of the organization to enable them to delve deep into processes and procedures. Performed correctly, internal audits can provide the greatest benefit in the audit program.

2. Second-Party Audits

Second-party audits are exactly what the name implies: audits conducted by one party on a second party. An example is an audit carried out by an organization on its suppliers or contractors to confirm compliance with applicable requirements of standards, contracts, or purchase agreements.

Second-party audits often involve members of the internal audit team and any other relevant discipline. For example, when auditing a potential supplier, the audit team may include internal auditors familiar with applicable standards as well as members of the functions who will be affected or interact with the supplier, such as engineering, fabrication, procurement, and so on.

3. Third-Party Audits

Third-party audits are conducted by independent external organizations to verify that the management system meets specific standards, regulations, or other legal requirements. Audits carried out by registrars who grant ISO certification are examples of third-party audits.

Third-party audits are carried out by accredited certification bodies. Third-party auditors must themselves be certified to perform the audits.

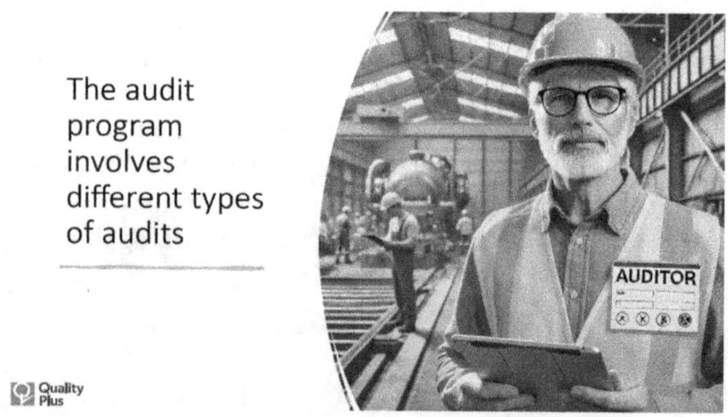
The audit program involves different types of audits
AUDITOR
Quality Plus

The audit program may include a mixture of audit types, within one or more of these groupings. For example:

1. Compliance Audits
   Purpose: Verify compliance with standards, regulations, laws, or other legal requirements.

2. System Audits
   Purpose: Evaluate the compliance and effectiveness of the entire management system in meeting performance expectations.

3. Performance Audits
   Purpose: Evaluate the operational performance of specific processes and acceptability of the outputs of the processes.

4. Process Audits
   Purpose: Examine specific processes within the management system to verify that they are effectively implemented and functioning efficiently. Process audits examine the process from start to finish and typically touch various requirements of the audit criteria.

5. Product Audits
   Purpose: Assess the quality of products to verify that they meet specifications and standards.

6. Element Audits
   Purpose: Examine the control of a discreet element of the management system and its application in various departments or areas. For example: while the procurement program is an element of the management system with its own controls and practices, purchasing activities can also occur within other processes, projects, or functions. Therefore, an element audit of procurement would examine both the core procurement system and controls, as well as purchasing activities conducted outside the department.

7. Contract Audits
   Purpose: Review a contract or job from start to final deliverable to confirm that all requirements have been met, determine the level of efficiency, identify lessons learned, or verify that the job is ready for closure.

8. Desk Audits
   Purpose: Review documentation and records without or prior to on-site verifications. Desk audits help identify whether documentation is adequate, procedures reflect the requirements of the applicable criteria, and are often used to establish readiness for an on-site assessment.

9. Gap Assessment / Gap Analysis
   Purpose: Compare current practices and performance against the audit criteria to identify gaps or shortcomings. Unlike standard audits which identify nonconformances and leave it to the process owner to plan the action to correct, gap assessments may also quantify the percentage of compliance or specify what is needed to close the gaps.

10. Integrated Audits
    Purpose: Examine the requirements of multiple systems or criteria (e.g., quality, health and safety, environmental) in one audit. Since management systems have many common clauses, integrated audits are efficient and effective for evaluating process interactions and isolating where requirements are addressed.

11. Joint Audits
    Purpose: Two or more auditing groups cooperate jointly to complete an audit of an organization or system which affects them both. For example, a client and its prime contractor carry out an audit of a subcontractor together. While they can be more stressful, integrated audits save time and resources.

12. Cold Eyes Review
    Purpose: Evaluate and identify issues, risks, or inefficiencies within a process or project. While a cold eyes review is not a typical audit, it is an excellent way to gain constructive feedback and recommendations based on unbiased analysis of the area being examined.

Each type of audit serves its own purpose. All of them help the organization comply and improve. The audit program will often, therefore, include several different types of audit, depending upon the specific needs and the available audit capabilities.

PROCESS APPROACH

ISO 9000 defines a process as a "set of interrelated or interacting activities that use inputs to deliver an intended result."

These days, the major management system standards have adopted a process approach. This approach recognizes that the management system and indeed, the organization itself, is comprised of a series of processes. Each process transforms inputs to outputs, and the output of one process becomes the input for the next.

For example, the process for "product delivery" may start with a request for a quote from the customer and end with delivery of the final product and documentation. All the activities in between are both individual processes in and of themselves, as well as steps in the overall process for "product delivery."

Process Interaction Flow

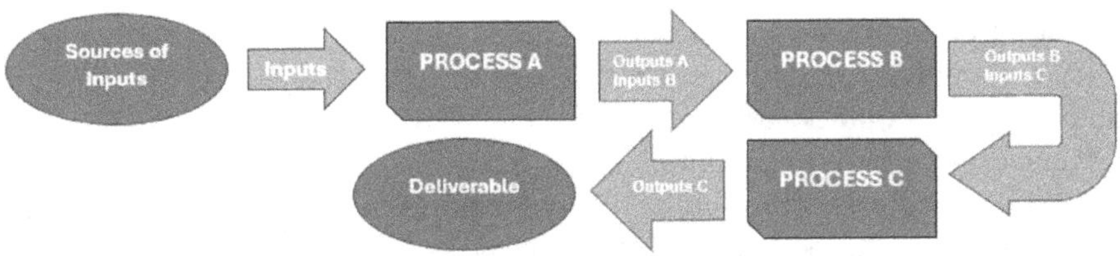

It makes sense, therefore, to take a similar approach to auditing. The process approach to auditing focuses on reviewing processes, their sequence and interaction, and their inputs and outputs.

A process audit traces the logical flow to determine whether the overall process is effectively meeting requirements, achieving objectives, and functioning smoothly. This enables the management system to be evaluated as an active system, identifying compliance, effectiveness in achieving objectives, inefficiencies, risks, and positive practices.

Process audits need to be planned considering the various business processes and performed across departmental boundaries. They provide insight into the flow of work and valuable information, including

- how processes work together to achieve goals;
- effectiveness of the management system and individual processes;
- handoffs and linkages between processes and departments;

- quality and timing of inputs and outputs;
- opportunities for internal improvement;
- risks within or between processes;
- inefficiencies and bottlenecks;
- extent to which objectives and key performance indicators are being met and how they affect other areas; and
- if operations are under control and resources are adequate.

Using the process approach allows findings to be evaluated more holistically. It provides continuity and context. It helps define the true depth of problems and solutions across the organization and focus action on areas of greatest organizational benefit.

This contributes to the achievement of organizational objectives, better efficiency, consistent compliance, and continual improvement.

AUDIT PROGRAM AND SCHEDULE

The audit program and the audit schedule are two parts of the auditing process. Although the terms are sometimes used interchangeably, they serve slightly different purposes.

An audit program is a comprehensive plan which includes the overall strategy, procedures, resources, and schedule for the organization's audits. It identifies what needs to be audited, types of audits, objectives, scope, auditors, and other factors. The audit schedule is a component of the audit program. It is the timetable outlining when various audits will occur.

The program focuses on "what" and "how," while the schedule addresses "when." The program defines the overall audit strategy and establishes the audit direction and approach. The schedule organizes the timing and sequence of the audit activities.

Audit Program

The management system audit program can include several types of audits, addressing one or more management system standards, conducted either separately or in combination. The extent of the audit program should be based on the size and nature of the organization, as well as the complexity, type, and history of the activity or process being audited.

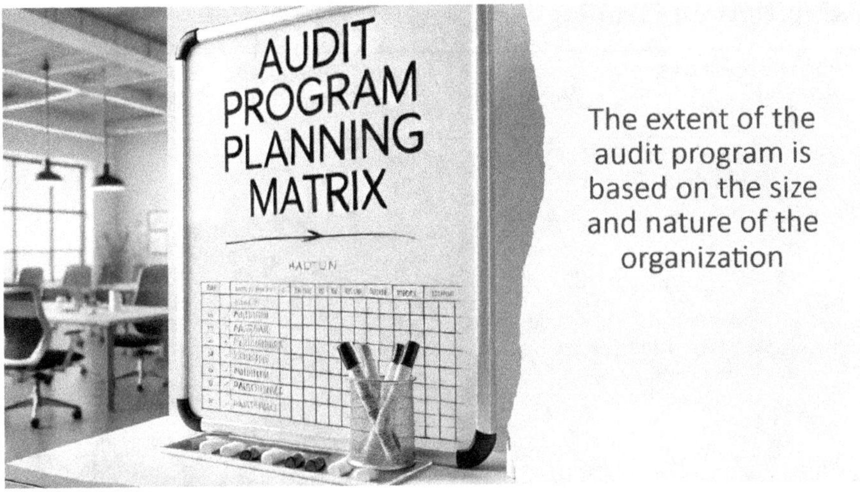

If the approach is to audit processes, projects or procedures, then care should be taken to ensure that those requirements of the applied standard which are not relevant to the processes, are covered elsewhere. For example, management systems based on the ISO Annex SL model will all have a section for leadership. The requirements of this section are specific to upper management and will not usually be reflected in product or service delivery processes. Therefore, a separate audit of leadership should be scheduled.

A common tool for establishing the audit program is an audit matrix which includes clauses of the audit criteria compared against processes to be audited. Using this matrix when planning audits helps ensure that nothing is missed.

Example: Audit Planning Matrix

Example: Audit Planning Matrix		*Leadership / Management*	*Sales and Marketing*	*Production Operations*	*Project 1: Design & Fab*	*HR Dept / Training*
4	**Context of the Organization**					
4.1	Understanding the Organization and its Context	Audit 1				
4.2	Understanding the Needs and Expectations of Interested Parties	Audit 1				
4.3	Determining the Scope of the QMS	Audit 1				
4.4	Quality Management System and Its Processes	Audit 1				
5	**Leadership**					
5.1.1	General	Audit 1				
5.1.2	Customer Focus	Audit 1				
5.2	Quality Policy	Audit 1				
5.2.1	Establishing the Quality Policy	Audit 1				
5.2.2	Communicating the Quality Policy	Audit 1				
5.3	Organizational Roles, Responsibilities, and Authorities	Audit 1				Audit 5
6	**Planning**					
6.1	Actions to Address Risks and Opportunities	Audit 1 (org)	Audit 2 (dept)	Audit 3 (dept)	Audit 4 (project)	Audit 5 (dept)
6.2	Quality Objectives and Planning to Achieve Them	Audit 1	Audit 2 (dept KPIs)	Audit 3 (dept KPIs)		Audit 5 (dept KPIs)
6.3	Planning of Changes	Audit 1				

Example: Audit Planning Matrix		*Leadership / Management*	*Sales and Marketing*	*Production Operations*	*Project 1: Design & Fab*	*HR Dept / Training*
7	**Support**					
7.1	Resources					Audit 5
7.1.1	General					Audit 5
7.1.2	People					Audit 5
7.1.3	Infrastructure					
7.1.4	Environment for the Operation of Processes					
7.1.5	Monitoring and Measuring Resources					
7.1.5.1	General					
7.1.5.2	Measurement Traceability					
7.1.6	Organizational Knowledge					Audit 5
7.2	Competence					Audit 5
7.3	Awareness					Audit 5
7.4	Communication					Audit 5
7.5	Documented Information					Audit 5
7.5.1	General					
7.5.2	Creating and Updating					
7.5.3	Control of Documented Information					
8	**Operation**					
8.1	Operational Planning and Control		Audit 2	Audit 3		
8.2	Requirements for Products and Services		Audit 2	Audit 3		
8.2.1	Customer Communication		Audit 2			
8.2.2	Determining the Requirements for Products and Services		Audit 2			
8.2.3	Review of the Requirements for Products and Services		Audit 2			

(*Continued*)

Example: Audit Planning Matrix		*Leadership / Management*	*Sales and Marketing*	*Production Operations*	*Project 1: Design & Fab*	*HR Dept / Training*
8.2.4	Changes to Requirements for Products and Services		Audit 2			
8.3	Design and Development of Products and Services				Audit 4	
8.3.1	General				Audit 4	
8.3.2	Design and Development Planning				Audit 4	
8.3.3	Design and Development Inputs				Audit 4	
8.3.4	Design and Development Controls				Audit 4	
8.3.5	Design and Development Outputs				Audit 4	
8.3.6	Design and Development Changes				Audit 4	
8.4	Control of Externally Provided Processes, Products, and Services					
8.4.1	General					
8.4.2	Type and Extent of Control					
8.4.2	Information for External Providers				Audit 4	
8.5	Production and Service Provision				Audit 4	
8.5.1	Control of Production and Service Provision			Audit 3	Audit 4	
8.5.2	Identification and Traceability			Audit 3	Audit 4	

Example: Audit Planning Matrix		*Leadership / Management*	*Sales and Marketing*	*Production Operations*	*Project 1: Design & Fab*	*HR Dept / Training*
8.5.3	Property Belonging to Customers or External Providers			Audit 3	Audit 4	
8.5.4	Preservation			Audit 3	Audit 4	
8.5.5	Post-delivery Activities			Audit 3	Audit 4	
8.5.6	Control of Changes			Audit 3	Audit 4	
8.6	Release of Products and Services			Audit 3	Audit 4	
8.7	Control of Nonconforming Outputs			Audit 3	Audit 4	
9	**Performance Evaluation**					
9.1	Monitoring, Measurement, Analysis, and Evaluation					
9.1.1	General					
9.1.2	Customer Satisfaction					
9.1.3	Analysis and Evaluation					
9.2	Internal Audit					
9.3	Management Review	Audit 1				
9.3.1	General	Audit 1				
9.3.2	Management Review Inputs	Audit 1				
9.3.3	Management Review Outputs	Audit 1				
10	**Improvement**					
10.1	General					
10.2	Nonconformity and Corrective Action					
10.3	Continual Improvement					

When developing the audit program, it is important to remember that in order to be considered compliant with most management system standards, all applicable requirements of the standard must be evaluated at least annually, and more often if needed. And while this is not necessarily explicitly stated, it is considered to be an implied requirement.

Audit Schedule

The audit schedule should reflect the strategic and audit objectives; risks; size and nature of the organization; complexity of processes; maturity of the management system; results of previous audits; and other relevant factors.

Audits should be planned and timed recognizing influencing conditions such as holidays, busy periods, shifts, and so on. For example, in extremely busy periods, an audit may be viewed as disruptive or unimportant and it may be more beneficial to schedule it for another time. Conversely, once in a while it can be helpful to schedule an audit when things are busy, since it is then that it will be evident if processes are still followed or if corners get cut. Balance is the key.

Remember that the audit schedule is fluid. If something occurs that will negatively influence the validity of the audit—reschedule.

Finally, ensure that all processes are audited at least annually, and more often if warranted.

AUDITING PRINCIPLES

ISO 19011, Guidelines for Auditing Management Systems, published by the ISO, identifies certain audit principles to help make audits effective, reliable, and consistent. Adherence to these principles ensures that the audit process is uncompromised and produces dependable and reproducible results. These seven principles are:

- Integrity
  Auditors must be worthy of trust. This means
  - performing their duties ethically with honesty and integrity;
  - only undertaking audit activities for which they are competent;
  - being independent of the area of audit and remaining unbiased and impartial; and
  - being sensitive to anything which could influence their judgment or compromise the audit.

- Fair Presentation
  Auditors have an obligation to report truthfully and accurately. Audit findings, conclusions, and reports must reflect the audit activities and evidence examined. Significant obstacles encountered during the audit or diverging opinions between the auditor and the auditee that remain unresolved must be reported. Communications must be truthful, objective, timely, clear, and complete.

- Due Professional Care
  Auditors must apply diligence and judgment in auditing which reflects the importance of the task they perform, and the confidence given to them by auditees and interested parties. To demonstrate due professional care, auditors must be competent and have the ability to make reasoned judgments based on the evidence provided.

- Confidentiality
  Auditors must exercise discretion in using information gained during the course of an audit. Information must not be disclosed without permission, used for personal gain by the auditor or the audit client, or handled in a manner that would negatively affect the rightful interests of the auditee. Auditees must be confident that confidential or sensitive information will be protected.

- Independence
  Auditor independence is the basis for impartiality and objectivity. Auditors should be independent of the activity being audited and free from bias or conflict of interest. It is imperative that auditors maintain objectivity throughout the audit process to ensure that findings and conclusions are based only on the objective evidence and not influenced by emotion, opinion, or other personal factors.

  For smaller organizations with limited resources, it may not be possible for auditors to be completely independent of the function being audited. Efforts should be made to maintain objectivity. For example, auditors may audit their own departments or functions, but refrain from auditing their own work or areas of responsibility. If auditors have firm opinions, conflicting interests, or interpersonal issues which could affect their judgment, they should not audit the associated area.

- Evidence-Based Approach
  Auditors reach their conclusions in consideration of verifiable, reproducible audit evidence. Findings are based on samples of information available

during the audit. Since audits are conducted in a finite period of time with finite resources, it is imperative that the use of sampling be appropriate.

Because something is not immediately available or evident at the time of audit, it does not mean it doesn't exist. Choosing the correct samples is as important as choosing enough. Auditors must be willing to delve deep and ask the questions needed to gain a true representation of the evidence.

- Risk-Based Approach
  Auditors employ an audit approach that considers risks and opportunities. This risk-based approach influences the planning, execution, and reporting of audits, focusing on areas of greatest significance and generating findings that can help prioritize actions reflecting the highest organizational risk or reward.

AUDITORS

An audit is only as good as the data collected and the auditor conducting it. A good internal auditor is

- an auditor primarily;
- a consultant;
- innovative; and
- a team player.

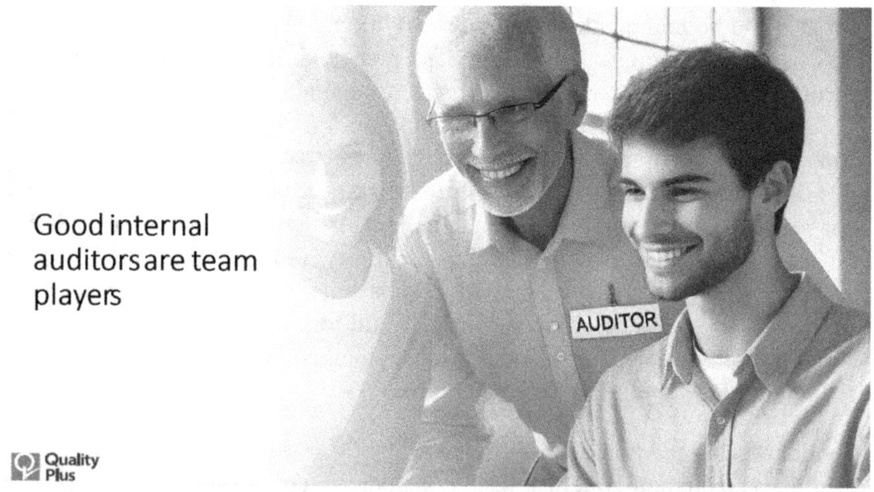

The primary job of an auditor is to do just that: audit. While auditors play several roles, first and foremost, they must be able to objectively collect the evidence and make informed, fair decisions. However, in some respects, auditors also function as consultants. Third-party auditors are restricted from advising auditees on how to fix issues or carry out activities, but they can offer insights and general observations which can be considered. Internal auditors have much more flexibility and can add great value. Once they have fulfilled their primary role—auditor—they can switch hats as part of the organizational team and participate in defining and implementing the necessary action.

Good auditors are innovative. Part of the auditor's role is to identify opportunities for greater efficiency, effectiveness, or other improvement. The ability to trace information and issues, and to problem solve, is a core skill of a good auditor.

Finally, a good auditor is a team player. Auditors who act as "police officers" are largely a thing of the past. Internal auditors are part of the same organization as the auditees, and it is in everyone's best interest to fix issues and make improvements together. Good external auditors are also team players. Their role is to help ensure compliance and drive improvement by highlighting risks and systemic issues. Together, auditors and auditees cooperate for the benefit of the organization.

WHO CAN BE AN AUDITOR

Anyone who has the necessary qualifications, opportunity to gain experience, and personal attributes can be an auditor.

At a minimum, management system auditors need to be trained as internal or lead auditors.

Often, auditors have degrees or certificates in relevant fields, auditor certifications, or other equivalent education. However, competency comes from a combination of education, training, and experience. Many excellent auditors come from an extensive work background where they have been trained on the job. The type and extent of formal education and certification is dependent upon the type of audit being conducted.

Industry and auditing experience is crucial. Familiarity with the industry relevant to the audit enables auditors to understand the processes, evaluate the risks and formulate conclusions. Practical audit experience is also important, and it is by auditing that auditors build this experience. For this reason, new auditors work with seasoned ones and carry out less complex audits until they gain experience and confidence.

Auditors need certain skill sets and abilities:

Communication Skills: Good verbal and written communication skills are essential. Auditors must be able to communicate effectively during the audit, asking direct questions, listening attentively, and initiating meaningful discussion. Often, the criteria to which the audit is being conducted is written in "standardeze." Where clarity is needed, the auditor must be able to explain the requirements in language that the auditee can understand.

Auditors must also be able to read and interpret records and documents and prepare audit reports and findings which are clear, unambiguous, and actionable.

Analytical and Problem-Solving Skills: Auditors must be able to analyze and evaluate data, detect anomalies and risks, and identify trends. They need to look beyond the immediate situation to the likely impacts on other areas or processes. Auditors identify problems, their potential impacts, and recommend practical solutions.

Inquisitive Nature and Attention to Detail: Not everyone is cut out to be an effective auditor. The best auditors are curious and genuinely interested in how things work. They are able to delve deep into processes and evaluate them in terms of compliance and effectiveness. Thoroughness is required to ensure that critical details are not missed.

Objectivity and Ethics: Integrity and adherence to ethical standards are primary if audits are to truly be impartial and fair. Auditors cannot be in a conflict of interest. They must also have the ability to separate how they expect or want to see things done from what is compliant and suitable for the organization.

Knowledge of Standards: Auditees are the experts in their processes. Auditors must be knowledgeable in the standards, regulations, or other criteria against which the audit is being conducted. They must remain up-to-date with changes in the criteria and best practices in the relevant industry or discipline. Ongoing professional development is a key factor.

AUDITING ROLES AND RESPONSIBILITIES

Depending upon the size of the organization, audits can be planned and carried out by one auditor or an entire team. Audit teams can include the team lead, auditors, technical experts, observers, or trainees. The responsibilities of the audit team members include:

Team Lead (Lead Auditor)

- Responsible for the audit overall.
- Determine the areas and processes to be audited (scope of the audit).
- Prepare or oversee preparation of the audit plan and checklists.
- Prepare audit notification.

- Chair opening and closing meetings.
- Represent the audit team.
- Authority for final decisions.
- Prepare and submit audit report.
- Raise findings.

Auditors

- Participate as required in the preparation of audit checklists.
- Plan and carry out assigned audit duties.
- Gather information.
- Document objective evidence and audit findings.
- Communicate effectively and clarify requirements.
- Report audit results.
- Verify effectiveness of corrective action from previous audits.
- Provide support to the team leader.

Technical Experts

- Provide specialized knowledge beyond the general auditing capabilities.
- Evaluate complex systems that require specialized expertise.
- Determine compliance to technical specifications or discipline-specific regulations or codes.
- Identify risks to technical operations that might not be generally apparent.
- Translate technical jargon.
- Contribute detailed findings, observations, and recommendations related to technical areas.

While the management system auditor can determine that there is a process, that it is consistently applied, and that it is compliant to the management system standard, the technical expert can judge whether the process is robust and correctly applied, and if results are reliable and accurate. In other words, the management system auditor determines if a compliant process is in place and the technical expert determines if it works.

Observers

Observers can be part of the audit team for various reasons. Observers do not interfere with the audit process or influence results. Their role is to observe, not to participate in the audit or contribute to decisions. Observers are bound by the same level of confidentiality as the auditors. Observers are included in audit teams for various reasons, such as:

- Assess the performance of auditors or to "recertify" them.
- Ensure that the audit process complies with established audit standards.
- Assure that the audit is thorough and unbiased.
- Represent the client or other interested party.
- Ensure transparency in sensitive audits.
- Provide feedback on the effectiveness of the audit.

Trainees

Audits can be excellent training opportunities. New auditors can participate in the audit, under the supervision of an experienced auditor, in order to develop their skills in a controlled situation. Potential auditors can learn how an audit actually works in preparation for their formal audit training. Process owners and personnel can be included in an audit in order to learn more about their processes or develop knowledge of others.

Regardless of the type of audit being conducted, auditors must all

- stay within the audit scope;
- remain objective;
- avoid giving opinions;
- observe, interview, and examine;
- manage time effectively;
- collect and analyze audit evidence;
- be alert for information that indicates the need for further investigation;
- verify if procedures and practices are available, implemented, and understood;
- verify that records are kept and are complete; and
- be ethical and protect the privacy of information.

Auditees also have certain obligations beyond mere involvement in the audit processes. Management must authorize and visibly place importance upon the audit, and ensure that action is taken upon audit findings in a timely fashion. All personnel must recognize and support the independence and integrity of the auditors and respect the audit process.

PHASES OF AN AUDIT

Effective audits have common characteristics:

- Audits must be planned.
- They must be performed by independent, qualified persons.
- Factual information must be gathered.
- Information must be analyzed and reported.

- Appropriate action must be determined and taken if required.
- Action must be followed up to verify it has been effective.

Audits can be broken down into five phases: Initiation, Preparation, Performance, Reporting, and Follow-Up. Some phases are the direct responsibility of the auditor, while some may involve other parties. All five must be completed with diligence if the audit is to be considered effective.

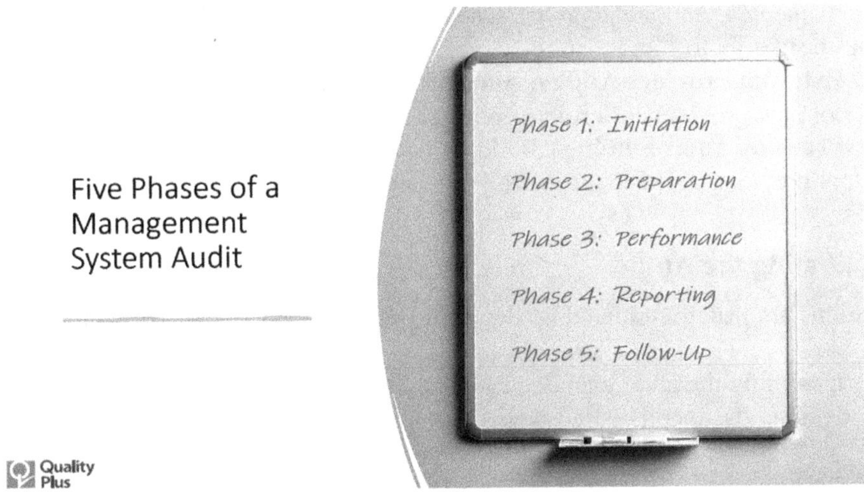

PHASE 1: INITIATION

Management system audits are triggered by a requirement or condition that initiates the need for the audit. The most common audit triggers are the audit schedule, a regulatory or customer requirement, or a problem which necessitates a close examination, but there can be many reasons why an audit needs to take place. Some include:

Regulatory or Certification Requirements: Audits may be required to maintain registrations or certifications, or to comply with regulatory and legal requirements.

Audit Schedule: The audit schedule, as defined in the audit program and procedures, drives the planning of audits included in that schedule.

Customer Requirements: Contractual agreements may require that the customer or its representatives be given the right to conduct audits of the organization, or that the organization provide copies of its own internal audits, to verify that it meets the contractual requirements.

Corrective Action or Incident Investigations: Specific issues such as process failures, safety or environmental incidents and other significant problems can trigger in-depth investigation through the audit process. Audits may also be initiated due to ongoing performance issues, such as recurring or increasing complaints, nonconformances or failures to meet objectives.

Management of Change: Significant planned or unplanned changes can necessitate an audit to determine readiness or effects of change, ensure that risks have been effectively managed, and to verify that changes have been successfully implemented.

New Implementations: When new projects, systems, or processes are implemented, an audit may be scheduled to verify that the implementation has been effective and that objectives are being met.

External Provider Audits: Audits can be carried out to verify the capability of new providers of critical goods or services or to review performance.

Previous Audit Findings: Follow-up audits might be triggered by findings from previous audits that require verification of corrective action.

Initiating the Audit

Audits are usually initiated by the audit program manager. This involves

- appointing the audit team leader or auditor;
- defining the specific audit objectives, scope, and criteria;
- determining the feasibility of the audit;
- selecting the audit team;
- establishing initial contact with the auditee; and
- following up with an audit notification.

Audit Objectives

Once an audit has been triggered, the objectives of the audit must be defined. There can be one audit objective or a combination. Some examples include:

- To determine conformance or nonconformance of the management system to specified requirements (including regulatory).
- To determine the effectiveness of the management system in meeting objectives.
- To identify potential improvements.
- To determine risks and appropriate mitigations.
- To demonstrate capability.
- To obtain acceptance as a contractor or supplier.
- To achieve certification or registration.

Once the audit has been initiated and the desired objective defined, the audit moves into the next phase.

PHASE 2: PREPARATION

The audit team lead assumes responsibility for audit preparations. Depending upon the complexity of the audit, this could involve a variety of activities but there are five that are common to every audit.

Review Basis for Audit: Research the basis for the audit and conduct relevant document review. For example: standards, regulations, policies, procedures, records, results of previous audits, past issues (e.g., NCRs), contract clauses, and so on.

Confirm Scope and Purpose: Determine the scope of the audit. The audit scope is the extent and boundaries of the audit. It generally includes a description of the physical locations, organizational units, activities, processes, and/or time period to be covered.

Prepare the Audit Plan: The audit plan identifies the topics, areas, interviews, and other specifics of the audit. The amount of detail in the audit plan will reflect the scope and complexity of the audit.

Schedule with the Auditees: The date and time of the audit will have been identified in the audit notification. The audit plan formalizes this date and specifies the schedule for the individual audit interviews.

Prepare Audit Checklist: Many organizations have standard audit checklists for long-standing criteria. These are helpful in preparing for audits, but should be reviewed and modified to reflect current activities, audit objectives, auditees, and scope. Asking exactly the same questions audit after audit will not always add value. Some questions must be asked to establish compliance. In the preparation stage, auditors should add additional items to the checklist if appropriate.

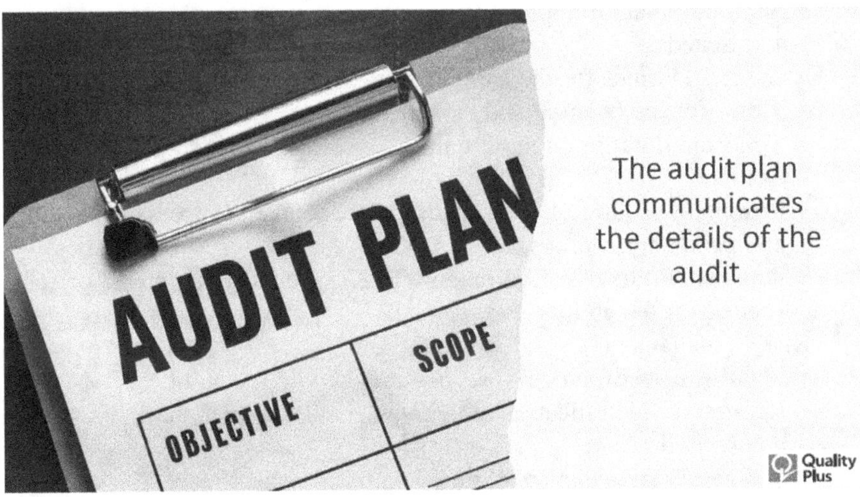
AUDIT PLAN
OBJECTIVE
SCOPE
The audit plan communicates the details of the audit

Audit Plan

When the details of the audit have been agreed upon, the audit plan is prepared. It provides the auditee and the audit team with the details of the audit. Audit plans can be simple or elaborate, as best suits the situation, but they typically include the following information:

1. Introduction
   - Purpose of the audit.
   - Scope of the audit, including the locations, departments, or processes to be audited.
   - Audit criteria, which may include standards, policies, procedures, or regulatory requirements.
2. Objectives
   - Clear statement of the objectives of the audit.
3. Audit Criteria
   - Standards, regulations, policies, or other references against which the audit will be conducted.
   - Documents or records to be reviewed.
4. Audit Team
   - Names and roles of the audit team members.
   - Responsibilities of the audit team, if applicable.
5. Audit Activities
   - Activities to be performed during the audit.
   - Processes, procedures, clauses to be audited.
   - Methods and techniques (e.g., interviews, document review, and observation).
   - Sampling plan, if applicable.
6. Audit Schedule
   - Dates and times for the audit activities.
   - Times for the opening and closing meetings.
   - Time and duration of audit units.
7. Resources
   - Resources required for the audit (e.g., documents, access to facilities and personnel, workspace).
   - Personal Protective Equipment (PPE), special equipment, or tools needed for the audit.
8. Risk Management
   - Identification of known risks associated with the audit.
   - Request for identification of unknown risks to which the auditor could be exposed.
   - Mitigation strategies to address identified risks, if needed.

9. Confidentiality and Security
   - Reference to or details of measures to ensure confidentiality and security of audit information.
10. Communication
    - Communication between the audit team, auditee, and other stakeholders during and after the audit.
    - Contact information for key personnel.
11. Audit Report
    - Information relating to the audit report content.
    - Timeline for report preparation.
    - Parties to whom the audit report will be distributed.
12. Follow-up Activities
    - Requirements for management of corrective action arising from the audit.
    - Requirements for follow-up, if applicable.
13. Appendices
    - Any additional information or documentation relevant to the audit plan.

A detailed audit plan helps ensure that the audit is thorough and that all requirements are understood and agreed upon between the audit team and the auditee.

Audit Checklist

A comprehensive audit checklist is a powerful tool when conducting a management system audit. There are several benefits to creating and using a formal checklist:

Ensured Preparation: Development of the checklist pushes the auditor to review and understand applicable audit criteria, past performance, and important relevant issues before starting the audit.

Anchors the Audit: Audits have a way of taking their own path. The audit checklist serves as an anchor point for the auditor, allowing the audit trail and discussions to progress, but ensuring that the audit returns to the objective and remains on track.

Comprehensive Evaluation: The presence of a checklist, ensures that all compliance requirements are checked and that the review is comprehensive and complete.

Flexibility: As noted above, sometimes audits must, by necessity, veer from the plan. For example, if a serious issue that could affect safety is uncovered in a health and safety audit, the prudent course of action is to deviate from the audit plan and resolve the issue. The audit checklist ensures that the auditor or another auditor can pick up the audit and see it to completion at another time.

Consistency: Different auditors bring different perspectives and sometimes place importance upon different areas. The presence of an audit checklist guarantees that the same questions will be asked and areas examined, regardless of the auditor.

Appropriate Sample Sizes: Audit checklists frequently include prompts such as "review three examples of . . ." In preparing the checklist, the auditor has the opportunity to consider the appropriate size sample and include a guidance note.

Focuses the Audit: The checklist focuses the audit on the requirements and the areas of greatest importance or risk. An effective audit does not rely on examining "what turns up," although it can certainly include information that presents during the audit. A checklist helps avoid a scatter gun approach, which relies as much on luck as it does on planning.

On preparing the audit checklist, some points to remember are:

1. Anticipate What Is Needed

Plan and define, as practical:

- What you want to see?
- Where you want to see it?
- Who you want to speak with?
- What you are looking for?
- How you are going to find it?

2. Plan What to Examine

Look at routine work, non-routine work, and what happens in a crunch. It is helpful to audit both routine and non-routine work to determine if the established controls are implemented and effective in both situations. It is also helpful to audit processes periodically during more extreme situations where unusual stresses are placed on the people or the processes. This will not likely be possible in one audit, but can be incorporated into the overall audit program.

3. Use an Effective Checklist Style

Different auditors have different styles. To a certain extent, the checklist style can be crafted to suit the auditor. Some auditors prefer step-by-step instructions, while others work well with statements of the requirements and formulate their own questions at the time of the audit. Whatever the approach, the audit notes must make it possible to determine what was asked and what was examined.

PHASE 3: PERFORMANCE

Once planned and scheduled, the audit moves into the Performance phase. There are three basic steps in performing the audit:

Step 1: Open the Audit

Open the audit with the auditee. For external or broad-scope audits, this can involve a formal opening meeting to review the audit plan, schedule, and details. For an internal process audit, it may simply mean taking a few minutes with the process owner to discuss the scope, reason, and audit approach. Taking the time to open the audit ensures that requirements are understood and gives all concerned the opportunity to provide information, ask questions and, above all, become comfortable with each other.

Step 2: Conduct the Audit

Gather the facts, make notes, and remember to tie answers to the questions asked. When conducting interviews, some points to remember are:

- **Relax**: Many auditees experience stress at the thought of being audited or "judged." It is important to start the audit in a way that helps alleviate that stress. It is also true that auditors, particularly new auditors, can feel some trepidation when being asked to examine a process with which they are unfamiliar. Taking the time to chat or ask some general questions, such as "explain what you do," gives both the auditee and auditor the time and space to get their bearings and establish a nonthreatening atmosphere.
- **Ask the Question:** Questions should be clear, unambiguous, and direct. If the auditee does not understand the question, rephrase it. And if the auditee answers a different question, allow them to continue as long as the information they are giving is helpful. Then rephrase the original questions and proceed.
- **Document the Answer:** This may be the most difficult part of auditing. When auditees are engaged, they speak rapidly and provide a lot of information. It is imperative that the auditor be able to capture this information for later review and evaluation. For this reason, it is a good practice to explain in the opening that you will be taking notes and may ask for a pause from time to time to do so. Auditors must not rely on memory or try to "fill in the blanks" after the fact.
- **Analyze:** Does the information collected indicate compliance, nonconformance, or an opportunity for improvement? To the extent possible, discuss

this during the audit. If you are not certain what the information represents, let the auditee know that you will investigate and follow-up.

- **Record the Result:** Record the objective evidence, and if possible, the findings in the audit notes.
- **Go to the Next Point:** Once a question has been asked, the evidence presented and the notes taken, proceed to the next point on the audit checklist.

Step 3: Close the Audit

Close off each interview by thanking the auditee for their time and cooperation, reviewing known audit results, and providing information on the communication of the audit report. At the end of external or broad-scope audits, a formal closing meeting may be conducted. Closing meetings should include representatives of upper management, including those responsible for the areas audited.

Conducting Interviews

Audits employ three general techniques:

1. Interviews
2. Observing people and processes
3. Reviewing records

All three techniques are utilized in the management system audit and have equal importance. The one which requires the highest level of interpersonal skills from the auditor is the interview. Audit interviews should be positive experiences.

When planning interviews, care must be taken to interview the people who can provide the information on the process under examination. Interviewing the wrong person is a waste of everyone's time. Points to remember when conducting audit interviews are:

- Interview persons from appropriate levels and functions. This includes people who perform the work, people who supervise or manage the work, and people who verify the work. This can happen in one audit or over time. Doing so provides different perspectives.
- Conduct interviews during normal working hours at the normal workplace. Audits are part of the job and it is unusual to ask auditees or auditors to participate in audits on their personal time. However, in the case of shift work, it is useful to audit each shift at some point in the overall audit program.

- Attempt to put the person at ease. This can be accomplished by having a brief conversation at the start of the audit interview about something that is non-audit related, or by explaining that the purpose of the audit is to examine processes, not people.
- Explain the reason for the interview and note-taking. It can be disconcerting for the auditee to see someone writing down everything they say. Let the auditee know that you must give details of the evidence provided and justify any findings of compliance or nonconformance with facts.
- Initiate by asking people to describe their work. This is a question that people will feel comfortable answering and the response can often answer other questions on the checklist.
- Avoid questions that bias the answer. This can be more of a risk for internal auditors who are familiar with the audit area than it is for external auditors who are not. Leading questions like: "I know the procedure wasn't followed for this job, but . . . " do not contribute to objectivity. Use direct questions like: "Please take me through the procedure that was followed for this job." Audits are not reviews of the auditor's knowledge.
- Summarize interview results before closing. Where possible, auditees should be informed of any nonconformances, opportunities, or positive practices which will be raised. Auditees should not be blindsided by findings they did not anticipate in audit reports.
- Thank the interviewed person. Regardless of whether the auditee is someone with whom the auditor interacts infrequently or daily, the fact remains that they have given their time and cooperation to the audit process and are deserving of the courtesy of thanks.

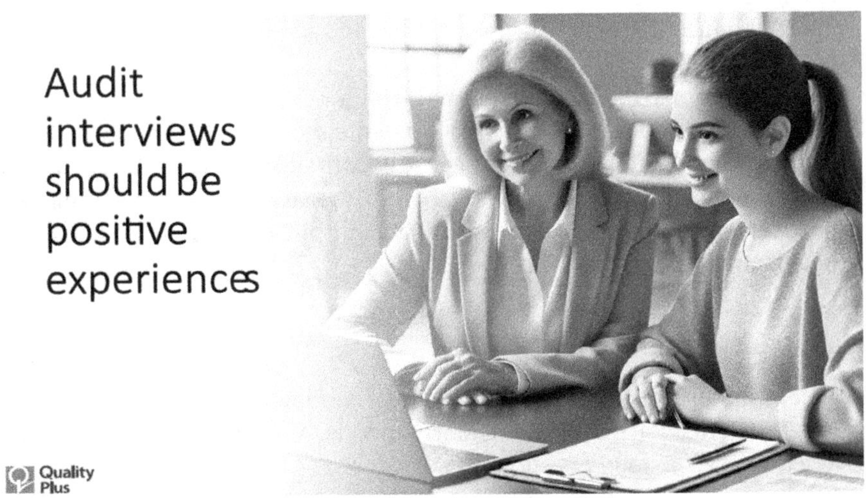

Basic Rules of an Audit Interview

Having established that part of the auditor's role is to make the auditee comfortable in order to smooth the interview process, there are some basic rules of an audit interview.

- **Accept a confession:** If an auditee says that they made an error, accept it. If an auditee says that a process is not implemented, it is likely a waste of time to continue searching. There are, of course, exceptions to this rule. For example, during an internal audit, the auditee may not know that there is a process, but the auditor may know otherwise. In this case, the finding is not that there was no process, but rather that the auditee was unaware of it.
- **Always verify a claim**: It is good practice to explain to the auditee at the outset that the auditor's responsibility is to gather objective evidence and for this reason will ask for it. This is not to question the auditee's integrity, but merely to fulfill the duty of an auditor.
- **Wait for the answer**: Sometimes people need time to think or the auditor knows the answer. This can sometimes be a challenge for internal auditors, especially. Audits are examinations of the auditees' knowledge and understanding, not that of the auditor.
- **Make sure the answer is to the question that was asked**: Conversations take wings. They can veer off in many directions for any number of reasons, intentionally or not. As long as the information is useful, allow the auditee to continue. Record the information and then circle back to the original question.
- **Confirm that a noncompliance is a noncompliance**: As previously noted, it is proper audit protocol to inform auditees of any noncompliances or potential noncompliances at the time of interview, if possible. The audit report or a meeting with their manager should not be the first time an auditee becomes aware of a problem.
- **Focus on improvement, not blame:** The job of the management system auditor is not to place blame or cast judgment on people. It is to examine processes and results. Where there are identified issues, the focus should always be on what failed, not who failed. By focusing on potential improvements, audits help establish trust in the audit process and add value to the organization.

What is a Good Question?

Any question that makes it possible to understand how well a process is controlled, how effective or useful documentation is, or communication, training, or other needs is a good question.

Open-Ended Questions

Accepted interview techniques dictate that open-ended questions are the most effective. They encourage detailed responses that provide deeper insight into processes and situations. For example:

Q:"Can you describe how materials and products are identified from the time you receive them to the point where you enter them into inventory?"
Q:"How do you ensure that all project requirements are defined before beginning work?"

The aim of the open-ended question is to elicit detailed, specific responses which enable the auditor to evaluate compliance, risk, effectiveness, and opportunities to improve.

Pointed Questions

Pointed, direct-answer questions can be answered with a "yes" or a "no." These questions can lead to dead ends in discussion if not used correctly, but there are times where they can be mixed into the audit interview to perform a specific purpose. For example, if an auditee appears uncomfortable or unsure, asking a series of direct-answer questions can help ease them into the audit, provided that they are followed up with a clarifier, such as "can you show me?" Mixing pointed and open-ended questions can help determine compliance and evaluate process.

Information must be coaxed out of some auditees. Others are quite willing and eager to talk to someone about their work. Stream of information can be very interesting and informative, but the auditor must be ready to interrupt, if necessary, to keep the audit on track.

Tried and true questions like "What do you do?" and "How do you do it?" will produce useful information on processes. Once the explanation has been given, it is important to follow up with "Show me." This will ensure that the anecdotal information is supported by objective evidence.

Finally, asking auditees if they have experienced any time wasters or frustrations can be useful in identifying inefficiencies or opportunities for improvement. In this case, the auditor must be mindful not to cross into the realm of emotion or human resources issues. The focus should always be on process improvement.

Summary

To summarize, when conducting the audit:

- Ask the questions.
- Consider: Do we have the necessary practices and procedures? Are risks being addressed? Is the process under control?
- Take notes.
- Use the checklist as long as the data is useful. Note any changes in direction.
- Record what you asked, what you were told, what you looked at.
- Report the facts as dictated by the **objective evidence**.
- Determine the findings and audit conclusion.

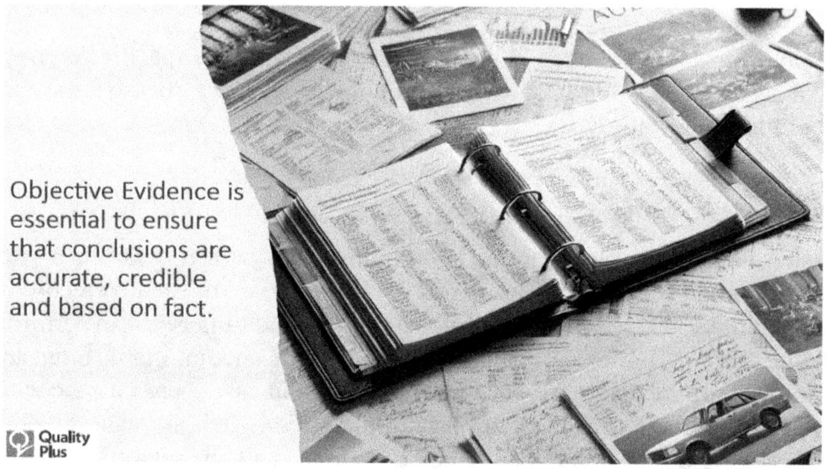
Objective Evidence is essential to ensure that conclusions are accurate, credible and based on fact.
Quality Plus

Objective Evidence

ISO 9000 defines the term *objective evidence* as "data supporting the existence or verity of something."

Objective evidence may be qualitative or quantitative. It includes information, records, or statement of fact, based on observation, measurement or test, which can be verified.

In the context of the management system, objective evidence is used to support the findings and conclusions of the audit. To be considered objective it must be factual, unbiased, and based on information gathered during the audit process. It is crucial to ensure that the conclusions and findings from the audit are accurate, reliable, credible, and based on fact rather than opinions, emotions, or assumptions.

To be considered objective, evidence must be:

- **Factual:** Based on actual data and observation.
- **Unbiased**: Free from personal opinion or subjectivity.

- **Verifiable**: Able to be independently verified or reproduced.
- **Relevant**: Directly related to the audit criteria and findings.
- **Sufficient**: Based on a sufficient sample size to support the audit's conclusions.

Fact versus Inference

We have stated that objective evidence is based on the collection of facts. However, in the auditing world, it can sometimes be difficult to distinguish fact from inference. Auditors must be aware of this challenge and take particular care to report the facts and avoid making inferences.

In some cases, such as the identification of potential risks, inferences may be required. If this is the case, the audit report must clearly identify that an inference is being made and state the data which supports it.

Definition of a Fact

A fact is a statement that can be proven based on evidence. A fact is objective, verifiable, concrete, and can stand alone as truth.

Definition of an Inference

An inference is a conclusion drawn from observations, evidence, or reasoning. An inference depends on an individual's interpretation and can, therefore, be subjective and can vary from person to person. An inference is based on facts or observations but is not itself observable or verifiable.

An inference may be the logical conclusion, but it may not be the only possible explanation. For this reason, auditors should limit the use of inference and strive to report fact.

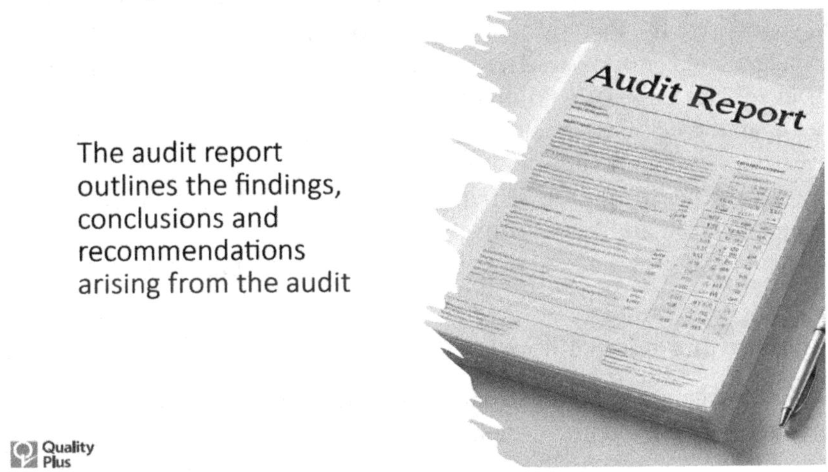

PHASE 4: REPORTING

It has already been stated that a good internal auditor must possess excellent oral and written skills. The quality of the audit report depends on the ability of the auditor to interpret the data gathered and to clearly communicate the evidence, findings, and recommendations in the audit report.

In preparing the report, some points to remember are:

- **Review the evidence and write up the findings**. If something has been missed or is unclear from the notes taken, the auditor must not rely on memory or fill in the blanks. External auditors may have to abandon potential findings if the required evidence is not available to them once they have left the auditee's premises. Internal auditors, on the other hand, may be able to clarify with the auditee or revisit the process.
- **Roll related items into the same statement**. If there are multiple nonconformances relating to the same process, roll them into one noncompliance statement with several examples.
- **List the findings.** Findings include noncompliances/nonconformances, observations, and opportunities for improvement.
- **Identify any nonconformances corrected during the audit.** In some cases, nonconformances can be corrected during the audit and a formal nonconformance or corrective action request may not be raised. In this case, the report should still list the nonconformance and the action taken to correct it. This will be useful information in trending and data analysis.
- **Determine the audit conclusion.** The findings and evidence examined in the audit may be summarized in a general conclusion relating to overall effectiveness of a process.
- **Complete the formal audit report.** Some organizations do not require formal audit reports. However, it is good practice to prepare this document to summarize the findings and important information from the audit, since management is responsible for reviewing audit outcomes. Providing copies of checklists and notes to management is generally ineffective, although notes and checklists should be maintained in order to provide details of evidence to support audit findings.
- **Close out the Audit and Distribute the Report.** Once the report has been completed, the audit is effectively closed. Make **note** of this in the audit schedule and program and distribute the audit report as planned.

Content of the Audit Report

Audit report templates vary from organization to organization. There are, however, common elements, including:

- Report Number
- Auditor(s)
- Auditee(s)
- Audit Date
- Audit Report Date
- Distribution
- Process, Entity, or Area Audited
- Location
- Scope of the Audit
- Purpose / Objective
- Audit Conclusion
- Findings (i.e., noncompliances/nonconformances, areas of concern/risk, observations, opportunities for improvement, nonconformances corrected in audit, positive observations).

Audit Findings

An audit is all about finding things, so we refer to what we found as a finding.

ISO 19011 defines a *finding* as "the result(s) of the evaluation of the collected audit evidence against audit criteria."

Audit findings can be positive, negative or neutral, although the term is usually used to refer to noncompliant conditions.

Common categories of audit finding are:

Noncompliance

If a number of problems associated with a single process are identified during an audit and the conclusion is that the process has not been effectively implemented, is out of control, or that the documentation describing it is inaccurate, then the process or the documentation is considered to be noncompliant.

The term "noncompliance" is usually associated with failure to meet a requirement of the applied standard, regulation, or other criteria. In some organizations, the term "major nonconformance" is used instead.

Nonconformance

When a process is found to be generally in control, but a single failure has been identified, that situation or result represents a nonconformance. Nonconformances, unless recurring, are systemic.

Area of Concern/Risk

This term is often used to draw attention to a process which may be compliant for the present but is at risk of becoming noncompliant if action is not taken. It is also used to report on an area where there was not enough objective evidence found at the time of audit to conclusively call a nonconformance, but where there is a strong concern that a nonconforming situation may exist.

Observation

Observations can be raised in the audit report to identify areas where there was not enough evidence or the auditor was not technically competent to come to a definitive conclusion, where the auditor wishes to raise an issue for follow-up by others, or to communicate something that is considered to be important information. The responsible individuals are not mandated to take action on observations, but the next audit will likely look into it again.

Improvement Opportunity

An opportunity for improvement identifies an area or process that has room to improve. Opportunities for improvement should be reported in adequate detail to enable the process owners to understand the conclusions and decide if action is necessary.

Positive Observations

Management system audits not only uncover problems but also positive performance. Raising positive observations in the audit report highlights best practices, allowing recognition and the possibility of migrating them to other areas of the organization.

Documenting Audit Findings

When documenting audit findings the auditor must

- describe succinctly, but comprehensively, the problem or opportunity;
- state the objective evidence leading to the finding;
- define the scope of the issue (sample size); and
- identify the requirement to which the finding applies.

Example Statement of Nonconformance

In a sample of forty purchases made in the first two quarters of the year, a total of twenty-seven had signed purchase orders. The remaining purchases resulted from telephone calls to suppliers with no follow-up documentation. This is noncompliant with Procedure 123 which requires that purchases may not be made without a purchase order or documented approval from an authorized member of management.

This example provides sufficient information to allow the responsible person to determine the extent of the issue (thirteen purchases were made without purchase orders), when it occurred (first two quarters of the year) and insight into the purchasing situation which gives rise to the nonconformance (purchases initiated through telephone calls.) Further investigation is, of course, needed to determine the true gravity (e.g., how many purchases were made in total during the two months), but the nonconformance statement provides sufficient information to make a preliminary decision on the need for root-cause analysis.

PHASE 5: FOLLOW-UP

In general, the auditor's role is finished once the audit report is submitted. However, depending upon the organization, the auditor may or may not be responsible for opening nonconformances or corrective action requests in the management system actioning system.

Further, in certain types of audits (e.g., gap analysis) or where auditors are part of the organization and have the requisite expertise, they may be asked not only to raise findings, but also to make recommendations for action to address those findings.

Where this is the case, recommendations often follow the SMART framework to ensure that actions are clear, actionable, and effective.

SMART stands for Specific, Measurable, Achievable, Relevant, and Timely.

- Specific
  Recommendations should be clear and unambiguous. For example, instead of saying "maintenance of equipment is required," the finding should specifically identify the equipment referenced and details of the maintenance needed.
- Measurable
  Recommendations should include information that allows progress tracking and measurement of completion. For example: "reduce production errors on shift #1 by 15% within 12 months."
- Achievable
  Recommendations should be realistic and attainable considering the organization's resources, current or accessible skills sets, or available resources.

- Relevant
  Recommendations should align with the organization's objectives and KPIs, and address the key issue identified in the audit.
- Timely
  Recommendations should include an appropriate and clear timeline for implementation and completion.

Applying the SMART framework helps prioritize and align actions with organizational objectives and makes it more likely that audit recommendations will be effectively implemented.

Follow-up Audits

Follow-up audits are usually conducted only in cases where there has been serious noncompliance or where legally or contractually required. In most cases, evidence that corrective actions have been effectively implemented and closed-out is accepted unless the activity or finding was critical enough to warrant reaudit.

The effectiveness of corrective action is also followed up in subsequent audits scheduled as part of the normal audit program.

SUMMARY

In summary, effective audits, regardless of the type of audit or the discipline involved, have common characteristics:

- They must be planned.
- They must be performed by independent, qualified persons.
- Factual information must be gathered.
- Information must be analyzed and reported.
- Appropriate action must be determined and taken, if required.
- Action must be followed up to verify that it has been effective.

Just as the early ship's audits did, modern-day management system audits help establish that requirements are being met; necessary capabilities and practices are in place; risks are managed; problems are caught and appropriately actioned; and improvements are made.

Auditors play an integral role in ongoing control and management of the relevant area or system, maintenance of operational integrity, and continuous improvement. Theirs is not always an easy job, but it is always important and gratifying.

REFERENCES

https://cdn.standards.iteh.ai/samples/70017/559078f9a2634aca84ff0a6aac1498f6/ISO-19011-2018.pdf.

https://cdn.standards.iteh.ai/samples/62085/4eb398f0e6dd4379a04fc7d5df82bab8/ISO-9001-2015.pdf.

Appendix F

ChatGPT-generated integrated HSEQ Audit Checklist

We spoke in an earlier chapter about how we are predicting that Artificial Intelligence (AI) has the potential to bring significant changes to the world of HSEQ auditing and auditing in general. If you look at the questions we asked ChatGPT regarding developing an integrated HSEQ audit checklist, you can see from the version we created below, developed with the baseline information that ChatGPT created for us, that the potential is unlimited. This is our example using ChatGPT. Use your own needs to help develop your own AI-generated audit checklist requirements.

Integrated HSEQ Audit Checklist

1. Context of the Organization	Conformance (Yes/No)	Finding	Action Required
Guidance: Identify internal and external issues relevant to the organization's purpose and strategic direction (ISO 9001: 4.1, ISO 14001: 4.1, ISO 45001: 4.1). Determine interested parties and their requirements (ISO 9001: 4.2, ISO 14001: 4.2, ISO 45001: 4.2). Objective evidence: Review documented procedures, policies, and records. Interview management representatives and relevant personnel.			
ISO 9001:2015			
Determine the internal and external issues relevant to the organization (4.1).			

Integrated HSEQ Audit Checklist			
Identify the needs and expectations of interested parties (4.2).			
Define the scope of the quality management system (QMS) (4.3).			
Documented information required by the standard (4.4).			
ISO 14001:2015			
Determine external and internal issues relevant to the environmental management system (EMS) (4.1).			
Identify the needs and expectations of interested parties (4.2).			
Define the scope of the EMS (4.3).			
Documented information required by the standard (4.4).			
ISO 45001:2018			
Determine external and internal issues relevant to the occupational health and safety management system (OHSMS) (4.1).			
Identify the needs and expectations of workers and other interested parties (4.2).			
Define the scope of the OHSMS (4.3).			
Documented information required by the standard (4.4).			
2. Leadership and Commitment	Conformance (Yes/No)	Finding	Action Required
Guidance: Verify top management commitment to the management systems (ISO 9001: 5.1, ISO 14001: 5.1, ISO 45001: 5.1). Ensure the establishment of policies for quality, environment, and occupational health and safety (ISO 9001: 5.2, ISO 14001: 5.2, ISO 45001: 5.2). Objective evidence: Review policy documents, organizational charts, and job descriptions. Interview top management and relevant personnel.			

Integrated HSEQ Audit Checklist			
ISO 9001:2015 Leadership and commitment (5.1). Quality policy (5.2). Organizational roles, responsibilities, and authorities (5.3). ISO 14001:2015 Leadership and commitment (5.1). Environmental policy (5.2). Organizational roles, responsibilities, and authorities (5.3). ISO 45001:2018 Leadership and worker participation (5.1). Occupational health and safety policy (5.2). Organizational roles, responsibilities, and authorities (5.3).			
3. Planning	Conformance (Yes/No)	Finding	Action Required
Guidance: Assess risk and opportunities that could affect the management systems (ISO 9001: 6.1, ISO 14001: 6.1, ISO 45001: 6.1). Verify objectives and planning to achieve them, including environmental and OH&S objectives (ISO 9001: 6.2, ISO 14001: 6.2, ISO 45001: 6.2). Objective evidence: Review risk assessment and opportunity analysis documents. Check alignment of objectives with strategic goals. ISO 9001:2015 Actions to address risks and opportunities (6.1). Quality objectives and planning to achieve them (6.2). ISO 14001:2015 Actions to address risks and opportunities (6.1).			

Integrated HSEQ Audit Checklist			
Environmental objectives and planning to achieve them (6.2). ISO 45001:2018 Actions to address risks and opportunities (6.1). Occupational health and safety objectives and planning to achieve them (6.2).			
4. Support	Conformance (Yes/No)	Finding	Action Required
Guidance: Check the provision of necessary resources (ISO 9001: 7.1, ISO 14001: 7.1, ISO 45001: 7.1). Review competence, training, and awareness programs (ISO 9001: 7.2, ISO 14001: 7.2, ISO 45001: 7.2). Verify communication processes (ISO 9001: 7.4, ISO 14001: 7.4, ISO 45001: 7.4). Objective evidence: Review training records, communication logs, and documented procedures. Interview personnel responsible for training and communication. ISO 9001:2015 Resources (7.1). Competence (7.2). Awareness (7.3). Communication (7.4). Documented information (7.5). ISO 14001:2015 Resources, roles, responsibilities, and authority (7.1). Competence, training, and awareness (7.2). Communication (7.4). Documented information (7.5). ISO 45001:2018 Resources, roles, responsibilities, and authority (7.1).			

Integrated HSEQ Audit Checklist			
Competence (7.2). Awareness (7.3). Communication (7.4). Documented information (7.5).			
5. Operation	Conformance (Yes/No)	Finding	Action Required
Guidance: Ensure operational planning and control, including emergency preparedness and response (ISO 9001: 8.1, ISO 14001: 8.1, ISO 45001: 8.1). Verify the processes for product/service realization and operational controls for environmental and OH&S risks (ISO 9001: 8.2, ISO 14001: 8.2, ISO 45001: 8.2). Objective evidence: Audit production processes, service delivery, and emergency response procedures. Review records of product/service conformity and emergency drills. ISO 9001:2015 Operational planning and control (8.1). Requirements for products and services (8.2). Design and development (if applicable) (8.3). Control of externally provided processes, products, and services (8.4). Production and service provision (8.5). ISO 14001:2015 Operational planning and control (8.1). Emergency preparedness and response (8.2). ISO 45001:2018 Operational planning and control (8.1). Management of change (8.2). Emergency preparedness and response (8.3).			

Integrated HSEQ Audit Checklist

6. Performance Evaluation	Conformance (Yes/No)	Finding	Action Required
Guidance: Review monitoring, measurement, analysis, and evaluation processes (ISO 9001: 9.1, ISO 14001: 9.1, ISO 45001: 9.1). Verify internal audit processes and their implementation (ISO 9001: 9.2, ISO 14001: 9.2, ISO 45001: 9.2). Ensure management review meetings are conducted and documented (ISO 9001: 9.3, ISO 14001: 9.3, ISO 45001: 9.3). Objective evidence: Review audit reports, management review meeting minutes, and performance indicators. Interview auditors, process owners, and management representatives. ISO 9001:2015 Monitoring, measurement, analysis, and evaluation (9.1). Internal audit (9.2). Management review (9.3). ISO 14001:2015 Monitoring, measurement, analysis, and evaluation (9.1). Internal audit (9.2). Management review (9.3). ISO 45001:2018 Monitoring, measurement, analysis, and performance evaluation (9.1). Internal audit (9.2). Management review (9.3).			
7. Improvement	Conformance (Yes/No)	Finding	Action Required
Guidance: Check processes for nonconformity and corrective action (ISO 9001: 10.2, ISO 14001: 10.2, ISO 45001: 10.2). Verify continual improvement processes (ISO 9001: 10.3, ISO 14001: 10.3, ISO 45001: 10.3). Objective evidence:			

Integrated HSEQ Audit Checklist
Review corrective action requests, improvement projects, and continual improvement records.
Interview personnel involved in nonconformance handling and improvement initiatives.
ISO 9001:2015
Nonconformity and corrective action (10.2).
Continual improvement (10.3).
ISO 14001:2015
Nonconformity and corrective action (10.2).
Continual improvement (10.3).
ISO 45001:2018
Nonconformity and corrective action (10.2).
Continual improvement (10.3).
Objective Evidence to seek for verification of conformance to the requirements of the Standards
Policies and Objectives: Documented policies, objectives, and targets.
Training Records: Attendance sheets and training certificates.
Audit Records: Internal and external audit reports.
Meeting Minutes: Records of meetings, decisions, and actions taken.
Performance Data: Monitoring results, performance metrics, and KPIs.
Risk Assessments: Risk assessment reports, hazard analysis.
Emergency Plans: Emergency preparedness and response plans, drill reports.
Compliance Records: Legal compliance registers and inspection reports.
Nonconformance Reports: Records of nonconformities and corrective actions taken.

Index

About the Authors

CO-PRINCIPAL AUTHOR—TERRI ANDREWS

Terri Andrews is a systems consultant with a focus on the development, implementation, improvement, and assessment of HSEQ Management Systems within a diverse range of industries. Terri is the coauthor of the book, *Integrated Management Systems: Leading Strategies and Solutions*. Terri has helped numerous organizations achieve registration or recognition of their management systems to various standards and requirements, including ISO 9001:2000, 2008, and 2015 (Quality), ISO 14001:2004 (Environmental), ISO 17025 (Laboratory Practices), CSA Z1000 and OHSAS 18001 (Health & Safety), ANSI/ASC Z1.13 (Quality for Basic and Applied Research), CWB, NVLAP, NQI Canadian Quality Criteria for Public Sector Excellence, and various medical and governmental regulatory approvals (FDA, GMP, etc.).

For almost twenty-five years, Terri has guided dozens of organizations through the design, management, and improvement of operational and management policies, procedures, and documentation across all organizational functions including strategic and upper management, human resources, procurement, design, construction and fabrication, service delivery, production, QHSE system management, and quality improvement (corrective action, incident management, lessons learned systems, auditing, etc.). Her work has spanned a wide range of private and public sectors including oil and gas, manufacturing, research and design, service, aviation, education, government, tourism, aquaculture, and medical and laboratory facilities.

Terri regularly develops and delivers a varied range of QHSE seminars and training sessions, including internal auditor courses, risk analysis and HSEQ tools. Terri is a Certified Safety Management Practitioner (CSMP) through the Institute for Safety and Health Management (ISHM). As a Certified Lead Auditor in both ISO 9001:2015 and ISO 14001:2004, she conducts registration audits on behalf of a number of registrars and third-party assessments for her clients. She is a senior member of ASQ and was one of the founders of ASQ in the Province of Newfoundland and Labrador.

CO-PRINCIPAL AUTHOR—WAYNE PARDY

Wayne Pardy is a graduate of Memorial University of Newfoundland and is currently the HSEQ manager with Quality Plus Inc. For the past thirty-five years, he has assisted many organizations develop and enhance their HSEQ management systems as a consultant, trainer, author, speaker, and auditor. Prior to joining Quality Plus Inc., Wayne was the vice president of safety and quality for Q5 Systems, helping bring that company from a high-tech start-up in 1999 to a multimillion-dollar high-tech safety and quality software and HSEQ service company with a global client base. Some of the Q5 audit software success stories are referenced in this book based on Wayne's international HSEQ audit experience with Q5.

Holder of an Advanced Safety Certificate from the National Safety Council in Chicago, a Certified Safety Management Practitioner (CSMP), a Canadian Registered Safety Professional (CRSP), an Accredited Quality Auditor (ISO 9001), and an Associate Member of the Institute of Industrial Accident Investigators (AIIAI), he has been a frequent speaker at national conferences and professional development seminars in Canada and the United States. His work has been featured in international conferences and studies in safety management in Canada, the United States, and Australia. He's also received additional audit training from the International Loss Control Institute.

A former Advisory Board member for the Safety Engineering Technology Program at CONA, Wayne has also guest lectured on safety for the School of Continuing Studies and Professional Development, Memorial University of Newfoundland, Simon Fraser University in British Columbia, and Dalhousie University in Nova Scotia. A past member of the Board of Directors of the Newfoundland and Labrador Construction Safety Association, Mr. Pardy is also the immediate past chair of the Minister's Advisory Council on Occupational Health and Safety for the province of Newfoundland and Labrador, a position he held for over ten years, and is currently an employer representative on the Board of Directors of WorkplaceNL.

Wayne is a member of the Technical Advisory Committee for the Occupational Health & Safety Management Systems (CSA Z1000) and Z1010, Management of Work in Extreme Conditions. Wayne is also a member of the CAC/ISO/PC 283 Committee advising the Standards Council of Canada on the development of the ISO standard for Occupational Health and Safety Management Systems, ISO 45001. An international award-winning safety professional, Wayne is the author of the book *Safety Incentives: The Pros and Cons of Award and Recognition Programs* and coauthor of the book *Integrated Management Systems: Leading Strategies and Solutions*, as well as a contributing author of the book *A Guide to Health and Safety Management: 20 Proven Programs*. This is his fifth HSEQ book as an author or contributing author.

www.ingramcontent.com/pod-product-compliance
Lightning Source LLC
LaVergne TN
LVHW011657200926
848484LV00004B/976

* 9 7 9 8 8 9 2 0 5 0 4 6 3 *